AF308112

Shock, Sepsis, and Organ Failure

Springer

Berlin
Heidelberg
New York
Barcelona
Budapest
Hong Kong
London
Milan
Paris
Santa Clara
Singapore
Tokyo

G. Schlag · H. Redl · D. Traber (Eds.)

Shock, Sepsis, and Organ Failure

Brain Damage Secondary
to Hemorrhagic-Traumatic Shock,
Sepsis, and Traumatic Brain Injury

Fifth Wiggers Bernard Conference 1996

With 91 Figures and 35 Tables

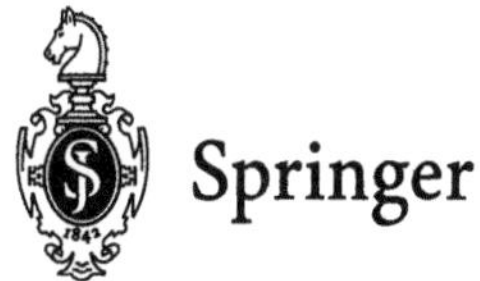

Springer

Univ.-Prof. Dr. GÜNTHER SCHLAG
Univ.-Prof. Dr. HEINZ REDL

Ludwig–Boltzmann–Institut
für experimentelle und klinische Traumatologie
Donaueschingenstraße 13, 1200 Wien, Austria

DANIEL TRABER, Ph.D.
Investigational Intensive Care Unit
Department of Anesthesiology
The University of Texas Medical Branch
Galveston, TX 77555-0833, USA

ISBN-13: 978-3-642-64513-6   e-ISBN-13: 978-3-642-60698-4
DOI: 10.1007/978-3-642-60698-4

Library of Congress Cataloging-in-Publication Data. Wiggers Bernard Conference (5th: 1996: Krumbach, Austria) Shock, sepsis, and organ failure: I brain damage secondary to hemorrhagic-traumatic shock; II brain damage secondary to sepsis: III brain damage secondary to traumatic brain injury/Fifth Wiggers Bernard Conference 1996; G. Schlag, H. Redl, D. Traber, eds. p. cm. Includes bibliographical references.
1. Brain damage — Pathogenesis — Congresses. 2. Septic shock — Complications — Congresses. 3. Hemorrhagic shock — Complications — Congresses. 4. Brain — Wounds and injuries — Complications — Congresses. I. Schlag, Günther. II. Traber, D. (Daniel), 1938- . III. Title. [DNLM: 1. Brain Damage, Chronic — etiology — congresses. 2. Brain Injuries — etiology — congresses. 3. Shock — complications — congresses. 4. Sepsis — complications — congresses. 5. Head Injuries — complications — congresses. 6. Brain Injuries — therapy — congresses. WL 354 W655s 1997]
RC387.5.W54   1996   617.4'81044 — dc21   DNLM/DLC   for Library of Congress   96-40408

The use of general descriptive names, registered names, trademarks, etc. in this publication does not imply, even in the absence of a specific statement, that such names are exempt from the relevant protective laws and regulations and therefore free for general use.

Product liability: The publishers cannot guarantee the accuracy of any information about dosage and application contained in this book. In every individual case the user must check such information by consulting other relevant literature.

Cover design: Design & Production GmbH, Heidelberg

Typesetting: Best-set Typesetter Ltd., Hong Kong

SPIN: 10560743   23/3020/SPS – 5 4 3 2 1 0 – Printed on acid-free paper

Preface

This book contains the proceedings of the Fifth Wiggers-Bernard Conference. The Wiggers-Bernard Conferences, named after two great physiologists, are biannual gatherings of the leaders in the field of shock. These meetings focus on specific areas of interest, where much new information is available. There are informal presentations during which a speaker can be interrupted in order to clarify a particular point. Formal discussions follow each presentation, and these are followed by informal gatherings in which discussion continues in a very relaxed environment.

The 1996 meeting took place in Krumbach again, a charming castle built during the eleventh century and restored and opened as a hotel in 1993. The frank beauty of this area and hospitable atmosphere acted as a catalyst to crystallize the thoughts of this interdisciplinary group of scientists as they discussed new findings pertaining to secondary brain damage after trauma, sepsis, and brain injury.

Severe traumatic shock with longer periods of hypotension may induce flow changes in the brain that can ultimately lead to cerebral infarction. This was shown experimentally in baboon models intended to reproduce traumatic shock. It is a well-known fact that patients with moderate or severe traumatic brain injury react diffently to secondary insults such as hemorrhagic shock. Therefore, it was quite interesting to discuss primary resuscitation after severe hypotension with hyperosmotic solutions.

Severe sepsis may also lead to often ignored changes in the peripheral and central nervous system that, in turn, may cause irreversible damage.

Isolated traumatic brain injury is often linked with secondary brain damage involving the blood–brain barrier. There are pathomechanisms similar to the reperfusion syndrome that may lead to secondary brain damage, sometimes inducing severe irreversible damage of the brain. A better understanding of these pathomechanisms may help to find new therapeutic approaches. Inflammatory events following head injury, even in the absence of systemic injuries, seem to be of particular importance. The role of cytokines in these inflammatory reactions is discussed as regards the possible deleterious outcome.

We would like to thank the participants of this conference for taking time away from their very productive and busy schedules and for their cooperation in preparing manuscripts and editing the discussions.

The conferences could never have taken place without the generous support of the Immuno Company of Vienna, Austria. The editors would especially like to thank Dr. Eibl, managing director and chief of Immuno AG, for his encouragement and advice.

We gratefully acknowledge the untiring efforts of Mrs. E. Hengsberger and Mrs. G. Schrodt who typed the discussions during the conference so that they could be corrected the following day. We also thank the editorial staff of Springer-Verlag for their cooperation.

GÜNTHER SCHLAG
HEINZ REDL
DANIEL TRABER

Contents

Brain Damage Secondary to Traumatic Brain Injury

List of Contributors

BAETHMANN, A.
Inst. Surgical Research, Klinikum Grosshadern, Marchioninistr. 15,
81366 München, Germany

BOLTON, C.F.
Victoria Hospital, 375 South Street, London, Ontario N6A 4G5, Canada

BOROVIC, S.
Ruder Boskovic Institute, Department of Experimental Biology and Medicine,
Bijenicka 54, 10000 Zagreb, Croatia

CARLOS, T.
Division of Hematology, North 811, Montefiore Hospital, Pittsburgh, PA 15213,
USA

CLARK, R.S.B.
Children's Hospital of Pittsburgh, One Children's Place, 3705 Fifth Avenue,
Pittsburgh, PA 15213, USA

CONROY, B.
Department of Anesthesiology, The University of Texas Medical Branch,
Galveston, TX 77555-0591, USA

CSUKA, E.
Division of Trauma Surgery, Department of Surgery, University of Zürich,
Medical School, 8091 Zürich, Switzerland

DEKOSKY, S.T.
Western Psychiatric Institute and Clinic, 3811 O'Hara St., Pittsburgh, PA 15213,
USA

DEWITT, D.S.
Department of Anesthesiology, The University of Texas Medical Branch, Suite 2A
John Sealy, 301 University Boulevard, Galveston, TX 77555-0591, USA

DEYO, D.J.
Department of Anesthesiology, The University of Texas Medical Branch,
Galveston, TX 77555-0591, USA

EIDELMANN, L.A.
Department of Anesthesiology and Critical Care Medicine, Hadassah-Hebrew
University Medical Center, The Hebrew University of Jerusalem, P.O. Box 12000,
91120 Jerusalem, Israel

ERISKAT, J.
Inst. Surgical Research, Klinikum Grosshadern, Marchioninistr. 15,
81366 München, Germany

GENNARELLI, T.A.
Department of Neurosurgery, MCP, Hahnemann University, Alleghery University
of the Health Sciences, Broad & Vine, Mail Stop 455, Philadelphia, PA 19102-1192,
USA

GRAHAM D.I.
Department of Neuropathology, Institute for Neurological Sciences,
Southern General Hospital, Glasgow G51-4TF, UK

HANS, V.H.J.
Division of Trauma Surgery, Department of Surgery, University of Zürich,
Medical School, 8091 Zürich, Switzerland

KEJLA, Z.
University Clinic of Traumatology, Draskoviceva 19, 10000 Zagreb, Croatia

KOCHANEK, P.M.
Safar Center for Resuscitation Research, University of Pittsburgh
School of Medicine, 3434 Fifth Avenue, Pittsburgh, PA 15260, USA

KOSSMANN, T.
Division of Trauma Surgery, Department of Surgery, University of Zürich,
Medical School, 8091 Zürich, Switzerland

LEHMANN, U.
Department of Trauma Surgery, Hannover Medical School,
Konstantin-Gutschow-Str. 8, 30623 Hannover, Germany

LENZLINGER, P.M.
Division of Trauma Surgery, Department of Surgery, University of Zürich,
Medical School, 8091 Zürich, Switzerland

MORGANTI-KOSSMANN, M.C.
Division of Trauma Surgery, Department of Surgery, University of Zürich,
Medical School, 8091 Zürich, Switzerland

OPPENHEIM, A.
Department of Anesthesiology and Critical Care Medicine, Hadassah-Hebrew
University Medical Center, The Hebrew University of Jerusalem, P.O. Box 12000,
91120 Jerusalem, Israel

PAPE, H.C.
Department of Trauma Surgery, Hannover Medical School,
Konstantin-Gutschow-Str. 8, 30623 Hannover, Germany

PLESNILA, N.
Inst. Surgical Research, Klinikum Grosshadern, Marchioninistr. 15,
81366 München, Germany

POHLEMANN, T.
Department of Trauma Surgery, Hannover Medical School,
Konstantin-Gutschow-Str. 8, 30623 Hannover, Germany

POLLARD, V.
Department of Anesthesiology, The University of Texas Medical Branch,
Galveston, TX 77555-0591, USA

PROUGH, D.S.
Department of Anesthesiology, The University of Texas Medical Branch, Suite 2A
John Sealy, 301 University Boulevard, Galveston, TX 77555-0591, USA

REDL, H.
Ludwig-Boltzmann Institute for Experimental and Clinical Traumatology,
Donaueschingenstr. 13, 1220 Vienna, Austria

REGEL, G.
Department of Trauma Surgery, Hannover Medical School,
Konstantin-Gutschow-Str. 8, 30623 Hannover, Germany

RICKELS, E.
Department of Neurosurgery, Hannover Medical School,
Konstantin-Gutschow-Str. 8, 30623 Hannover, Germany

SCHLAG, G
Ludwig-Boltzmann Institute for Experimental and Clinical Traumatology,
Donaueschingenstr. 13, 1220 Vienna, Austria

SHACKFORD, S.R.
Department of Surgery, University of Vermont, Fletcher 301, FAHC,
Burlington, VT 05401, USA

SPRUNG, C.L.
Department of Anesthesiology and Critical Care Medicine, Hadassah-Hebrew
University Medical Center, The Hebrew University of Jerusalem, P.O. Box 12000,
91120 Jerusalem, Israel

STAHEL, P.F.
Division of Trauma Surgery, Department of Surgery, University of Zürich,
Medical School, 8091 Zürich, Switzerland

STOFFEL, M.
Inst. Surgical Research, Klinikum Grosshadern, Marchioninistr. 15,
81366 München, Germany

THIBAULT, L.E.
MCP, Hahnemann School of Medicine, Allegheny University of the Health Sciences,
Broad & Vine, Mail Stop 455, Philadelphia, PA 19102-1192, USA

TRABER, D.
Department of Anesthesiology, The University of Texas Medical Branch,
Galveston, TX 77555-0591, USA

TRABER, L.
Department of Anesthesiology, The University of Texas Medical Branch,
Galveston, TX 77555-0591, USA

TRENTZ, O.
Division of Trauma Surgery, Department of Surgery, University of Zürich,
Medical School, 8091 Zürich, Switzerland

TSCHERNE, H.
Department of Trauma Surgery, Hannover Medical School,
Konstantin-Gutschow-Str. 8, 30623 Hannover, Germany

WAEG, G.
Institute of Biochemistry, Karl Franzens University of Graz, Schubertstr. 1,
8010 Graz, Austria

WHALEN, M.
Children's Hospital of Pittsburgh, One Children's Place, 3705 Fifth Avenue,
Pittsburgh, PA 15213, USA

WILDBURGER, R.
University Clinic of Traumatology, LKH-Graz, Auenbruggerplatz 7a, 8036 Graz,
Austria

YOUNG, G.B.
Department of Clinical Neurological Sciences, London Health Sciences Centre,
375 South Street, London, Ontario N6A 4G5, Canada

ZARKOVIC, K.
Rudjer Boskovic Institute, Department of Experimental Biology and Medicine,
Bijenicka 54, 41001 Zagreb, Croatia

ZARKOVIC, N.
Rudjer Boskovic Institute, Department of Experimental Biology and Medicine,
Bijenicka 54, 41001 Zagreb, Croatia

ZORNOW, M.H.
Department of Anesthesiology, The University of Texas Medical Branch, Suite 2A
John Sealy, 301 University Boulevard, Galveston, TX 77555-0591, USA

Brain Damage Secondary to Hemorrhagic-Traumatic Shock

Brain Damage Secondary to Hemorrhagic Traumatic Shock in Baboons*

G. Schlag, K. Zarkovic, H. Redl, N. Zarkovic, and G. Waeg

Introduction

Trauma and hemorrhage in experimental models should closely mimic human polytrauma to create a valid basis for drawing definitive conclusions about the pathomechanisms and pathophysiology of polytrauma.

The baboon is the only large animal (e.g. dog, pig, sheep) that is able to maintain spontaneous respiration under general anesthesia in the supine position for hours with normal gas exchange parameters. It is therefore ideally suited for the study of post-traumatic events in a setting similar to that of human trauma victims. The baboon offers a multitude of other similarities to humans, e.g., its cross-reactivity with several human antibodies.

In order to simulate the condition of traumatic shock within the scope of polytrauma in the baboon and the resulting organ damage corresponding to the human condition, the animals have to be exposed to severe shock for a certain time. It is well known [1,4,22,23] that decreasing the cerebral blood flow to about 40% of normal or below will result in the development of ischemic brain edema with increased water accumulation in the brain parenchyma. In addition, the development of irreversible tissue damage such as infarction may be possible. Such brain infarction can occur as disseminated hemorrhagic infarction and be of importance for the outcome of the experiment. Animals thus affected cannot be used for the evaluation of treatment and the results of shock, and must therefore be removed from the study.

Traumatic shock is associated with the release of numerous mediators via hemorrhage, soft tissue trauma, and fractures of the long bones. Within a few hours these mediators may provoke a generalized nonbacterial inflammatory reaction, especially in vital organs such as the lung, liver, kidney, and gut, a condition we refer to as "organ in shock."

Most mediators released in traumatic shock originate from the complement and other humoral systems (coagulation, fibrinolysis, kallikrein-kinin) and cellular systems, in particular from activated polymorphonuclear neutrophil (PMN), such as the neutrophil elastase, a marker of PMN activation. Many of these released mediators can be detected in plasma and tissue and cast light on the pathomechanisms of organ damage in baboons.

* This study was supported by a grant from Lorenz Böhler Fond and in part supported by Croation Ministry of Science.

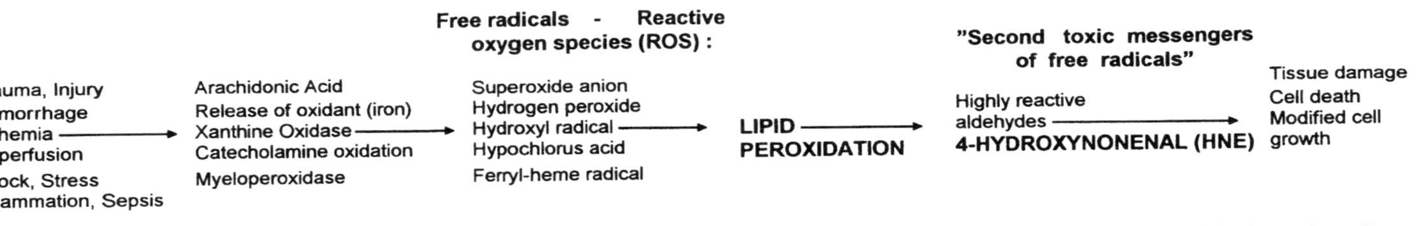

Fig. 1. Biochemical pathways in a cascade of events inducing production of 4-hydroxynonenal (HNE) as a marker and biological mediator of oxidative stress. HNE produced in this manner is highly reactive and forms relatively stable conjugates with different macromolecules, particularly proteins

To cope with the problem of species differences we performed several in vitro investigations to test, for example, whether there are differences in neutrophil oxygen radical release between humans and baboon (unpublished data). Reactive oxygen species (ROS) released by phorbol myristic acid (PMA) and endotoxin in baboons is comparable to that in humans. These preliminary data convinced us to employ the baboon as a model to study traumatic shock. This model was designed to produce new insights into the pathomechanisms involved in trauma and to provide a highly useful tool to investigate the efficacy of pharmacologic interventions in traumatic shock.

Proteinase release is accompanied by the release of toxic oxygen radicals, both of which account for tissue damage during shock, particularly to tissue susceptible to ischemia and oxidative stress [7,8,16–19,27]. The tissue-damaging effect of toxic oxygen radicals can be seen in lipid peroxidation products [e.g., formation of conjugated dienes, malondialdehyde, loss of vitamin E, SH groups of albumin etc.]. Various pathophysiological conditions (induced and mediated by different biochemical pathways) generate ROS and thus induce lipid peroxidation (Fig. 1). Highly reactive aldehydes are also produced as a consequence of lipid peroxidation [10,11,24]. Because of their toxicity, they are considered "secondary toxic messengers" of free radicals which cause secondary tissue damage [11,24,32]. One of the most important products of lipid peroxidation is highly reactive aldehyde 4-hydroxynonenal (HNE) [9–11]. There are data indicating that HNE and related aldehydes are involved in ROS-induced damage to various organs, particularly the brain, after different pathological events [3,11,17,29,32]. However, cascade(s) of events leading to oxidative damage in the brain under different pathological conditions such as stroke, trauma, and sepsis can not be analyzed from a morphological point of view. The reason is that the data indicating involvement of ROS and their secondary toxic messengers in different diseases were obtained by biochemical analysis of the activity of enzymes involved in ROS production or detoxification, or from the presence of HNE or related aldehydes in serum, CSF or the tissue homogenates [10,12,29]. Consequently, morphological evaluation of the tissue and cellular distribution of the mediators of oxidative stress that would show probable differences between the different types of cells or parts of organs involved in pathological events were not possible. Very recently [28], specific monoclonal antibodies have been developed against HNE-protein (or peptide) conjugate(s) that allow morphological analysis of the tissue distribution of the aldehyde. The results obtained using anti-HNE monoclonal antibodies for the immunohistochemical analysis of HNE distribution in the brain of baboons exposed to experimental hemorrhagic shock will be presented.

Materials and Methods

Animals

Adult male baboons (*Papio ursinus*) weighing between 20 and 23 kg were studied. The animals had been caged at the nonhuman primate unit of Biocon Research Ltd Laboratories in Pretoria, South Africa, for a mean period of at least 3 months. The clinical condition of the baboons had been checked prior to their entry into quarantine. At the beginning of the study all the animals had been found to be free of diseases.

Anesthesia

The baboons were fasted for 12 h before each experiment and had water ad libitum. The animals were sedated and immobilized on the morning of the experiment with intramuscular ketamine hydrochloride [8–10 mg/kg body weight (BW)].

The animals were anesthetized with intravenous pentobarbital sodium administered via an electroencephalogram (EEC) controlled closed loop feedback system as previously described [10,11]. The animals received between 1–3 mg pentobarbital/h per kilogram BW.

The baboons were spontaneously ventilated throughout the experiment with a positive end expiratory pressure (PEEP) of 0–2 mm Hg to keep the alveoli open with a controlled end expiratory CO_2 measurement.

For this purpose the animals were intubated (tube no. 8–9) and connected to a servoventilator C900 with a continuous positive airway pressure (CPAP) device for spontaneous breathing. The FiO_2 (inspiratory O_2 concentration) was adjusted to about 25% ± 2%.

The administration of pentobarbital was automatically discontinued whenever the end expiratory CO_2 exceeded 55 mm Hg.

Instrumentation

Following exposure of the right femoral vein, an introducer with a heparinized 7F Swan-Ganz catheter was positioned. The Swan-Ganz catheter was placed in a pulmonary artery branch to measure cardiac output (CO) and pulmonary wedge pressure (PWP), right atrial pressure (RAP), and also to sample mixed venous blood. A triple lumen catheter was inserted into the left brachial vein for infusions, anesthesia, medication, and blood sampling. The arterial blood pressure was monitored via a 20-gauge catheter in the left brachial artery, and in addition the line served for blood sampling for gas analysis for bacterial blood cultures. Ipsilateral to the Swan-Ganz catheter a larger catheter (14–16 F) was placed in the femoral artery for fast blood removal during the hemorrhage period.

To determine the hourly urine quantity during the acute phase of the experiment only, a catheter was placed in the bladder via the urethra. The animals were warmed with an ultra-red lamp to maintain the core temperature (monitored via the Swan-Ganz catheter) at no less than 37°C. The lamp was turned off when the temperature increased to more than 37.5°C.

Experimental Protocol (Traumatic Shock)

The experimental protocol was reviewed and approved by the Institutional Animal Care and Use Committee of Biocon Research Laboratories, Pretoria, South Africa.

After the instrumentation a period of 60 min was given for stabilization of the animals.

Traumatic shock was produced first by a simulation of trauma (soft tissue injury, fractures) with complement activation. Recent clinical studies have shown that complement activation occurs very early in traumatic shock [12–14]. For ethical reasons, fractures and soft tissue trauma are only justifiable in acute shock models where the animals are killed at the end of the experiment. In our subchronic model the animals recover from anesthesia and shock and may survive. Complement activation was achieved by the administration of cobra venom factor (10 U/kg) at the beginning of the experiment and 1 h after the start of reperfusion (5 U/kg).

A total of 30 min after the bolus application of cobra venom factor the hemorrhage was activated. Blood was withdrawn from nonheparinized animals into blood bags containing 70 ml CPDA (sodium citrate, sodium dihydrophosphate, glucose, adenine).

The amount of blood removed was varied until the mean arterial pressure (MAP) reached 35–45 mm Hg and the cardiac output was reduced by about 50%–60%. If the pressure dropped below 35 mm Hg, the animals received a bolus of Ringer solution (20–30 ml). In the absence of response, shed blood (uptake of blood) was reinfused. The time point of shed blood reinfusion and the overall quantity of supplied blood was documented. The overall blood loss (including the samples) was defined as the total quantity of removed blood. Usually about 50%–60% of the total blood volume was removed (total blood volume is approximately 8%–9% of the BW).

The start of complement activation and the subsequent blood removal take no more than 3 h (time-limited hypotension model) (Fig. 1). After the hypotension period (low flow stage), the reperfusion of the shed blood with the same amount of Ringer solution was started, which takes 4 h. During the reinfusion period the mean pulmonary pressure (PAP) must not exceed the threshold value of 25 mm Hg. At the same time, cardiac output was monitored several times in addition to the hourly measurement and should not exceed an amount 15%–20% above baseline.

After the shock procedure and the reperfusion period, the triple lumen catheter in the left brachial vein and the Swan-Ganz catheter were removed, leaving the introducer in place. Both the arterial catheter (left brachial artery) and the Swan-Ganz introducer were filled with diluted heparin solution (500 U/10 ml) and placed in a subcutaneous pouch. The subcutaneous pouch had been opened under sterile conditions. Then the wounds were closed with stitches. During the subchronic period of the experiment for the hemodynamic measurements, a Swan-Ganz catheter was again positioned via the introducer and catheters (including the arterial line) were reconnected to the measurement lines. After the measurement the catheters were removed and wounds reclosed. These procedures were repeated for all of the measurements and blood samplings during the subchronic phase of the experiment (24, 32, 48, 72 h).

Special Postmortem of the Brain

Brain Fixation and Morphological Analysis

The brain was examined by subserial consecutive paraffin section as modified by Grcevic [15]. The brain was removed by autopsy within 1h after death and fixed in 10% formalin. Upon fixation, the brain was grossly inspected and cut by consecutive coronal section into slabs about 5mm thick. After detailed examination, the material was photographed. The samples of brain tissue fixed in 10% buffered formalin were dehydrated in graded ethanol and embedded in paraffin.

Paraffin blocks of different sizes, corresponding to the sizes of the brain slabs, were cut subserially by the large Tetraner-Jung microtome into 5-μm sections and used for histological and immunohistochemical analysis.

Monoclonal Antibodies Against HNE

Monoclonal antibodies to detect HNE-modified proteins were obtained from the culture medium of the clone "HNE 1g4" which was derived from a fusion of Sp2-Ag8 myeloma cells with B-cells of a BALBc mouse immunized with HNE-modified keyhole limpet hemocyanine [28]. The antibody is specific for the HNE-histidine epitope in HNE-protein (peptide) conjugates. HNE-lysine and HNE-cysteine give 5% and 4% cross-reactivity with HNE 1g4.

Immunohistochemical Analysis

For immunohistochemical detection of HNE adducts, the immunoperoxidase technique was used, with secondary rabbit-anti-mouse antibodies (Dako, Denmark). Nonspecific binding was prevented by the use of normal, nonimmunized rabbit serum while endogenous peroxidase reaction was abolished by H_2O_2 treatment of the sections using 1% bovine serum albumin (BSA) solution as scavenger for the slide washing (three times). Affinity for HNE 1g4 antibody was determined by testing the serial dilution of the antibody on the 4% buffered paraformaldehyde fixed HeLa cells treated by HNE in vitro for 1h with a range of aldehyde concentrations ($0.1-100\,\mu M$). The specificity of HNE 1g4 monoclonal antibody was previously verified by adsorption with its primary antigen (HNE-histidine epitope) in the form of a HNE–BSA conjugate ($100\,\mu M$ HNE/25 mg BSA/ml saline solution). The HNE–BSA conjugate was washed, removing excess free aldehyde by filtering on an Amicon membrane ultrafiltration system using 0.5 kDa membrane (Amicon, Ireland) under pressure of nitrogen, with constant stirring of the sample. An immunohistochemically positive reaction to HNE was stained by 3,3′-diaminobenzidine tetrahydrochloride (DAB, Dako, Denmark) and nickel chloride ($NiCl_2$, Kemika, Croatia). Contrast staining was done using 1% Acridine orange solution (Sigma, USA) and 1% Safranin-O-stock solution (Sigma, USA). Positive immunostaining thus produced a dark gray-to-black color with contrast light yellow-to-orange staining.

Results and Discussion

It is well known that circulatory failure and hemorrhagic shock are extremely important extracerebral factors which strongly influence the mortality of severe head injuries [25]. In our polytrauma baboon model in connection with hemorrhage, a period of profound arterial hypotension developed, causing a blood pressure of around 40 mm Hg mean aortic pressure for 2 h. Brierley et al. [4] demonstrated the influence of various hypotension procedures (trimetaphan, shed blood or combination, tilted head position) on the cerebral perfusion pressure in *Macacus rhesus* monkeys, which was reduced to below 25 mm Hg and kept at this level for different periods of time (up to 58 min). Brain damage did not occur when the cerebral perfusion pressure remained above 25 mm Hg. Brain damage was also dependent on the onset of hypotension: the faster the hypotension was achieved, the more severe the resulting brain damage. In our model the fall in blood pressure was produced slowly (30–40 min). Arterial hypotension at about 40–50 mg Hg was achieved about 40–50 min after the onset of blood withdrawal. The hypotension period lasted 90–130 min. In very rare cases apnoea was observed, which was managed by controlled ventilation. During the entire experiment the animals were on CPAP to prevent atelectasis during spontaneous ventilation. After a short while – as soon as the reperfusion of the shed blood with Ringer solution was started – the animals started to breathe on their own. Similar to Brierley's studies [4,5], a failure of spontaneous respiration occurred in animals with brain damage but was also seen in some without histological evidence of brain damage.

Overly high arterial pressure should be avoided at retransfusion and reperfusion. Brierley et al. [4] observed significantly increased intracranial pressure that significantly decreased the perfusion pressure causing areas of the brain to have decreased blood flow. Apnoea was observed after the peak level of intracranial pressure, as we also noted in one case after complete retransfusion of the shed blood, including Ringer solution. Clinical apnoea caused severe damage (multiple infarction). These neurological and neuropathological changes were a complication in our traumatic

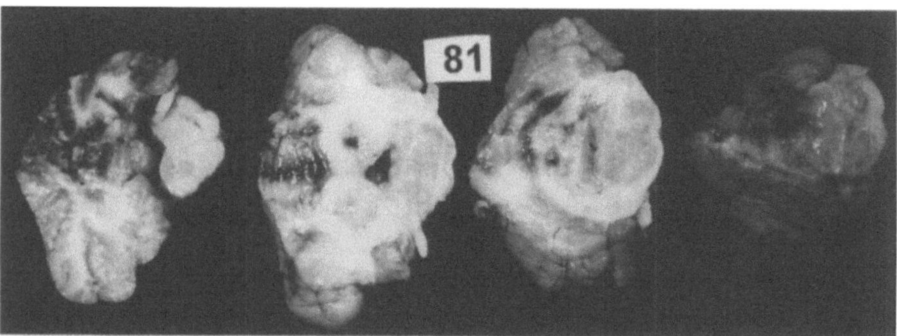

Fig. 2. Macroscopic view of the horizontal section at the level of middle pons and cerebellum. Recent hemorrhagic infarction (hemorrhage 11 h before death) of the left hemisphere of cerebellum was evident

Table 1. Histological evaluation of the brain damage induced by hemorrhage in baboon

Type of cells or tissue	Brain structure/region	Immunohistochemical positivity to HNE[c]
Inflammatory cells – monocytes and neutrophils[a]	Blood vessels[b]	Moderate to strong
Blood vessels (the wall)	Meninges	Moderate
	Subarchnoidal space	Moderate
	White matter	Weak
	Gray matter	Weak
Astrocytes	White matter	Rare[d] and moderate
	Gray matter	Negative
Neurons	Cortex	Often[e] and strong
	Midbrain	Often[e] and strong
	Cerebellum	Often[e] and moderate
Ependimal cells	Plexus chorioideus	Often[e] and strong
White matter	Subependimal region	Strong[f]
Pio-glial border		Strong[f]
Astrocytes around the blood vessels	Blood–brain barrier	Often[e] and strong
Infarction, necrosis	Cerebellum	Negative, both in neurons and astrocytes

HNE, 4-hydroxynonenal.
[a] Only monocytes and neutrophils were noticed.
[b] Inflammatory cells were seen only within the blood vessels, not in the brain tissue.
[c] Positivity of reaction depending on the intensity of immunohistochemical staining and the incidence of positive cells on high magnification field microscopy.
[d] Between one and two HNE-positive cells per high magnification field.
[e] More than ten HNE-positive cells per high magnification field.
[f] Diffuse and intensive immunostaining.

shock model in the baboon and were responsible for our wish to further examine these clinical casualties on a neuropathological basis.

On the coronal section of the brain, ventricular tissue was reduced in size due to the evident brain edema. On the horizontal section through the brain stem and cerebellum, acute hemorrhagic infarction with perifocal edema was noticed in the rostral part of the left cerebellar hemisphere (Fig. 2). According to the morphology of the tissue damage, the infarction occurred only a few hours before death. As a result, only a few inflammatory cells, monocytes, and neutrophil granulocytes were noticed in and around the blood vessels of the affected region. Interestingly, neurons and glial cells in the damaged tissue did not show a presence of HNE, indicating that the oxidative processes associated with lipid peroxidation and generation of HNE did not accompany acute tissue necrosis after infarction (Table 1). However, moderately diffuse HNE positivity was observed in the surrounding cerebellar white matter and in the astrocytes near the necrotic tissue (Fig. 3). On the other hand, soft membranes and subarachnoidal and cerebral blood vessels showed marked immunopositive reaction to HNE (Table 1, Fig. 4). Although it cannot be definitely determined if the

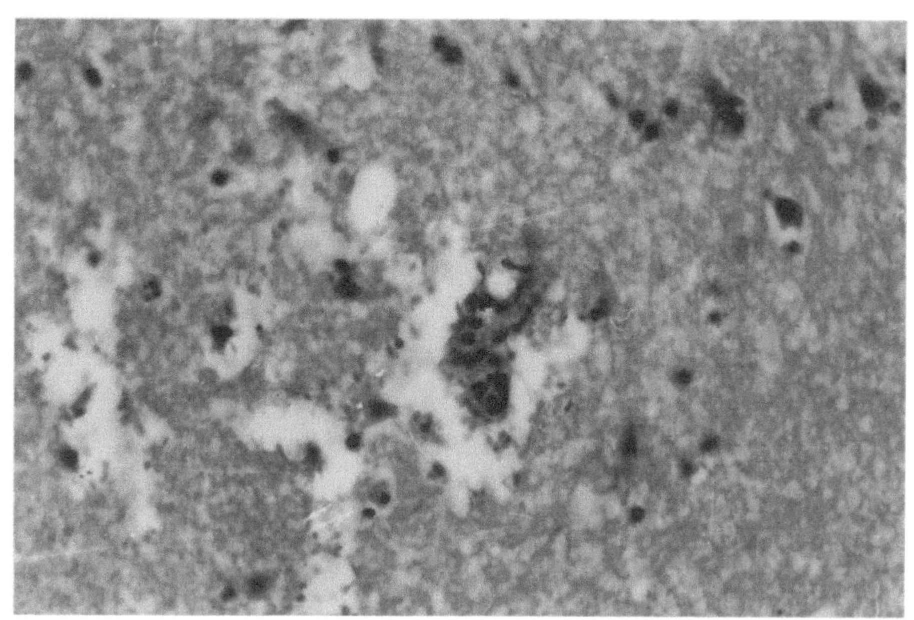

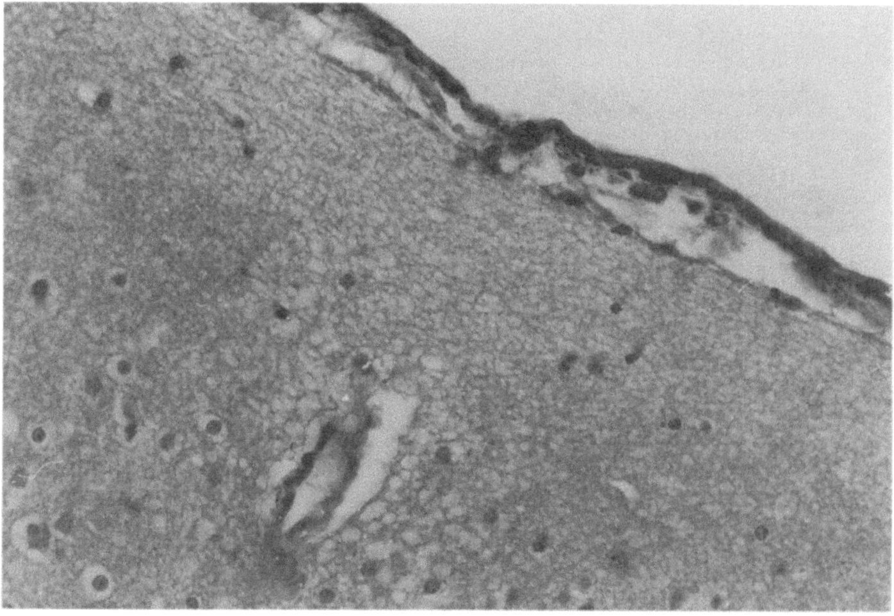

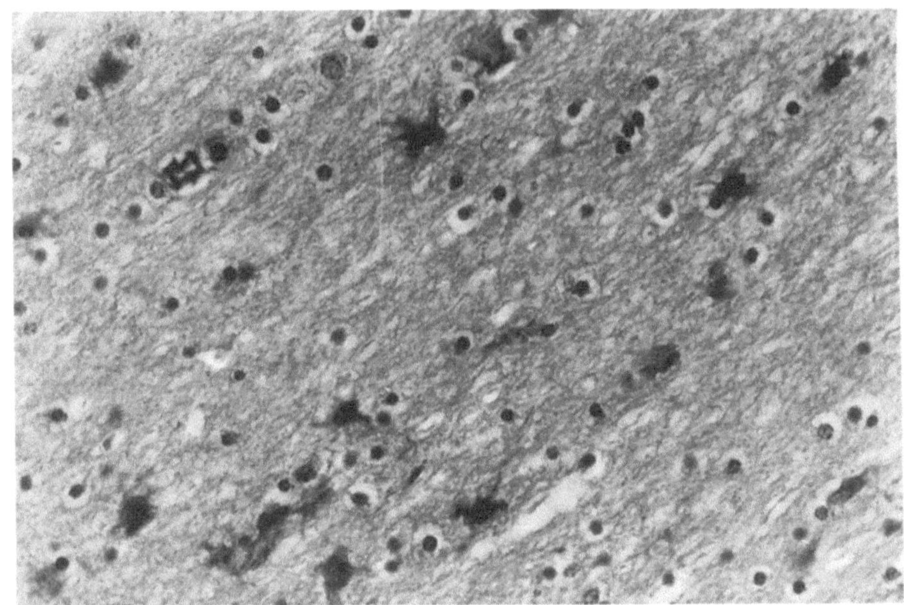

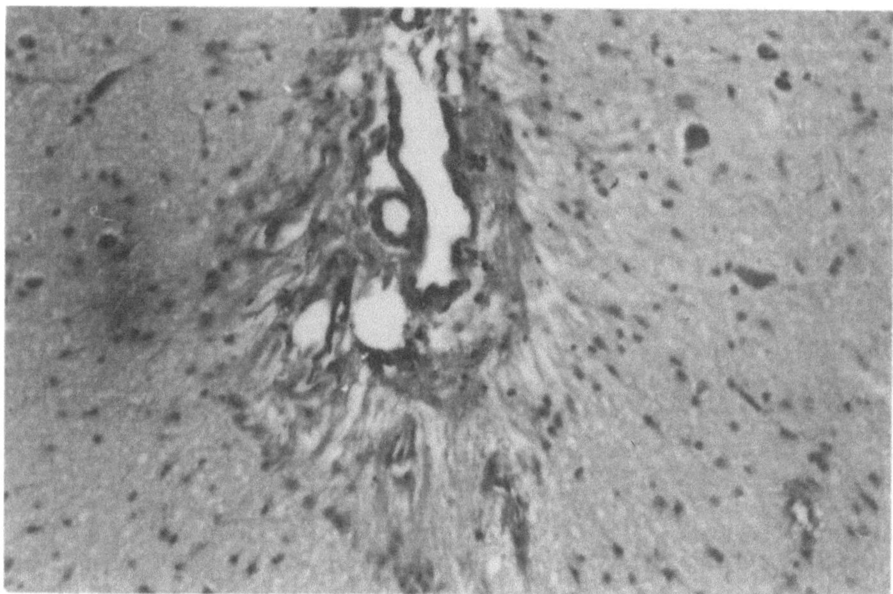

Fig. 6. Around the blood vessels astrocytes comprising the blood–brain barrier showed 4-hydroxynonenal (HNE)-positive immunohistochemical staining (×400)

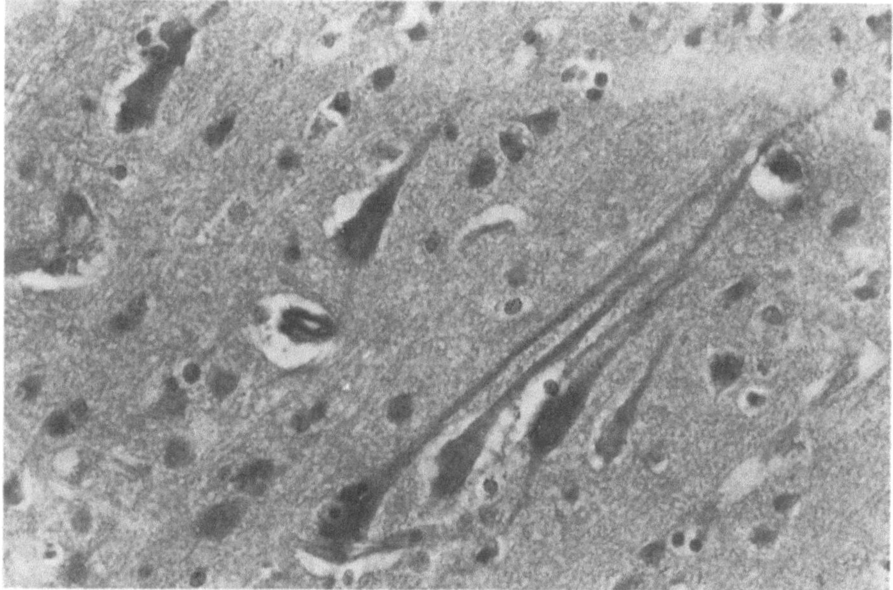

Fig. 7. In the frontal parasagital cortex (arterial boundary zones), neurons, astrocytes, and blood vessels were 4-hydroxynonenal (HNE)-positive (×400)

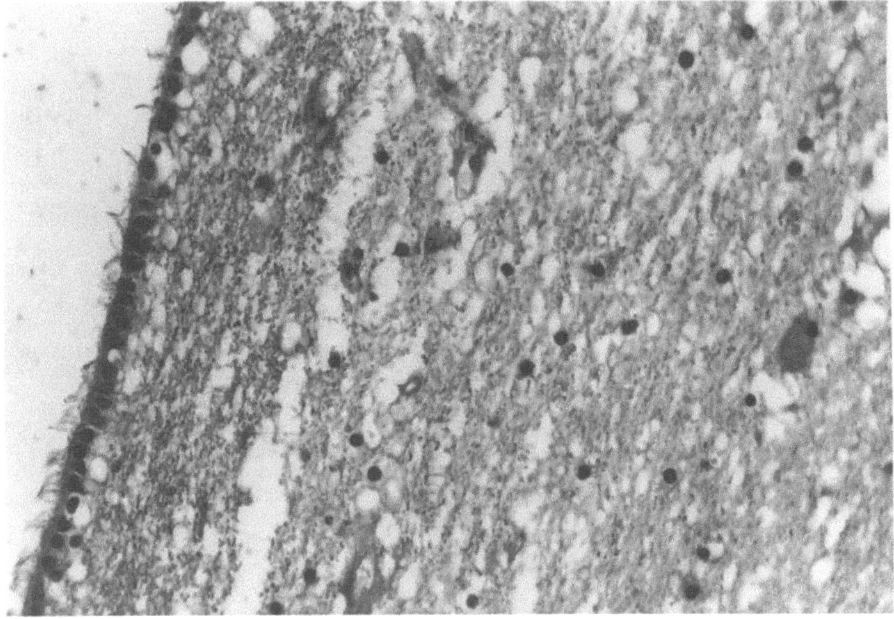

Fig. 8. Strong immunohistochemical reaction of the ependimal cells to 4-hydroxynonenal (HNE) (×400)

these territories which are the most remote from stable blood supply falls to a critical level. Furthermore, hypoxic damage may be limited to certain layers of the cortex after occlusion of the carotid or middle cerebral artery, as reported in the gerbil [6,8,13] and nonhuman primates [20]. This seems to be a consequence of greater reduction of cerebral blood flow in the "deep" parts of the brain than in the more superficial layers of the cortex. The parietal and occipital neocortex is usually damaged to a greater extent than the temporal and frontal parts. The damage is also usually more severe in the depths and side of the sulci than over the crests and gyri. Within the hippocampus, CA1 (Sommners sector) and CA3 to CA4 are the most vulnerable parts of the allocortex, while CA2 is much more resistant to hypovolemic-ischemic damage. The most vulnerable elements of subcortical gray matter are the outer halves of the head and body of the caudate nucleus and the outer half of the putamen, while the most vulnerable elements in cerebellum to be Purkinje's and basket cells.

Damage to the brain appears to depend not only on the severity of hemorrhagic shock, but also on: (1) selective vulnerability of the different brain regions, (2) anatomical features of the blood supply of the brain, (3) permeability of the blood–brain barrier, (4) the "drain" of the secondary toxic messengers of free radicals such as HNE (its protein or peptide adducts) from the tissue and blood vessels into the CSF, causing particularly prominent HNE immunostaining in the plexus chorioideus, ependimal cells, and adjacent white matter (Fig. 8).

Finally, it should be mentioned that while HNE could contribute to the development of the tissue damage, it might on the other hand also be involved in the recovery of the damaged tissue since HNE can also act as regulator of cellular growth [30,31]. Of importance in this regard would be not only the content of HNE within the tissue but also the nature of the local tissue and the humoral, blood-originating factors present at the site of damage which would be related to the histological and anatomical features of the brain.

Conclusions

1. Oxidative stress and the resultant secondary toxic messenger of free radicals, HNE, play a role in the cascade of events determining the brain damage induced by hemorrhagic shock.
2. HNE present in the brain tissue seems to be of vascular origin and could play a role in the function of the blood–brain barrier and the regulation of the cerebral blood flow.
3. As a result, HNE could be of relevance for determining the outcome of the hemorrhagic shock, or at least its consequences for the brain.

References

1. Baethmann A, Kempski O (1991) The brain in shock. Secondary disturbances of cerebral function. Chest 100:205S–208S
2. Bahrami S, Schlag G, Yao YM, Redl H (1994) Involvement of endotoxin, tumor necrosis factor, and nitric oxide in hemorrhagic shock-related alterations. In: Schlag G, Redl H, Traber DL (eds) Shock, sepsis and organ failure-nitric oxide, Fourth Wiggers Bernard Conference. Springer, Berlin Heidelberg New York, pp 59–76
3. Braughler JM, Hall ED (1989) Central nervous system trauma and stroke I. Biochemical considerations of oxygen radical formation and lipid peroxidation. Free Radic Biol Med 6:289–301
4. Brierley JB, Brown AW, Excell BJ, Meldrum BS (1969) Brain damage in the rhesus monkey resulting from profound arterial hypotension. I. Its nature, distribution and general physiological correlates. Brain Res 13:68–100
5. Brierley JB, Excell BJ (1966) The effects of profound systemic hypotension upon the brain of M. rhesus. Physiological and pathological observations. Brain 89:269–298
6. Brierley JB, Prior PF, Calrerley J, Jackson SJ, Brown AW (1980) The pathogenesis of ischemic neuronal damage along the cerebral arterial boundary zones in Papio ursinus. Brain 103:929–965
7. Chaudry IH, Ayala A, Meldrum A, Ertel W (1993) Hemorrhage-induced alterations in cell mediated immune function. In: Faist E, Meakins J, Schildberg FW (eds) Host defense dysfunction in trauma, shock and sepsis. Springer, Berlin Heidelberg New York, pp 149–160
8. Cole G, Cowil VA (1987) Long term survival after cardiac arrest – case report and neuropathological findings. Clin Neuropathol 6:104–109
9. Esterbauer H (1993) Cytotoxicity and genotoxicity of lipid-peroxidation products. Am J Clin Nutr 57 [Suppl]:779S–786S
10. Esterbauer H, Weger W (1967) Über die Wirkungen von Aldehyden auf gesunde und maligne Zellen; Synthese von homologen 4-Hydroxy-2-alkenalen. Chemical Monthly 98:1884–1891

11. Esterbauer H, Schaur RJ, Zollner H (1991) Chemistry and biochemistry of 4-hydroxynonenal malonaldehyde and related aldehydes. Free Radic Biol Med 11:81–128
12. Freeman BA, Topolosky MK, Crapo JD (1982) Hyperoxia increases oxygen radical production in rat lung homogenates. Arch Biochem Biophys 216:477–484
13. Graham DI, McGeorge A, Fitch W, Jones JV, Mac Kerzil ET (1984) Ischemic brain damage induced by rapid lowering of arterial pressure in hypotension. J Hypertens 2:297–304
14. Graham DI, Menedelow AD, Tuor U, Fitch W (1990) Neuropathologic consequences of internal carotid artery occlusion and hemorrhagic hypotension in baboons. Stroke 21:428–434
15. Grcevic N (1982) Topography and pathogenic mechanisms of lesions in "Inner cerebral trauma". Rad JAZU 402:265–331
16. Haglund U (1993) Hypoxic damage. In: Schlag G, Redl H (eds) Pathophysiology of shock, sepsis, and organ failure. Springer, Berlin Heildelberg New York, pp 314–321
17. Hall ED, Braughler JM (1989) Central nervous system trauma and stroke II. Physiological and pharmacological evidence for involvement of oxygen radicals and lipid peroxidation. Free Radic Biol Med 6:289–301
18. Katusic ZS, Schugel J, Consentino F, Vanhoutte PM (1993) Endothelium-dependent contractions to oxygen-derived free radicals in the canine basilar artery. Am J Physiol 257:H859–H864
19. Levy DE, Brierley JB, Plum F (1975) Ischemic brain damage in the gerbil in the absence of no-reflow. J Neurol Neurosurg Psychiatry 38:1197–1205
20. Little JR, Sundt TM, Kerr FWL (1974) Neuronal alteration in developing cortical infarction. An experimental study in monkeys. J Neurosurg 39:186–198
21. Martinez MC, Bosch-Morell F, Raya A, Roma J, Aldasoro M, Vila J, Lluch S, Romero FJ (1994) 4-Hydroxynonenal, a lipid peroxidation product, induces relaxation of human cerebral arteries. J Cereb Blood Flow Metab 14:693–696
22. Meldrum BS, Brierley JB (1969) Brain damage in the rhesus monkey resulting from profound arterial hypotension. II. Changes in the spontaneous and evoked electrical activity of the neocortex. Brain Res 13:101–118
23. Murr R, Berger S, Schürer L, Kempski O, Staub F, Baethmann A (1993) Relationship of cerebral blood flow disturbances with brain oedema formation. Acta Neurochir Suppl (wien) 59:11–17
24. Redl H, Gasser H, Hallström S, Schlag G (1993) Radical related cell injury. In: Schlag G, Redl H (eds) Pathophysiology of shock, sepsis, and organ failure. Springer, Berlin Heidelberg New York, pp 92–110
25. Siegel JH, Gens DR, Mamantov T, Geisler FH, Goodarzi S, Mackenzie EJ (1991) Effect of associated injuries and blood volume replacement on death, rehabilitation needs, and disability in blunt traumatic brain injury. Crit Care Med 19:1252–1265
26. Stratakis CA, Chrousos GP (1995) Neuroendocrinology and pathophysiology of the stress system. Ann NY Acad Sci 771:1–18
27. Strieter RM, Colletti LM, Metinko AP, Rolfe MW, DeMeester SR, Standiford TJ, Kunkel SL (1993) The role of cytokine networks mediating inflammation and ischemia-reperfusion injury. In: Schlag G, Redl H, Traber DL (eds) Shock, sepsis and organ failure, Third Wiggers Bernard Conference, Springer, Berlin Heidelberg New York, pp 205–227
28. Waeg G, Dimsity G, Esterbauer H (1996) Monoclonal antibodies for detection of 4-hydroxynonenal modified proteins. Free Radic Biol Med 25:149–159
29. Waterfall AH, Singh G, Fry JR, Marsden CA (1995) Detection of the lipid peroxidation product malondialdehyde in the rat brain in vivo. Neurosci Lett 200:69–72
30. Zarkovic N, Ilic Z, Jurin M, Schaur RJ, Puhl H, Esterbauer H (1993) Stimulation of HeLa cell growth by physiological concentrations of 4-hydroxynonenal. Cell Biochem Funct 11:279–286
31. Zarkovic N, Schaur RJ, Puhl H, Jurin M, Esterbauer H (1994) Mutual dependence of growth modifying effects of 4-hydroxynonenal and fetal calf serum in vitro. Free Radic Biol Med 16:877–884
32. Zollner H, Schaur RJ, Esterbauer H (1991) Biological activities of 4-hydroxyalkenals. In: Sies H (ed) Oxidative Stress. Academic, London, pp 337–369

Discussion

Baethmann:
As far as traumatic-hemorrhagic shock without any primary involvement of the brain is concerned, I think there are few data available of what is actually going on in the brain unless systemic hypotension is so severe that cerebral blood flow is affected. Then one may expect ischemic damage of the brain in the selectively vulnerable areas. My question is concerned with the specific effects of activating the complement system, or what would occur in the brain then without inducing hemorrhagic shock in addition? In other words, what is more damaging for the brain: complement activation or hemorrhagic hypovolemia?

Schlag:
We did these same studies in hemorrhagic shock without complement activation and we saw exactly the same results. First we thought the complement activation has some influence on this event, and therefore we did five animals with hemorrhagic shock and in two animals we also found this encephalomalacia.

Baethmann:
Did blood pressure drop under these circumstances below the lower threshold of the cerebrovascular autoregulation? And for how long was the period of hemorrhagic shock maintained?

Schlag:
Yes, I think so. Because in the future we will measure the cerebral blood flow, but right now we are not able to do this.
The maximum period is about between 2 and 3 h. The mean arterial blood pressure is 40 mm Hg. But as you know the baboon is quite resistant, and I know Dr. Shackford is doing his studies in pigs with hemorrhagic shock. We also did studies in pigs; they are even more resistant because they can remain with 30 mm Hg for 3–4 h without showing any change in the basic sets. The baboon is really very similar to humans.

Baethmann:
Altogether the changes you are observing in the baboons with hemorrhagic hypovolemia are quite similar to the findings of Brown and Brierley published in the late 1960s (or early 1970s) in baboons also surviving periods of severe arterial hypotension (~20–40 mm Hg) of 20–40 min duration for a couple of days to weeks. In these studies also the selectively vulnerable parts of the brain were injured, such as the boundary zones of the arterial supply territories.

Traber:
Günther, did you confirm that you did not have a complement activation in the hemorrhage animals?

Schlag:
Of course!

Kossmann:
I just want to make a comment on this very nice study. There is actually a clinical correlation to your study in the case of patients with traumatic aortic rupture. When

they are actually operated there is brain ischemia for some time. Some of these patients actually show some similarities to what you have shown in your study. There is a clinical importance to our study and, knowing this, I think the substances should be tested to protect such brain damage. Your model is ideal for that because you could actually give it preoperatively, trying to avoid brain damage.

Kochanek:
I have one other comment related to that. There is one other correlation to your study. Peter Safar in his research with the US Army and the US Navy has frequently discussed how the families of the survivors of sustained hemorrhagic shock often complain that these people are just not the same person after the episode. In particular, their memory is often disturbed. Related to this, I was intrigued to see the hippocampal injury; it would be what you would expect to see if hemorrhagic shock were actually producing brain injury.

Young:
I was interested in your thoughts about where the presumed free radicals are produced. To follow up on Dr. Baethmann's question, I was wondering if you did find similar damage with HNE positivity in other organs, or do you think there was a disruption of blood–brain barrier and activated free radical production intrinsically within the brain rather than in the vascular system?

Schlag:
I have to give this question to Dr. Zarkovic: Could you answer this?

N. Zarkovic:
The pattern of oxidative or free radical-induced damage during ischemia-reperfusion injury is quite general. Whether this happened in these baboons I really do not know; we analyzed the brain so far. However, one could assume that it probably happened throughout the body.

Redl:
We have a lot of systemic evidence for radical action from previous baboon studies where we have done extensive monitoring of plasma antioxidants and lipid peroxidation parameters. The source of oxygen radicals are ischemia-reperfusion events and in addition activation of phagocytic cells.

Young:
So you think it probably is a systemic thing that causes free radical damage to the brain?

Redl:
I would believe it is both local ischemia-reperfusion and, in addition, what you have seen around these hemorrhage areas when the phagocytes come in.

N. Zarkovic:
One could in fact assume it particularly to happen wherever there are collaterals to be activated, because then this is a real ischemia-reperfusion kind of damage that could make a local focal damage based on the general principle.

Redl:

We see similar effects actually in the liver where the injury is also very focal.

Schlag:

I just want to show you a few slides. You see, here we measured the neuron specific enolase in the serum of these baboons and we see an increase at about 24 h; the green line is a group of baboons in which we used an antiselectin for treatment, and this group had a significant survival compared to the control group, the red line. One baboon showed really severe brain damage which we showed in the histology. We see the severe increase of the neuronic specific enolase so that it would be a nice predictor, but mostly it is too late because we do this retrospectively. So the point is, what we are looking for is to have a predictor to say when it is enough hypotension and we have to start with the reperfusion, otherwise you get this severe damage. So we are looking for a continuous measurement of cerebral blood flow and also of PO2 in the brain tissue.

Fluid Resuscitation of Brain Injury and Shock: Preventing Secondary Injury

S.R. SHACKFORD

Summary

Head injury remains the leading cause of traumatic death. Secondary insults, such as hypoxia or hypotension, occur in up to one-third of head-injured patients. When secondary insults occur they increase the incidence of adverse outcome. Of the two insults, hypoxia or hypertension, hypotension appears to have the greatest impact upon outcome. Because hypotension has such a disastrous effect on outcome, it is apparent that hypovolemia must be treated aggressively in patients with head injury.

There are currently no methodologies available to determine the presence of secondary injury in patients who have suffered head trauma. Surrogates, such as ICP, CBF and cortical water content are currently felt to be adequate indicators of secondary injury.

Laboratory and clinical evidence would suggest that administration of solute "free" water to head-injured patients increases the ICP, decreases intracranial compliance and increases cortical water content. Hypertonic solutions appear to decrease ICP, improve intracranial compliance and maintain or elevate CBF. Hemoglobin substitutes are currently under evaluation.

Introduction: The Problem of Secondary Brain Injury

Head injury remains the leading cause of traumatic death in the United States (Shackford et al. 1993). Traumatic brain injury (TBI) causes between 50000 and 75000 deaths annually and disables over 80000 persons per year (Sosin et al. 1995; Kraus 1993). Of the 450000 head injures admitted to the hospital annually in the United States, 90000 (20%) are either moderate (Glasgow Coma Scale 9–12) or severe (Glasgow Coma Scale $\leq$ 8). The direct costs of medical treatment for TBI are estimated to be more than \$4 billion annually (Max et al. 1991).

The outcome following TBI is dependent not only on the *primary* injury, but also on subsequent events which can produce a *secondary* injury. Examples of the primary injury are skull fracture, cerebral contusion, and subdural hematoma (Graham et al. 1995). Pressure necrosis, uncal herniation, and ischemic damage are considered to be secondary injuries. The primary injury can disrupt the blood–brain barrier (BBB) and produce cerebral edema and brain swelling which raise the intracranial pressure

(ICP). Prolonged elevation of the ICP can result in pressure necrosis and herniation. Transient elevation of the ICP will reduce the cerebral perfusion pressure (CPP, which is calculated by subtracting the ICP from the mean arterial pressure [MAP]) and lead to ischemia (Graham et al. 1978).

Pathologic evidence of secondary injury is very common in patients dying of TBI. Graham and coworkers (1978, 1989), in compulsively done postmortem examinations utilizing histologic analysis, found evidence of elevated ICP (sufficient to produce hippocampal necrosis) in 86% of patients with TBI. Ischemic brain damage was present in 90%. They found that secondary injury was significantly more common in patients who had a documented episode of either hypoxia or hypotension. They concluded that ischemia was an important cause of mortality in patients who survive the primary injury. Surprisingly, areas of ischemic damage were often remote from the area of injury – occurring in the "boundary" zones between major arteries, the so-called watershed areas of the cerebral circulation. This suggested that the injured brain might be particularly sensitive to reductions in cerebral blood flow (CBF).

Secondary insults, such as elevated ICP, hypoxia, and hypotension, are common in patients with moderate and severe TBI and appear to worsen the outcome. Miller and associates (1978) noted hypotension in 15% of 100 consecutive patients admitted with severe TBI and found that secondary insults doubled the frequency of adverse outcome (severely disabled, vegetative or dead). Chestnut and coworkers (1993) documented the presence of hypotension in 34.6% of 717 patients during the interval from injury to resuscitation and found, similar to Miller et al. (1978), that it doubled the incidence of adverse outcome. Chestnut et al. also analyzed the independent effects of hypoxia and hypotension on outcome and found that, of the two, hypotension was more detrimental. Marmarou et al. (1991) found that elevated ICP and hypotension were major factors in determining outcome in patients surviving a TBI. Our group has made similar observations regarding the effect of hypotension on outcome. Wald et al. (1993) demonstrated that the presence of prehospital hypotension doubled the incidence of adverse outcome following severe TBI. Pietropaoli (1992) demonstrated a three-fold increase in mortality when intraoperative hypotension occurred in patients with severe TBI undergoing operation for an associated injury.

Increased ICP (>20 mm Hg) is associated with an increase in poor outcome. In brain injured patients without a mass lesion who had slight elevations in the initial ICP (11–20 torr), Miller et al. (1977) showed a significant increase in poor outcome (25% mortality, 11% severely disabled or vegetative) compared to patients whose initial ICP was 0–10 torr (8% mortality, 7% severely disabled or vegetative, $p < 0.02$). In a subsequent series, Miller and coworkers (1981) demonstrated a significant correlation between raised ICP and poor outcome ($p < 0.001$) and observed a universal mortality in those patients in whom the ICP could not be controlled. Controlling intracranial hypertension has historically been a major focus of therapeutic efforts during the acute stages of managements of patients with TBI (Becker et al. 1977; Pacult et al. 1989).

Aggressive resuscitation of patients with TBI can prevent secondary insults and improve outcome. Klauber et al. (1981, 1985) reported a 24% decline in deaths due to

TBI in San Diego, California over a 10-year period. This decline was primarily the result of a reduction in deaths at the scene of the injury and a reduction in the number of patients with TBI who were dead on arrival at the hospital. This trend was observed as San Diego improved its trauma system and provided advanced prehospital care. The authors suggested that the decline in mortality was due to improvements in prehospital care – better airway control and treatment of hypotension associated with the head injury. Carrel and coworkers (1994) have shown that advanced prehospital care of patients with TBI effectively prevented secondary insults and doubled the frequency of a good outcome (normal or moderate disability). In the aggregate, these autopsy and clinical studies emphasize the vulnerability of the injured brain to even brief periods of hypoperfusion. Furthermore, these studies suggest that rapid treatment of hypovolemia is an important factor in improving the outcome of patients with TBI.

The treatment of hypovolemia in TBI requires the rational and judicious use of blood volume expanders. Overzealous infusion or infusion of an "inappropriate" fluid could lead to increased ICP and a reduced CPP. Inadequate fluid infusion could lead to a reduction in MAP and a reduced CPP. In order to understand the factors that contribute to increased ICP and, therefore rationally resuscitate patients with head injuries, it is important to understand the principles of transcapillary fluid exchange and the factors controlling normal cerebral blood flow and metabolism and to have an appreciation of how this physiology is altered by brain injury.

Determinants of Intracranial Pressure

It is useful to consider ICP as a function of the relative space occupied by the brain, the cerebrospinal fluid and the cerebral blood volume.

$$ICP = V_{Brain} + V_{Blood} + V_{CSF} + V_{ECF} + V_{ICF} + V_X$$

where ICP, intracranial pressure; V, volume; CSF, cerebrospinal fluid; ECF, extracellular fluid; ICF, intracellular fluid; X, hematoma, edema, swelling (engorged blood vessels), etc.

An increase in the volume of one must be accompanied by a reduction in one or more of the other volumes or there will be an increase in the ICP. For example, the volume of brain tissue can be increased by edema, due to a disruption of the blood brain barrier, or brain swelling, both of which accompany brain injury. The increased volume of brain will result in intracranial hypertension if there is no compensatory reduction in either the cerebrospinal fluid volume or the cerebral blood volume. ICP can also be increased by expansion of the cerebral blood volume, such as occurs with vasodilatation of cerebral vessels. Ischemia, severe enough to cause a shift from aerobic to anaerobic metabolism, generates lactate, a potent cerebral vasodilator. The resultant increase in cerebral blood volume can increase the ICP. An increase in ICP, in turn, results in diminished cerebral perfusion pressure and a decrease in cerebral blood flow resulting in a further decrease in delivery of both oxygen and glucose.

Transcapillary Fluid Exchange

In general, transcapillary fluid exchange is governed by capillary permeability and the hydrostatic and oncotic pressure gradients that exist between the capillary and the interstitium. The relationship of these forces in determining net fluid movement across the capillary membrane is described by the Starling equation (Starling 1896; Civetta 1979):

$$Q_f = K_f S\left[\left(P_c - P_t\right) - r\left(p_c - p_t\right)\right]$$

where Q_f is net fluid flux across the membrane; K_f is the filtration coefficient of the membrane; S is the surface area of the membrane; P_c is the capillary hydrostatic pressure; P_t is the tissue hydrostatic pressure; r is Staverman's coefficient of reluctance (Staverman 1952); p_c is the oncotic pressure of plasma proteins; and p_t is the oncotic pressure of the interstitial fluid proteins.

Under normal conditions, edema is prevented by a combination of a low hydrostatic gradient between the capillary and interstitium and the relatively high reflection coefficient of albumin, the major colloid in serum and the primary determinant of the colloid osmotic pressure (COP). Normally, these hydrostatic and oncotic gradients favor net fluid movement out of the arterial end of the capillary. Fluid accumulation in the interstitium is prevented by the lymphatics, which have a great capacity for fluid removal (Zarins et al. 1978).

Based on these normal relationships, one would expect that electrolyte solutions without colloid or protein would result in greater fluid movement out of the capillary (Q_f) at any given hydrostatic pressure (P_c) because they dilute plasma proteins and reduce the COP. Colloids, by raising the albumin concentration (increased p_c), would be expected to sustain the COP, resulting in a lower Q_f at a given P_c.

Interpretation of the Starling equation, as Civetta (1979) points out, depends on a number of factors, including the methodologies for measuring both hydrostatic and oncotic pressures, the physiological state of the organism, and the specific capillary bed in which fluid movement is studied. In the cerebral capillary bed, endothelial cells have extremely tight intracellular junctions, are devoid of fenestrae, and contain few microvesicles for transport. These attributes, in the aggregate, constitute the BBB (Fenstermacher 1984; Fenstermacher and Johnson 1966), which has an extremely low filtration coefficient (equal to 1/30th of the filtration coefficient of the muscle capillary). The intact BBB, therefore, has a very low hydraulic conductivity which abrogates, to a large extent, the effects of any changes in either hydrostatic or oncotic pressure. As a result, the brain is protected from edema formation which might occur as a result of an increase in mean arterial pressure or a decrease in COP. The integrity of the blood brain barrier in preventing edema formation or increased Q_f, is quite important because the brain, unlike muscle or lung, lacks lymphatics. The lack of lymphatics compromises mobilization of fluid from the brain interstitium when the BBB is disrupted as occurs in TBI. Thus, when treating patients with head injury it is important to consider not only the volume of fluid given, but also its composition.

Table 1. Acute effects of changes in plasma sodium and proteins on osmotic pressure in the cerebral capillaries from Zornow and Prough (1995)

Physiologic state	Site (cerebral capillary lumen or interstititum)	Osmolality (mOsm/kg)	Osmotic pressure (mm Hg)	Change in osmotic pressure differences (mm Hg)
Baseline (sodium, protein, and nonprotein osmoles)	Plasma	282	5443	
	Interstitium	282	5443	
Plasma [Na+] acutely increased by 1.0 mEq/l	Plasma	284	5482	
	Interstitium	282	5443	39
Baseline protein osmoles	Plasma	1.2	23	
	Interstitium	0	0	
Plasma protein acutely doubled	Plasma	2.4	46	
	Interstitium	0	0	23

[Na+], sodium concentration.
Colloid osmotic pressure = oncotic pressure.

Oncotic and Osmotic Pressure

Solutes in solutions separated by semipermeable membranes exert a pressure gradient capable of moving water between the compartments. The magnitude of the pressure gradient is dependent upon many factors including the number and type of solute particles and the permeability of the membrane to the solutes. *Osmolality* quantifies the number of solute particles per kilogram of solvent. The solute particles may be small charged ions, such as sodium and chloride, or large protein molecules, such as albumin. *Osmolarity* quantifies the number of particles per liter of solution. Both osmolarity and osmolality are characteristics of a solution and do not describe the magnitude of the pressure gradient since the permeability of the membrane is unknown. Rather, *tonicity* is a measure of the number of osmotically active particles. An osmotically active solute cannot passively cross a semipermeable membrane. Because most solute particles are excluded by the BBB, they generate an osmotic gradient between the capillary lumen and the brain interstitium.

The osmotic effect of even low molecular weight ions acting on the intact BBB is significant. A hydrostatic pressure gradient of 19.3 torr can be generated for each milliosmole difference between the brain's interstitial space and the intravascular space. Changes in COP exert much less of a gradient (Table 1).

Normal Cerebral Blood Flow and Metabolism

An in-depth review of normal circulatory physiology (Siesjo 1984; Heistad et al. 1983; Prough et al. 1989; Kontos 1981) is beyond the scope of this chapter, but certain points deserve emphasis.

Cerebral Metabolic Requirements

The brain, relative to its size, has an immense requirement for energy (Prougn and Rogers 1989). To understand this need, recall that the neuron has a large membrane surface area relative to its volume and that axons and dendrites extend for considerable distances away from the cell body (Siesjo 1984). Energy is required by the neuron to maintain ionic gradients for depolarization and to regulate cellular volume over the large membrane area. Energy is also required to synthesize phospholipids for maintenance of membrane integrity, and to transport proteins (excitatory and inhibitory transmitters) to axon terminals. Prough and Rogers (1989) have suggested that 40%–50% of substrate consumed by the brain is needed to maintain cellular integrity while the rest is used to perform electrophysiologic work.

It is estimated that the oxygen requirement of the "resting" brain is approximately 3.5 ml per 100 g/min. The average adult brain weights approximately 1400 g and would, therefore, consume about 50 ml of oxygen per minute in the "resting" state or 20% of the oxygen consumed by the entire body. To provide this large amount of substrate, the brain requires a high blood flow (approximately 700 ml/min) and has a high oxygen extraction ratio (approximately 0.35). Because of the large energy requirement and a limited capacity to store substrate, the brain is extremely vulnerable to ischemia or hypoxia.

Regulation of Cerebral Blood Flow

Regulation of the CBF occurs through alteration in cerebral vascular resistance (CVR). CVR is influenced by the CPP, the cerebral metabolic rate and the chemical milieu. There may also be direct neural influences, especially on the larger branches of the cerebral arteries, but these are of relatively little consequence and are not considered to play a major role in controlling CVR (Heistad et al. 1983; Kontos 1981; Wei et al. 1980).

Pressure Autoregulation

Pressure autoregulation is the normal homeostatic mechanism which maintains a constant CBF as CPP varies. Between a MAP of 50 and 150 torr, CBF is relatively constant. Within this range of MAP, CBF is maintained by changes in CVR; as MAP increases CVR increases (vasoconstriction) and as MAP decreases CVR decreases (vasodilation). As MAP falls below 50 mm Hg, CBF decreases because vasodilation is maximal; similarly, elevation in MAP above 150 mm Hg is accompanied by a corresponding elevation in CBF because vasoconstriction is maximal. It had been thought that alterations in cerebrovascular tone were mediated by effects of stretch on the arterial wall (i.e., "myogenic") (Heistad et al. 1983). Recent work, examining the relationship between venous pressure and CBF (Wagner et al. 1983), has shown that an increase in central venous pressure (CVP) results in a decrease in venous return, and an increase in CBF. The opposite would have been expected if the myogenic hypothesis were true since a decrease in venous return would cause vascular congestion and dilatation of the capacitance vessels, thus increasing their "stretch". Increased stretch, in the myogenic hypothesis, should initiate reflexic vasoconstriction and reduced CBF, not increased CBF. Pressure autoregulation, therefore, appears to be mediated by the local concentration of vasodilator metabolites (see below) (Kontos 1981).

Metabolic Regulation of Cerebral Blood Flow

There is a linear relationship between functional activity of the brain and the regional CBF (Prough and Rogers 1989; Kontos 1981). Any neuronal activity in the brain increases oxygen consumption and results in an increase in CBF. Similarly, systemic motor activity will increase the oxygen requirements of the motor cortex and increase CBF to that area. It is now generally accepted that the cerebral metabolic rate for oxygen ($CMRO_2$) and CBF are directly and positively coupled.

Chemical Regulation of Cerebral Blood Flow

Changes in the arterial blood gases have profound effects of CBF (Siesjo 1984; Heistad et al. 1983; Prough and Rogers 1989; Kontos 1981). A direct and positive relationship exists between CBF and the carbon dioxide tension of blood (pCO_2) within the range of 20–80 torr (Reivich 1965; Greenberg et al. 1978). The effects of pCO_2 are mediated through changes in the concentration of hydrogen ions in the extracellular fluid (Kontos 1981).

There is an inverse relationship between the oxygen tension in blood (pO_2) and CBF. This appears to be due, in large part, to the dependency of the hemoglobin saturation on the pO_2 and their combined effects on arterial oxygen content. Brown and coworkers (Brown and Marshall 1982, 1985; Brown et al. 1985) have elegantly shown that hemodilution, with reduction of the arterial oxygen content, increases CBF. These changes were not explained by changes in blood viscosity.

Table 2. Regulation of cerebral blood flow (CBF)

	Change	CBF
PCO_2	Increased	Increased
	Decreased	Decreased
Arterial Oxygen Content	Increased	Decreased
	Decreased	Increased
$CMRO_2$	Increased	Increased
	Decreased	Decreased
MAP	Increased	No change[a]
	Decreased	No change

MAP, mean arterial pressure.
[a] When the MAP is between 50–150 torr.

The regulation of CBF in the uninjured brain is summarized in Table 2.

Cerebral Blood Flow and Metabolism After Head Injury

A considerable volume of clinical and experimental information exists about CBF and metabolism after isolated head injury. Much less is known about changes in CBF and metabolism when hypotension or hypoxia accompany head injury.

As previously discussed, the regulation of CBF is a function of both MAP and local cerebral metabolism. Severe head injury, however, may lead to ischemia or hyperemia suggesting that, in some patients, normal regulation of CBF may be lost (Bruce et al. 1973; Marion et al. 1991; Mendelow et al. 1985; Muizelaar et al. 1989; Obrist et al. 1984). It is now felt that many patients with severe head injury exhibit an early reduction in cerebral blood flow. Jaggi et al. (1990) conducted acute CBF determinations in 96 patients with severe head injury, 70% of whom were studied within 48 h of the injury. Forty-four (46%) patients were found to have reduced CBF which was significantly related to adverse outcome. Marion and coworkers (1991) were able to perform CBF studies on 43% of a series of 32 patients during the first 24 h. Reduced CBF was evident in the group of patients without mass lesions during the first hours after the injury. By 24 h, however, global blood flow had returned to nearly normal levels. It has been suggested on the basis of these studies and others that the first few minutes to hours after a severe head injury are characterized by a significant reduction of CBF, both globally and regionally, followed by a period of relative hyperemia (Bruce et al. 1973; Marion et al. 1991). Although many investigators have attempted to correlate CBF with outcome following head injury (Overgaard et al. 1981; Marshall et al. 1975; DeSalles et al. 1987), most of these studies have failed to conclusively demonstrate a direct correlation.

Laboratory evaluation would seem like an ideal setting for the observation of acute changes in CBF produced by brain injury. The graded fluid-percussion model of head injury has received the widest attention although few experiments have been done combining shock with this model of head injury. Fluid percussion injury, without shock, produces an abrupt rise of MAP followed by brief periods of hypotension (DeWitt et al. 1981, 1986; McIntosh et al. 1989). The time course of this immediate rise in blood pressure suggests that it is mediated by both direct neural influences and humoral effects, specifically catecholamine release. DeWitt et al. (1986) noted an elevation of CBF 1 min after both high and low levels of impact. Within 30–60 min CBF returned to normal values. Using the same model, Muizelaar et al. (1983) reported that cortical CBF increased within seconds after injury but dropped to levels of 50% of normal at 1 h after the injury. These results were similar to those reported by Yuan et al. (1988) and by Pfenninger et al. (1989), using different techniques to measure CBF. Schmoker and associates (1993) have shown that lesion volume has an effect on CBF following head injury. In a porcine model of cryogenic brain injury they showed that small lesions have hyperemic flow and that large lesions have reduced flow. Both large and small lesions caused a loss of cerebral autoregulation following hemorrhage. These experiments support the concept of impaired control of the cerebral circulation after head injury although the evidence of early and significant posttraumatic ischemia is not compelling. We believe that these early changes in circulatory control lay the ground work for future ischemic changes to neurons and initiate the complex metabolic and chemical changes which may further damage the brain.

If cerebral energy requirements for glucose and oxygen cannot be met by compensatory flow or pressure changes, the brain will revert to anaerobic metabolism to meet its energy needs. In temporary ischemia and stroke models, it has been shown that increased production of lactate, the marker for anaerobic metabolism, occurs during both the hypoperfusion period as well as during the reperfusion period. It is assumed that the continued increase in anaerobic metabolism during the reperfusion period, when oxygen and glucose delivery have returned to normal, is due to derangement of aerobic pathways (Jenkins et al. 1989). Elevated levels of lactate in the CSF have been reported in many clinical studies of head injury (DeSalles et al. 1987; Bakay et al. 1985; Sood et al. 1980). CSF lactate concentration is probably a direct reflection of intracellular lactate accumulation. Lactic acidosis would be expected to result in a lowering of the pH, which may lead to further cell deterioration and edema. Using ^{31}P magnetic resonance spectroscopy, Ishige et al. (1988) demonstrated a statistically significant fall in intracellular pH of rats subjected to a cranial impact injury and systemic hypotension compared to groups subjected to only one of these insults. Rango et al. (1990), however, were unable to demonstrate intracellular acidosis in 22 head-injured patients, although the earliest studies were done 36h after injury.

The information from experimental isolated head injury studies provides an important reference for reviewing results from experimental studies of head injury combined with either shock or hypoxia. It is only logical to speculate that the addition of hypotension would result in further degradation of neuronal function.

Using a porcine model of cryogenic injury and hemorrhagic shock, Schmoker et al. (1991) demonstrated a decrease in cerebral oxygen delivery which occurred immediately after shock and persisted for 24h despite the restoration of cardiac output, MAP, and CVP. This study suggested that the current clinical parameters of resuscitation inadequately represent cerebral oxygen delivery and may account for the significantly worse outcome of patients with combined head injury and hemorrhagic shock. This experimental work is supported by the clinical observations made by Bouma et al. (1990) who found no relationship between cardiac output and CBF in 35 patients with severe head injury, regardless of the status of autoregulation. Jenkins et al. (1989) subjected animals to an initial concussive injury followed by a global ischemic insult, neither of which by themselves would have produced cell death. The combination of injuries, however, resulted in an isoelectric EEG and histological evidence of diffuse neuronal death with early cerebral edema. Ishige et al. (1988) studied the effect of hypotension on cerebral metabolism in rats subjected to head injury. Magnetic resonance spectroscopy revealed a marked reduction in high-energy phosphates following head injury and hypotension which was significantly greater than that seen with head injury alone. These data support the concept that the traumatized brain appears to be more vulnerable to hypotension or hypoxia than does the normal brain. The detrimental effect of this combination of events clearly underscores the need for vigorous and active resuscitation after head injury.

Resuscitation of Shock and Brain Injury

Based on our knowledge of the metabolic requirements of the brain and what happens to the normal physiology after injury, it is obvious that cerebral resuscitation must be a high priority in the multiply injured patient. Furthermore, the vulnerability of the brain to even brief periods of hypoperfusion suggests that short delays in airway control and volume restitution may result in irreversible neuronal damage with permanent adverse outcome. The goal of fluid resuscitation is restoration of CPP.

Restoration of the CPP is achieved by expansion of the intravascular volume with asanguinous solutions followed by blood products if the deficit is persistent and physiologically significant (Shackford 1987a).

There is controversy regarding the constituents of the optimal asanguinous fluid for the patient with a head injury (Shackford 1990). Obviously, the best fluid would be one which limits the degree of secondary ischemic injury. Since there is currently no accurate way to measure or estimate the degree of secondary cerebral injury, surrogates, such as ICP, cortical water content, and CBF are used to assess the efficacy of fluid resuscitation of following brain injury. The ideal fluid should be effective in restoring CBF and CPP with small volumes and have little effect on either ICP or cerebral water content in the uninjured area of the brain.

Some of the clinical and much of the laboratory work evaluating fluid management of patients with TBI has been done in the setting of *isolated* brain injury, rather than in the setting of brain injury combined with hemorrhagic hypotension. Nevertheless, the investigations to date have added immensely to our understanding of the effect that fluid resuscitation has on ICP, CBF and cerebral edema formation.

Fluid Restriction

Fluid and salt restriction have been advocated to control ICP in an attempt to reduce vasogenic edema formation in areas of BBB disruption (Bakay et al. 1954; Shenkin et al. 1964). Since edema formation is driven by the capillary hydrostatic pressure acting at the site of injury (Reulen 1976), it is logical to attempt to minimize the hydrostatic gradient between the capillary and cerebral tissue whenever possible. Fluid restriction or active diuresis can lower the capillary hydrostatic pressure and, theoretically, reduce edema formation.

Despite the theoretical advantages of fluid restriction, there have been no controlled studies which demonstrate its benefit. In fact, several studies have shown that no relationship exists between fluid balance and ICP or cerebral water content (Walsh et al. 1990; Wisner et al. 1989; Wilkinson et al. 1983; Morse et al. 1985; Schmoker et al. 1992). Morse and associates (1985) specifically examined this question by comparing the effects of fluid restriction to *over*hydration in animals with a brain injury. Control animals received maintenance fluid while fluid restricted animals received 66% of the maintenance volume and overhydrated animals received 133% of the maintenance volume. There was no difference in cerebral water content between the groups despite the fact that the overhydrated group had a 13% gain in body weight. Similar results were obtained by Feldman et al. (1995) using a weight drop model of TBI and volumes of intravenous infusion exceeding three times the blood volume of the experimental animals. Schmoker and coworkers (1992) studied 57 consecutive patients admitted to their hospital with TBI. They found that sodium administration was directly related to fluid retention (positive fluid balance) during the first 72 h of hospitalization, but that neither sodium administration or fluid balance was related to the ICP and outcome. In a carefully done laboratory study, Ramming and associates (1994) found no relationship between the amount of sodium administered and either the ICP or the cerebral water content.

Fluid Administration: Endpoints of Resuscitation

It is often not possible to restrict fluids in patients sustaining head injury in association with other injuries, especially if they are hypotensive (Davis et al. 1988) or require operative therapy. Asanguinous fluid and blood are necessary, often in volumes which exceed the amount of blood lost (Shackford 1987a; Davis et al. 1988). In fact, restricting fluids in hypovolemic patients could lead to hypotension and decreased perfusion to vulnerable areas of injured brain.

The apparent controversy regarding whether or not to restrict fluid in the head injured patient can be rectified by understanding that the *volume of fluid* administered to a patient is not a surrogate for the capillary hydrostatic pressure in the brain. On the other hand, MAP, CVP or pulmonary capillary wedge pressure (PCWP) may be more appropriate surrogates. It is important to remember that resuscitation should be driven by *physiologic endpoints* which reflect the adequacy of perfusion rather than by arbitrary estimates of hydration. Since the capacity to measure CBF at the bedside in the head-injured patient is limited, it is appropriate to use surrogates of perfusion, such as MAP, cardiac output, base deficit (Davis et al. 1988) or jugular venous oxygen saturation (Cruz 1988). The physician treating a hypotensive patient with a severe head injury must rapidly restore perfusion, avoid excessive elevations in the capillary hydrostatic pressure and control ICP in order to prevent secondary injury.

Asanguinous Fluids: Crystalloids

Crystalloids are solutions of either ionizing or nonionizing solutes. Dextrose in water is a crystalloid with nonionizing solute while Ringer's lactate (RL) is a crystalloid with ionizing solutes.

Crystalloids: Hypotonic

Hypotonic crystalloids solutions are those with a tonicity (osmolarity) less than serum (i.e., <285 mOsm/l). Examples of hypotonic solutions are dextrose in water and $^1/_2$ normal saline (Table 3). Hypotonic solutions contain solute "free" water. Solute

Table 3. Asanguinous crystalloid fluids: compositional differences

Fluid	Na(%)	Na (mEq/l)	K (mEq/l)	Cl (mEq/l)	Ca (mEq/l)	Lactate (mEq/l)	Osmo (mOsm/l)	COP (mmHg)
D5W	0	0	0	0	0	0	227	0
1/2NS	0.45	77	0	77	0	0	154	0
RL	0.7	130	4	109	3	28	274	0
HSL	1.6	250	4	180	3	77	514	0
NS	0.9	154	0	154	0	0	308	0
HS	7.5	1200	0	1200	0	0	2400	0

COP, colloid osmotic pressure; RL, Ringer's lactate; NS, normal saline; HSL, hypertonic sodium lactate; HS, hypertonic saline.

"free" water is equivalent to the water that must be extracted from a hypotonic solution to make it an isotonic solution. Hypotonic solutions will decrease the serum osmolarity and the solute "free" water will distribute itself equally between the extracellular and intracellular compartments. Dextrose in water will eventually result in a greater decrease in the serum osmolarity because the dextrose is metabolized to carbon dioxide and water. The administration of "free" water would be expected to increase the intracellular and interstitial volume (McManus et al. 1995) and the ICP. This appears to be valid. Tranmer et al. (1989), using a controlled overhydration model, infused dextrose in water into dogs with a cryogenic lesion. This infusion resulted in 141% increase in the ICP which was substantially greater than the ICP rise following isotonic or colloid infusions. Shapira and coworkers (1992) infused distilled water into rats following a weight drop cerebral injury. The infusion significantly lowered the serum osmolarity and increased the cerebral water content compared to control injured animals and injured animals receiving isotonic and hypertonic fluids. Bakay and coworkers (1954) studied patients in chronic coma and found that the administration of dextrose in water resulted in a 14%–100% *increase* in the cerebrospinal fluid pressure. Kaieda and colleagues (1989) examined the relationship of serum osmolarity to cortical water content in a cryogenic injury model. They administered a hypotonic solution to lower the osmolarity and found that a significant inverse relationship existed between osmolarity and water content in the uninjured brain. Ramming and associates (1994) studied the relationship between serum osmolarity and ICP. They found that the volume of "free" water administered was significantly related to the ICP and that the ICP was inversely related to the serum osmolarity. Feldman et al. (1995) documented a significantly higher mortality rate in head injured animals receiving dextrose in water compared to those receiving isotonic fluids. Based on these investigations, hypotonic fluids should not be used in the resuscitation or fluid management of patients with TBI.

Crystalloid Solutions: Isotonic

Management of hypotension in the head injured patient has conventionally been achieved by the infusion of RL (Table 3). Conventionally considered an isotonic solution, RL contains approximately 100 ml of "free" water and is, therefore, a slightly hypotonic solution. RL has been recommended for the replacement of volume deficits until blood is available (Ali et al. 1993). RL has been shown to be effective in restoring MAP and cardiac output following hemorrhage, but it must be given in volumes equivalent to three to six times the volume of blood lost (Shackford 1987a; Wisner et al. 1989; Yuan and Wade 1992, 1993). Because it is effective, inexpensive, and safe, RL is the prototype asanguinous solution for early resuscitation and the solution to which all other intravenous resuscitative fluids area compared.

Infusion of RL in the volumes necessary to treat hemorrhagic shock will increase the ICP. In models of brain injury alone (without associated hemorrhagic shock), hemorrhage alone (without associated brain injury) or head injury combined with hemorrhagic shock, RL infusion has been associated with a 1.5 to 5-fold increase in the ICP – the greatest increases being observed when head injury and shock are combined (Poole et al. 1987; Prough et al. 1986; Wisner et al. 1989; Zornow et al. 1989; Battistella and Wisner 1991; Schmoker et al. 1991; Walsh et al. 1991; Shackford et al. 1992, 1994). RL has been shown to increase the cortical water content of uninjured areas of the brain (Zornow et al. 1989; Wisner et al. 1990; Battistella and Wisner 1991; Walsh et al. 1991; Shackford et al. 1992). Following severe hemorrhagic shock (associated with a loss of approximately 50% of the blood volume) RL is effective in elevating the CBF above the depressed levels seen in shock (Shackford et al. 1994), but it does not consistently return CBF back to baseline or control values. Furthermore, the effect of RL on CBF is not maintained. In studies lasting over 12 h (Walsh et al. 1991; Shackford et al. 1992) CBF gradually decreases compared to control animals.

The increase in ICP observed following RL infusion is due to a number of factors. First, RL is slightly hypotonic and increases the water content of the uninjured brain reducing intracranial compliance. Second, RL infusion in large volumes produces a significant hemodilution which will increase CBF because it lowers blood viscosity and reduces arterial oxygen content (Brown et al. 1982; 1985a,b). The increased CBF results in an increase in cerebral blood volume which will increase the ICP. Finally, the large volumes of RL necessary to restore hemodynamic stability increase the central venous pressure. This reduces venous return from the brain which also reduces intracranial compliance (Hariri et al. 1993).

Crystalloid: Hypertonic Solutions

Hypertonic salt solution would seem to be ideal for the treatment of head injured, hypovolemic patients. It restores blood pressure and cardiac output with significantly less volume and at a lower capillary hydrostatic pressure than does RL (Shackford et al. 1987a, 1988; Velasco et al. 1980; Nakayama et al. 1984). Hypertonic fluids achieve this by having a positive inotropic effect (Kreimeier et al. 1990; Wildenthal et al. 1969; Rowe et al. 1972; Kien et al. 1989, 1991) and by extracting water from the intracellular space to restore intravascular losses (Mazzoni et al. 1989, 1990). It also appears that hypertonic fluids may act to lower vascular resistance and improve blood flow to the brain, kidney, and gut (Wahl et al. 1973; Manningas et al. 1987; Gazitua et al. 1971;

Silva et al. 1986; Shackford et al. 1994). Whether hypertonicity induces active vasodilation or simply increases the size of the capillary lumen by reducing the volume of endothelial cells is, at this time, unknown. Mazzoni and coworkers (1990) have emphasized the importance of the latter mechanism (i.e., reduction of endothelial cell volume resulting in a decrease in hydraulic resistance) in improving blood flow after resuscitation from hypovolemic shock. Using intravital microscopy of a skeletal muscle bed, they observed a 20% reduction in capillary lumenal diameter after shock. Resuscitation with RL caused only a transient increase in flow and no change in the lumenal diameter. Resuscitation with a hypertonic solution resulted in a persistent in flow with return of the lumenal diameter to the control value.

The use of *very hypertonic* fluids (1.8%–7.5%) to treat laboratory models of head injury with and without associated hypovolemic shock has resulted in significantly lower ICP, improved CBF and a significantly lower cerebral water content than treatment with either hypotonic or isotonic fluids (Wisner et al. 1989, 1990; Gunnar et al. 1988; Ducey et al. 1989; Todd et al. 1985; Prough et al. 1985, 1986; Shackford et al. 1992). Gunnar and coworkers (1988), using a canine model of hemorrhagic shock combined with an epidural balloon to simulate an intracranial injury, compared 0.9% normal saline (NS, Table 4), 3% hypertonic saline (HS), and 10% dextran. After resuscitation, the ICP increased rapidly in the NS and dextran groups to 46 and 45 torr, respectively, but decreased to levels lower than baseline in the group resuscitated with 3% HS. Ducey and colleagues (1989) compared 0.9% saline, 6% saline, and hetastarch in a porcine model of shock and head injury (epidural balloon). Hypertonic resuscitation resulted in a significantly lower ICP and a significantly lower cerebral elastance (the reciprocal of compliance) compared to the other fluids. Wisner et al. (1989), using an ovine model of cryogenic injury and hemorrhagic shock, compared RL to 7.5% HS (Table 3). RL and the 7.5% HS equally restored hemodynamic parameters, but the RL group required significantly more fluid (48 ± 17 ml/kg) than the hypertonic group (9 ± 4 ml/kg) to achieve hemodynamic stability ($p < 0.0002$). The ICP rose in all RL animals and decreased in all hypertonic animals. The mean ICP at the conclusion of the study (2 h after insult) was significantly greater in the RL group ($p < 0.002$). Similar observations have been made by Hartl and colleagues (1995) using a rabbit model of cryogenic injury with and with out shock and by Berger and coworkers (1995) using a rabbit model of cryogenic injury *combined* with an inflatable epidural balloon used to increase ICP. Both investigations demonstrated a reduction in cortical water content in the uninjured brain associated with a hypertonic-hyperoncotic infusion (7.2% saline with 10% dextran 70) and Berger and coworkers demonstrated a significant reduction in intracranial hypertension with the hypertonic-hyperoncotic infusion. The possible role of the hyperoncotic dextran in producing these results will be discussed in the section on colloid solutions.

The studies demonstrating the efficacy of hypertonic solutions in head injury cited in the previous paragraphs utilized relatively short periods of study, usually less than 6 h, which may limit their applicability to the clinical situation. Observations of ICP during the first 6 h after insult may be irrelevant since major increases in ICP after injury, shock and resuscitation do not occur until between 18 and 24 h (Pitts et al. 1980; Hermann et al. 1972).

We have made similar observations in animals exposed to shock alone (Shackford et al. 1988; Schmoker et al. 1991), animals exposed to shock and a focal cryogenic brain injury (Walsh et al. 1991), and animals exposed to a focal cryogenic brain injury without shock (Shackford et al. 1992). We used a porcine model and a study paradigm which allowed for 24 h of observation after the insult. We selected a porcine model because the neurohumoral and cardiovascular responses of swine to hemorrhage are similar to those of man and because swine have a relatively large brain which facilitates study (Bustad et al. 1986). To determine the safety and efficacy of hypertonic resuscitation of hypovolemic shock in terms of its effects on systemic parameters in anticipation of future clinical trials with trauma patients, we studied awake animals hemorrhaged of 40% of their blood volume and resuscitated with either RL or hypertonic sodium lactate (HSL, Table 3) (Shackford et al. 1988). The animals were studied hourly for 24 h and then daily for 3 days. Resuscitation with RL required significantly more fluid and produced a significantly greater rise in ICP than HSL. HSL produced significant increases in serum sodium and osmolality which resolved within 48 h. Hypernatremia and hyperosmolality were not associated with either cerebral dysfunction (by physical exam and EEG analysis) or renal dysfunction. Increases in serum sodium and osmolality as a result of hypertonic resuscitation resolved spontaneously by increased renal sodium clearance, free water intake and a negative free water clearance. There was no late rise in ICP suggesting that late onset of edema does not occur after resuscitation with hypertonic solution.

To determine the effects of hypertonic resuscitation on cerebral perfusion in a model of hypovolemic shock without brain injury, we studied anesthetized swine for 24 h after hemorrhagic shock and resuscitation with either HSL or RL (Schmoker et al. 1991). Both fluids restored MAP to baseline, the RL group requiring significantly more fluid ($p < 0.01$). When compared to RL, HSL significantly increased CBF and cerebral oxygen delivery (cO_2del) for the 24 h after shock ($p < 0.05$) (Fig. 1). ICP and cerebral water content were significantly lower in the HSL group ($p < 0.05$). We attributed these effects to hypertonic dehydration of the brain parenchyma resulting in a decrease in ICP and to dehydration of the cerebrovascular endothelium resulting in a decrease in vascular resistance and improved CBF. These data suggest that by decreasing ICP and increasing CBF, hypertonic resuscitation might be useful in decreasing secondary brain injury. To determine the early and late effects of hypertonic resuscitation on the injured brain after shock, we used a porcine model of focal cryogenic injury and hemorrhagic shock and compared RL, 7.5% HS with 6% dextran (HSD) and HSL (Walsh et al. 1991). Shock and injury significantly reduced CBF to the penumbra (the "halo" area surrounding the injured brain) in all experimental animals. Hypertonic resuscitation resulted in an improved CBF and a lower ICP than RL. It appeared that the early benefits of lowered ICP and improved CBF derived from the bolus of HSD were abrogated by further resuscitation with RL. Continued hypertonic resuscitation with HSL, however, prolonged the period of improved CBF and low ICP (Fig. 2). At 24 h, CBF had deteriorated to the penumbra in all animals and to the uninjured cortex in animals receiving RL. These data suggest that hypertonic resuscitation of hemorrhagic shock and brain injury, by maintaining CBF without elevating the ICP, could effectively prevent secondary brain injury when focal contusion and shock occur together.

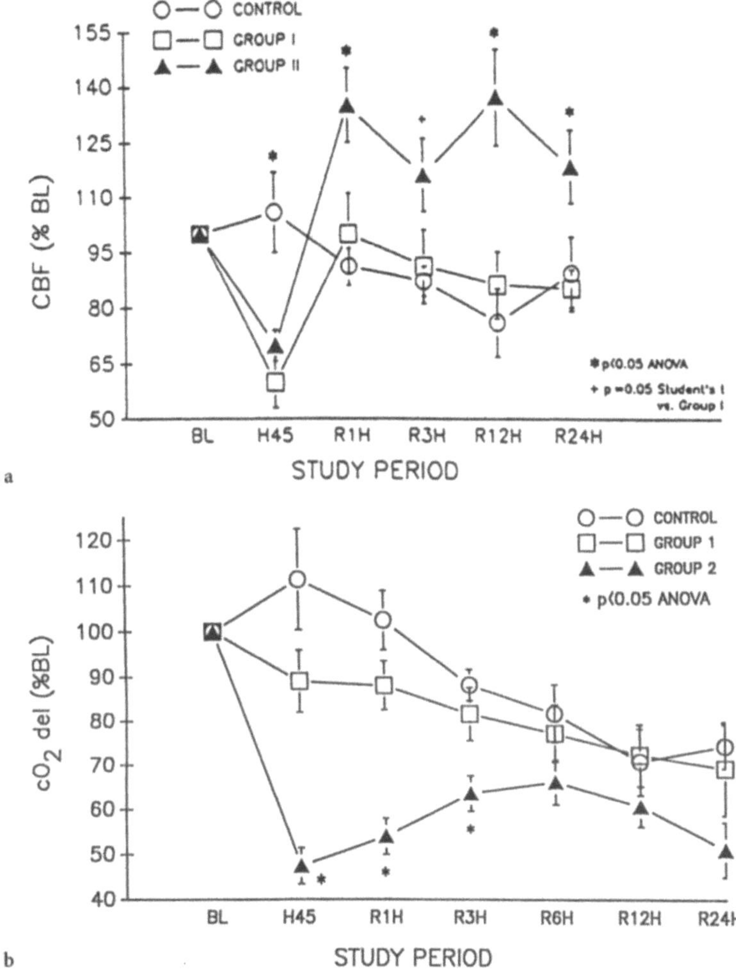

Fig. 1. a Cerebral blood flow (CBF) during shock and resuscitation in a porcine model without a head injury. Group I animals were resuscitated with Ringer's lactate (RL), and Group II animals were resuscitated with hypertonic sodium lactate (HSL). Hemorrhage significantly reduced CBF in both groups. HSL resuscitation resulted in a significantly greater CBF compared with RL throughout the resuscitation period. **b** Cerebral oxygen delivery during the study. Hemorrhage significantly reduced the cerebral oxygen delivery in both experimental groups compared with controls. HSL resuscitation (group II) restored cerebral oxygen delivery to values no different than controls at 1 h. In contrast, cerebral oxygen delivery in group I (RL) animals remained significantly below control and group II at 1 h. By 3 h, and for the remainder of the study, cerebral oxygen delivery in group II remained significantly greater than in group I and controls. *BL*, baseline; *H45*, at the end of hemorrhage; *R1H, R3H, R12H,* and *R24H* represent 1, 3, 12 and 24 h after the start of resuscitation. (From Schmoker et al. 1991)

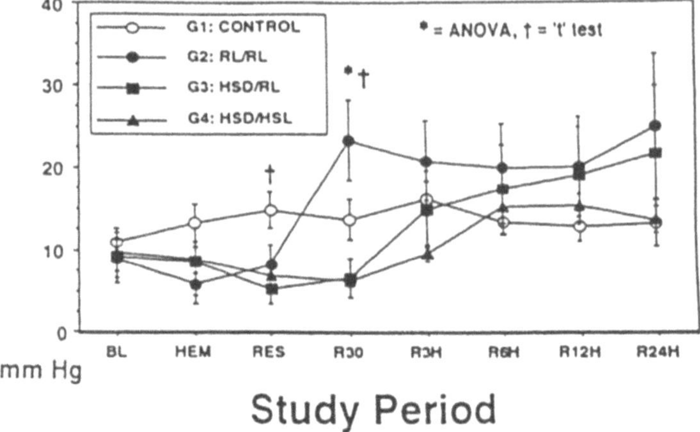

Study Period

Fig. 2. Intracranial pressure (ICP) after shock, head injury, and resuscitation in a porcine model. This study compared the use of bolus HSD followed by Ringer's lactate (RL) (group 3, *G3*) with either bolus hypertonic saline with 690 dextran (HSD) followed by hypertonic sodium lactate (HSL) (group 4, *G4*) or RL alone (group 2, *G2*). Resuscitation with RL alone increased the ICP significantly. A small bolus infusion of HSD did not increase the ICP, but continued resuscitation with RL increased the ICP. Resuscitation with HSD followed by HSL increased the ICP slightly, but the increase was not significant and was no greater than in uninjured controls. *BL*, baseline; *HEM*, immediately after hemorrhage; *RES*, immediately after the bolus infusion; *R30*, 30 min after *RES*; *R3H, R6H, R12H*, and *R24H*, 3, 6, 12, and 24 h after *HEM*. (From Walsh et al. 1991)

To investigate the role of intravenous fluid tonicity in determining ICP and CBF after isolated brain injury without shock, we compared maintenance infusions of RL and HSL in a porcine model of focal cryogenic injury alone studied for approximately 30 h after injury (Shackford et al. 1992). The cryogenic injury produced a significant increase in ICP and a significant decrease in CBF to the penumbra as we had previously observed. Maintenance infusion of HSL resulted in a significantly lower ICP and higher CBF than RL (Fig. 3). Cortical water content in the area of the lesion was similar in both groups, but cortical water content in the uninjured hemisphere was significantly lower in the HSL group. As in all of our previous studies we measured lesion volume (all animals had been injected with Evan's blue dye to ascertain areas of blood–brain barrier disruption). While lesion volumes were not significantly different between groups, the area of Evan's blue staining was always larger in the animals resuscitated with or maintained on HSL. Similar observations had been made by others in animals receiving hypertonic solutions (Gunnar et al. 1988; Waters et al. 1986), leading them to suggest that hypertonic solutions were *increasing* the size of the lesion. Rather, it is our belief that the area of staining was increased because movement of edema fluid (and Evan's blue dye) away from the injury was being facilitated by the hypertonic fluid. Edema formation, as previously stated, is dependent on the creation of a hydrostatic gradient; the same should be true of edema resolution. That is, since hypertonic fluids extract water from cells and decrease ICP, they logically reduce the intracellular volume. Reduction of the intracellular volume

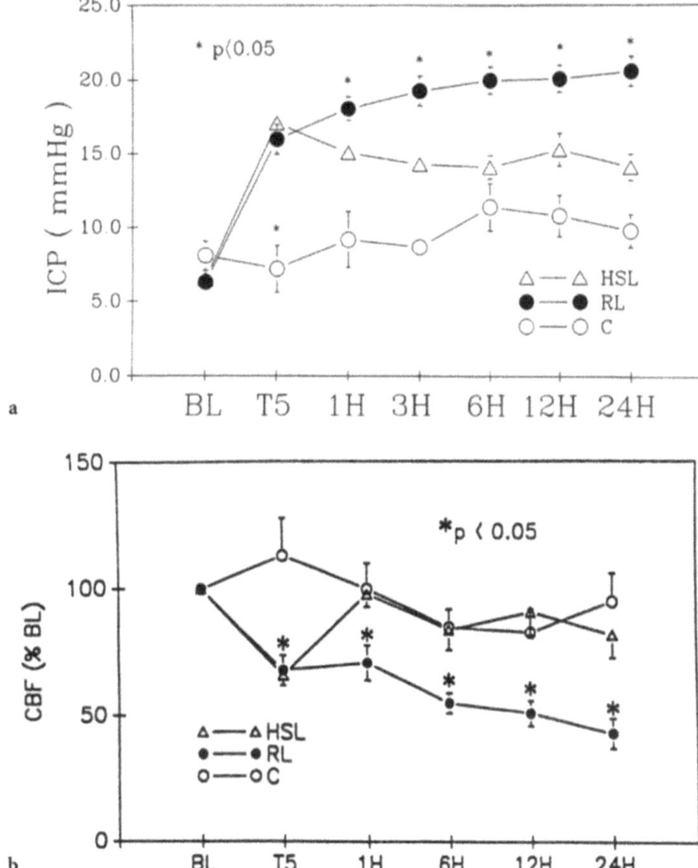

25.0
20.0
15.0
10.0
5.0
0.0
ICP (mmHg)
* p<0.05
HSL
RL
C
BL T5 1H 3H 6H 12H 24H
a
150
100
50
0
CBF (% BL)
*p < 0.05
HSL
RL
C
BL T5 1H 6H 12H 24H
b

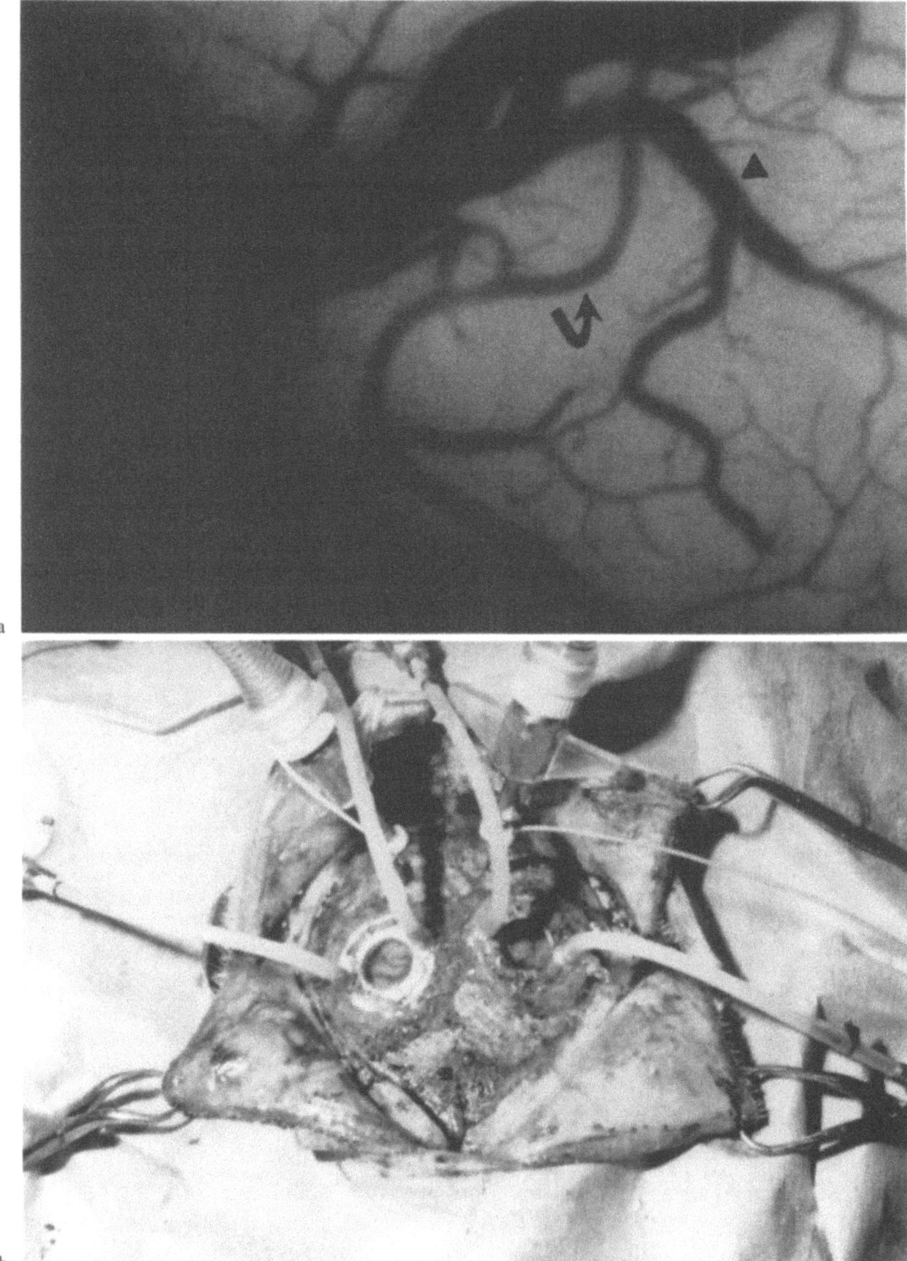

Fig. 4. a Cranial preparation during an experiment looking down on to the surface of the calvaria. Cephalad on the exposed calvaria is at the bottom of the photo, caudad is at the top. Notice the pial vessels distinctly visible through the cranial windows. **b** Microscopic view (×40) of the pial circulation demonstrating both pial arterioles (*curved arrows*) and pial venules (*arrowheads*)

attribute the observed increase in Evan's blue staining to the more expeditious movement of edema fluid through the white matter toward the ventricle. Rapid resolution of edema may represent another mechanism by which ICP is controlled or reduced with hypertonic resuscitation.

To investigate the mechanism of improved CBF following hypertonic resuscitation, we studied changes in the pial vessel diameter following cryogenic brain injury and hemorrhagic shock in a porcine model using a cranial window (Shackford et al. 1994). The cranial window technique (Fig. 4) allowed observation and measurement of changes in pial arteriolar during the entire 5-h experiment. We found that the cryogenic injury was associated with vasomotor dysfunction and a loss of pressure autoregulation. We also found that hypertonic resuscitation produced a significant and sustained elevation in cerebral perfusion pressure, pial arteriolar diameter and CBF when compared to RL ($p < 0.05$). These data suggested to us that hypertonic resuscitation following brain injury and shock improves CBF, at least in part, by causing vasodilatation of cerebral resistance vessels.

Despite the demonstrated efficacy of hypertonic solutions in achieving systemic resuscitation with less volume than isotonic fluids while increasing CBF and reducing cortical water content and ICP, there is no evidence that hypertonic solutions reduce secondary ischemic injury following shock and brain trauma. There is, however, suggestive evidence that they may limit neuronal death. Following global cerebral ischemia and reperfusion, Hamaguchi and Ogata (1995) studied the hippocampal CA1 subfield (a layer of cells in the hippocampus known to be extremely vulnerable to ischemia) in the gerbil following carotid occlusion and subsequent reperfusion. One group of animals was given 10% saline and the other an isotonic balanced salt solution. Animals were euthanized 5 days after the insult and the CA1 subfield was examined histologically. Animals receiving the isotonic solution had neuronal degeneration or death in 95% of cells which was significantly greater than the 7.1% degeneration or death rate observed in animals receiving hypertonic saline.

In summary, the mechanism proposed for the reduction of ICP and cortical water content by hypertonic fluids is the extraction of intracellular water from uninjured cerebral tissue down an osmolar gradient. The extraction of water from the cerebrovascular endothelium and from erythrocytes combined with dilatation of pial vessels are the probable mechanisms for improvement of CBF. The reduction in intracellular volume may also aid in edema resolution. Concerns that mild hypertonicity is injurious to the brain or that return of the osmolarity to the normal range would result in an increase in intracellular volume and a late increase in ICP appear unwarranted. These laboratory data suggest that hypertonic resuscitation, by improving intracranial compliance and CBF, may reduce secondary brain injury after trauma and hemorrhage.

The potential benefits of hypertonic resuscitation must be balanced against the risks of hypernatremia, hyperosmolarity and an induced hypokalemia. The hypernatremia and hyperosmolarity result from the infusion of the hypertonic solutions, but are only temporary (Shackford et al. 1988). The hypokalemia results from the kaliuresis associated with the large filtered renal tubular sodium load being presented to the distal convoluted tubule (Shackford et al. 1987b). The concern about intracellular dehydration as a result of the hyperosmolarity is justified. However, cells have the capacity to control their volume in response to increases in osmolarity by rapid ion and solute shifts and the accumulation of organic osmolytes which are considered to be "compatible" or "nonperturbing" (McManus et al. 1995). Recent clinical work has demonstrated that a serum osmolarity of 320–330 mOsm/l after hypertonic resuscitation is well tolerated (Shackford et al. 1983, 1987b; Holcroft et al. 1987). Nevertheless, the concerns about intracellular dehydration remain and current clinical recommendations are to stop hypertonic resuscitation when the serum osmolarity exceeds 350 mOsm/l. There are no data to support the presumption that exceeding a serum osmolarity of 350 mOsm/l will result in cellular dysfunction. In fact, the upper limit of osmolarity which can be tolerated by cells is unknown. To determine the effects of severe hyperosmolarity on cellular viability and function we exposed bovine aortic endothelial cells to hypertonic media under conditions of normoxia, hypoxia, and hypoxia-reoxygenation (Luh et al. 1996). The hypoxia and the hypoxia-reoxygenation were done to simulate a shock like state in these in vitro experiments. Cell viability and function were ascertained utilizing trypan blue exclusion, lactate dehydrogenase enzyme release, and cell replating assays. Endothelial cells exposed to media of 460 mOsm/l demonstrated no significant decrease in either viability or function compared to cells exposed to normal control media. A 6-h anoxic insult followed by 24 h of reoxygenation in media of 530 and 570 mOsm/l resulted in significantly *increased* viability and replating efficiency compared to 30 h of normoxia. These data indicate that in vitro endothelial cells tolerate media osmolarity of up to 460 mOsm/l without apparent decrement in viability or replating efficiency even in adverse conditions of anoxia and reoxygenation. Our data also suggest that exposure to anoxia may induce tolerance of endothelial cells to hyperosmotic media. These experimental data suggest that, during hypertonic resuscitation, exceeding a serum osmolarity of 350 mOsm/l may not be unsafe.

While hypertonic resuscitation has been used in the treatment of patients with burn injury (Monafo et al. 1984; Bowser-Wallace et al. 1985), there have been few published trials of hypertonic resuscitation in trauma patients with and without head injury (Mattox et al. 1991; Manningas et al. 1989; Holcroft et al. 1987; Vassar et al. 1991). Unfortunately, all of these trials evaluated a single bolus of 250 ml of 7.5% HS in 6% HSD followed by resuscitation with conventionally used crystalloid solutions. Therefore, these studies were not a true evaluation of hypertonic resuscitation since serum osmolarity and serum sodium were normalized very shortly after admission to the hospital. All of the studies have shown, however, that administration of HS to severely injured trauma patients is safe and at least as effective in initial resuscitation as conventional crystalloid. In each of the studies, the bolus of HSD resulted in a greater increase in blood pressure than did an equivalent volume of isotonic crystalloid. The HSD patients tended to require less blood and fluid than did the RL patients. Furthermore, in the largest study to date, there were trends indicating improved survival and fewer complications in patients receiving HSD (Mattox et al. 1991). Holcroft and colleagues (1987), in their initial study of 20 patients, observed significantly better survival in the HSD group ($p < 0.05$). Holcroft and coworkers expanded their experience to 166 patients (Vassar et al. 1991). While overall survival was similar in both the RL and HSD groups in this expanded study, survival after severe head injury was greater in patients treated with HSD (32%) than in patients treated with RL (16%) and approached statistical significance ($p = 0.07$).

Based on solid laboratory data and an early clinical experience, it appears that the use of hypertonic fluid for the resuscitation of head injured patients is justified (Eornow and Prough 1995). The early clinical experience with HSD followed by RL may not be a valid evaluation of hypertonic resuscitation since the patients eventually received large volumes of solute free water in the RL. Rather, the use of HSD as a bolus injection followed by continued hypertonic resuscitation compared to RL resuscitation would seem to be a more reasonable paradigm to evaluate hypertonic resuscitation. Additional investigation of hypertonic resuscitation is required to determine the levels of serum sodium and osmolarity which can be safely tolerated in this patient group.

Crystalloid: Mannitol

Hyperosmolar solutions containing nonionizing solutes such as urea or mannitol have been shown to decrease ICP and cerebral water content in the normal brain. Because these are low molecular substances which are filtered but not reabsorbed by the kidney, they induce an "osmotic" diuresis (Stahl 1965; Gennari et al. 1974). The capacity of hyperosmolar nonionizing solutes to reduce ICP and cerebral water content has long been attributed to this diuretic property. Reed and Woodbury (1962), performing studies of urea in nephrectomized rats, demonstrated that these changes were independent of a forced diuresis. The decrease in ICP occurred rapidly (within 20–30 min) and returned to baseline within 2 h owing to compensatory increases in the volumes of the other intracranial contents. The decrease in cerebral water content occurred within 1 h and returned to normal by 8 h as urea crossed the blood–brain barrier and entered cells. Kassell and associates (1982) demonstrated a transient increase in CBF associated with mannitol administration in the normal brain and postulated that the beneficial effects of hyperosmolar therapy were due to a reduction in endothelial and perivascular cell volume, reduced blood viscosity, and an increase in cardiac output. Muizelaar and colleagues (1983), using a cranial window technique to directly observe pial arterioles, demonstrated a reduction in pial arteriolar diameter associated with a reduction in blood viscosity and a decrease in ICP. They postulated that reduced viscosity improves flow (by Poiseuille's law), which increases oxygen delivery and improves the removal of cerebral metabolites, which are thought to reduce cerebral vascular tone. They suggested that the improved flow causes pial vasoconstriction which led to a reduction in cerebral blood volume and ICP. Whatever the mechanism of the rapid decrease in ICP, it has been shown by Nath and Galbraith (1986) that even low-dose mannitol (0.28 gm/kg) decreases the water content of the white matter, suggesting that dehydration plays some the role in the reduction of ICP by hyperosmolar solutions in the normal brain.

Mannitol and urea have also been shown to consistently decrease ICP and cerebral water content in the presence of a brain injury. Mannitol appears to have a variable effect on CBF in brain injury, causing an increase when autoregulation is lost and no charge when autoregulation is intact. Bruce and colleagues (1973) found that mannitol decreased the ICP in 11 of 13 patients, increased the CBF in 12 of 13 and increased the metabolic rate in 10 of 13. They found that the increase in CBF appeared to be independent of the effects of ICP. Further, mannitol was equally effective in patients with and without a mass lesion. Similar results were obtained by Mendelow and colleagues (1985). The magnitude of the decrease in ICP appears to be affected by two factors: the ICP itself (higher pressures tend to have greater decreases), and the dose of mannitol (McGraw et al. 1983). Marshall and coworkers (1978) suggest that doses as low as 0.25 g/kg are effective in lowering the ICP, but the larger doses (1.0 g/kg) are associated with a more persistent reduction.

Most of the studies involving mannitol have been performed in hemodynamically stable patients with supposedly normal blood volume. Mannitol has not been advocated for reduction of ICP in hypovolemic subjects because it can cause or exaggerate hypotension. Cote and associates (1979) have suggested that the hypotension due to mannitol infusion is a result of vasodilation in skeletal muscle and is proportionate to the dose and rate of administration. Even with maximal doses and rapid administration, the hypotension is transient and self-limited, with blood pressure returning to normal in 85–115 s. Brown and co-workers (1979) observed an increase in MAP, CPP, and CBF when animals with a penetrating brain injury were given mannitol. They attributed the improved hemodynamics to a positive inotropic effect and to decreased blood viscosity, suggesting that mannitol could be used early as a resuscitative therapy.

The consistent reduction in ICP and, in some studies, improved CBF rekindled interest in mannitol for the treatment of hypovolemic shock associated with a head injury. Israel and associates (1988) compared 25% mannitol to normal saline in dogs that were hemorrhaged 25 ml/kg (approximately 35% of the blood volume). The dogs were also subjected to a brain injury by the inflation of an epidural balloon that created a mass effect and intracranial hypertension. Both solutions restored MAP and no hypotension was observed after mannitol infusion. In the dogs resuscitated with mannitol the ICP was significantly lower and left ventricular stroke work index, cardiac index, CPP, and urine output were significantly higher than in dogs resuscitated with NS ($p < 0.01$).

Based on these studies it would appear that mannitol may be useful in maintaining cerebral perfusion and decreasing ICP after head injury. The work of Israel and colleagues (1988) suggests that it may also be useful in head injury associated with hypovolemic shock, but this will require further study.

Asanguinous Fluids: Colloids

Colloid solutions contain large molecular weight solutes (>60 000 daltons) that generally exceed the pore size of most capillaries and are retained, at least temporarily, in the vascular compartment. The administration of a colloid solution will increase the colloid osmotic pressure and, according to Starling's hypothesis, should reduce the transcapillary fluid flux at a given hydrostatic pressure provided there is no increase in capillary permeability. Colloid solutions have been shown to be very effective in the resuscitation of hypovolemic shock, adequately restoring perfusion with a smaller volume of fluid than is necessary with isotonic salt solution. Studies comparing colloids and electrolyte solutions have focused primarily on the lung (Virgilio et al. 1979) where edema formation can be detrimental to function.

A few studies have examined the effects of colloid administration on the injured brain. Clasen and associates (1957) compared hypertonic glucose (50%, 50 ml) to albumin (25%, 50 ml) in normovolemic dogs with a cryogenic brain injury. The authors postulated that an oncotic gradient might reduce cerebral water content and lower ICP. Treatment with albumin lowered the cisternal pressure, but not significantly, whereas hypertonic glucose therapy resulted in a significant drop in the ICP. Postmortem cerebral water content was not affected by either treatment. The authors concluded that the solutions decreased ICP by a mechanism other than interstitial dehydration. One has to wonder, however, if the small dosages of albumin and glucose were sufficient to establish oncotic or osmotic gradients capable of dehydration. Albright and Phillips (1982) compared 25% albumin (1 g/kg) to an electrolyte solution in normovolemic dogs with a cryogenic lesion, also postulating that the oncotic gradient produced by the infusion would result in the withdrawal of cerebral interstitial water and lower the ICP. They found no difference between study groups in the cerebral water content in either the injured hemisphere or in the contralateral hemisphere and concluded that the dosage of albumin was insufficient to produce the desired oncotic effect. In a subsequent investigation Albright and colleagues (1984a) studied three groups of normovolemic dogs subjected to a cryogenic lesion. A control group was given a crystalloid solution and experimental groups received either 12% hydroxyethyl starch (a synthetic colloid) or 24% hydroxyethyl starch and furosemide. At the end of the 6-h study period the dogs receiving starch had a significantly higher COP and significantly lower ICP than the group receiving crystalloid ($p < 0.05$). Cerebral water content in the area of the lesion was significantly lower in the dogs receiving hydroxyethyl starch than in those receiving crystalloid. In the group treated with 24% hydroxyethyl starch and furosemide the water content of the *contralateral* uninjured hemisphere was also significantly lower than control ($p < 0.05$). In another study, Albright and coworkers (1984b) compared five groups of normovolemic dogs with a cryogenic lesion treated with either crystalloid (control), mannitol (20%, 1.5 g/ kg), furosemide, albumin (25%, 2 g/kg), or albumin and furosemide. Albumin alone failed to decrease the mean ICP compared to control, whereas albumin and furosemide did lower the mean ICP significantly ($p < 0.05$). The water content in the lesioned area of the albumin treated dogs was significantly lower than in control animals ($p < 0.05$). The water content of the uninjured cortex in the experimental groups was lower than control, but the difference was not statistically significant. The authors point out, however, that small differences in cerebral water content can result in significant volume displacement within the cranium and could have been responsible for the observed difference in the ICP. They conclude from this and their previous studies that colloid therapy, especially when combined with furosemide, is effective in lowering ICP through normovolemic dehydration of the lesioned area and the uninjured brain.

Zornow and colleagues (1988) induced normovolemic hemodilution with either crystalloid or colloid (hydroxyethyl starch) in rabbits without a brain injury and studied ICP and cerebral water content. There were no significant differences between the groups for either variable despite a significantly reduced COP in the crystalloid group. The authors concluded that the pivotal factor in water movement across the BBB was independent of the COP. Wisner and coworkers (1989), using an ovine model of combined trauma (crush injury of the leg) and hemorrhagic shock, compared the effects of colloid (4% albumin) and crystalloid resuscitation in groups of animals with and without a cryogenic brain injury. In the animals without a brain injury, the crystalloid group required significantly more fluid to achieve resuscitation than did the colloid group ($p < 0.01$). ICP increased with resuscitation in both groups but was not significantly different from baseline in either group, nor was there any difference between the groups in cerebral water content. Similar results were obtained when the cryogenic brain injury was added to traumatic hemorrhagic shock: ICP rose with resuscitation in both groups, but it was not significantly different than baseline values and there was no difference between the groups in cerebral water content in either the area of the lesion or the uninjured brain tissue. The authors concluded that maintaining the COP had no beneficial effect on ICP or cerebral water content. Further, they believe their data demonstrate that the large volume of crystalloid necessary to restore baseline hemodynamic function does not adversely affect either the ICP of the cerebral water content. The volume of hemorrhage in this study was relatively small (approximately 14 ml/kg or 20% of the blood volume), and the results might have been different had the shock been more severe. The duration of study was only 2h after completion of shock and the delayed effects of resuscitation could not be evaluated. Nevertheless, this well controlled study does suggest that colloid resuscitation offers no advantage over isotonic crystalloid in the resuscitation of brain injury with or without hemorrhage.

Warner and Boehland (1988) studied the effects of iso-osmolal 6% starch and crystalloid in a murine model of hemorrhage and ischemia at intervals up to and including 24h. Edema was noted in animals killed within 1.5h of injury, independent of the type of fluid used. At 24h there was no difference between the groups in cerebral water content. They concluded that the magnitude of edema was independent of the fluid used, provided osmolality was kept constant. Based on their data it seems unlikely that COP plays a substantial role in preventing edema formation.

Tranmer and colleagues (1989) compared crystalloid to colloid therapy in a model of cryogenic injury without hemorrhage. Animals received excessive amounts of fluid (up to 30 ml/kg per hour, equivalent to 2100 ml/h in a 70-kg person). Although no statistical analysis was performed to compare the groups, the greatest increases in ICP following fluid infusion occurred in the animals receiving crystalloid. In addition, a deterioration in the power ratio index of the EEG was noted in the crystalloid groups. Unfortunately, the authors did not measure either COP or osmolarity and it is difficult to determine the significance of the observed EEG changes.

Many of the previous studies have been flawed because important variables were either not controlled (i.e., osmolarity of the colloid solutions) or not measured (i.e., COP) or agents known to reduce ICP were used in conjunction with colloid therapy (i.e., diuretics). To clarify the relative importance of COP and osmolarity, Kaieda and associated (1989), in a well controlled experiment, infused fluids of varying oncotic and osmotic pressure in a model of focal cryogenic brain injury in which the animals had undergone plasmapheresis; experimental fluids were given to maintain the MAP and the CVP. Animals receiving hypo-osmolar fluids, regardless of the oncotic pressure of the fluid, had significant increases in ICP and cerebral water content in the uninjured cortex. The COP had no effect on either the ICP or the cerebral water content by regression analysis. On the other hand, there was a significant inverse relationship between the osmolarity of the fluid and the water content of the uninjured brain. Similar results were obtained by Zornow and coworkers (1988) in a model of cryogenic brain injury and isovolemic hemodilution. Despite a 53% reduction in COP and a significantly increased fluid requirement to maintain hemodynamic stability, animals receiving NS had a similar ICP and a similar cerebral water content to animals receiving 5% albumin or 6% hetastarch. We compared 6% dextran 70 to RL in a porcine model of cryogenic injury and found no difference between the groups in ICP, CBF or cerebral oxygen delivery (Zhuang et al. 1995).

In summary, colloids, while effective in restoring hemodynamic parameters with significantly less fluid than crystalloid, do not decrease either ICP or cerebral water content. This is not surprising given that the BBB, with a pore size of 8 Å, is not permeable to sodium, but is permeable to water. The possibility, therefore, exists for large osmotic gradients with significant absorptive power (Table 2). Thus, osmotic (not oncotic) forces are the major factors determining water movement in the brain. Such is not the case in the peripheral muscle capillary (pore size 19 Å) which is freely permeable to sodium and to water, but not to large protein moieties. Thus, a large oncotic gradient exists between the intravascular and the extravascular spaces and is the determining factor in water movement between those spaces.

The lack of consistency in reducing either ICP or cerebral water content, combined with the increased cost (Metildi et al. 1984), a small risk of anaphylaxis (Ring et al. 1977), and the potential for increased bleeding (Johnson et al. 1979) limit the usefulness of colloids as a primary choice in the resuscitation of head injury.

Hemoglobin Substitutes

Asanguinous solutions are given to trauma patients to expand intravascular volume until blood is available for transfusion. The major advantage of red blood cells in treating shock is that they carry oxygen. The major disadvantage is that blood is not always immediately available and typing and crossmatching can take up to an hour. Ideally, a solution which is capable of carrying and delivering oxygen to ischemic tissues would be of benefit in treating the shock victim, particularly one with an associated head injury.

Hemoglobin substitutes carry and deliver oxygen and are immediately available since they require no typing and crossmatching. Unfortunately, many of the previously used hemoglobin substitutes had very short plasma half lives and had P50's (the partial pressure of oxygen at which hemoglobin is 50% saturated) which were significantly lower than blood resulting in increased oxygen–hemoglobin affinity at low tissue PO_2 (Greenburg et al. 1979). Diaspirin crosslinked hemoglobin (DCLHb) is a hemoglobin tetramer made from human blood. During its production the α subunits are covalently bound, creating a stable tetramer that has a plasma half-life of 20–30 h

(Synder et al. 1979). The P50 of DCLHb is 29–32 torr which is slightly greater than whole blood (P50 = 27 torr). DCLHb has been shown to elevate MAP and reduce ischemic changes in the uninjured rodent brain following shock (Przybelski et al. 1990). The pressor effect of DCLHb is a result of the release of endothelin and the scavenging of nitric oxide. By elevating the MAP, DCLHb should increase the CPP, thereby potentially limiting the extent of secondary ischemic brain injury. Since DCLHb carries oxygen it should increase cerebral oxygen delivery when compared to a balanced salt solution. In support of this, Cole et al. (1993) have demonstrated that hemodilution with DCLHb significantly reduced infarct volume and edema formation in a rodent model of global cerebral ischemia.

Since hemodilution has been used effectively in occlusive ischemic models, we evaluated it in a porcine model of head injury and shock (Chappell et al. 1995). We compared hemodilution to a standard resuscitation paradigm using RL and shed blood. Resuscitation with DCLHb was achieved with significantly less volume. The hemoglobin concentration in the hemodiluted, DCLHb animals was significantly lower than the animals receiving RL and shed blood (8.5 ± 0.4 vs 12.1 ± 0.3, $p < 0.05$). During the initial phases of resuscitation animals receiving DCLHb had a significantly higher CPP and a significantly lower ICP. There were no differences between the groups in CBF or lesion volume. These data suggested to us that DCLHb might be beneficial in the early treatment of shock and head injury. We subsequently compared DCLHb combined with shed blood (no hemodilution) to RL and shed blood in a porcine model of head injury and shock. DCLHb animals had a significantly higher MAP and CPP, but required significantly less fluid to maintain hemodynamic stability. The ICP was lower in the DCLHb animals, but the difference was not significant. These results were obtained with only a single bolus of DCLHb (250 ml) leading us to believe that repetitive doses might be more efficacious.

In summary, these early investigations suggest the DCLHb is effective in elevating and maintaining CPP in a model of head injury and shock. This can be achieved with significantly less fluid and a trend toward a lower ICP when compared to RL. These data suggest that further investigation of DCLHb, probably in a multidose paradigm, is warranted.

Acknowledgments. This research was supported in part by grants P20 NS30324-03 and RO1 NS28637-02 from the National Institutes of Neurologic Diseases and Stroke.

References

Albright AL, Phillips JW (1982) Oncotic therapy of experimental cerebral edema. Acta Neurochir (Wien) 60:257

Albright AL, Latchaw RE, Robinson AG (1984a) Intracranial and systemic effects of hetastarch in experimental cerebral edema. Crit Care Med 12:496

Albright AL, Latchaw RE, Robinson AG (1984b) Intracranial and systemic effects of osmotic and oncotic therapy in experimental cerebral edema. J Neurosurg 60:481

Ali J, Aprahamian C, Brown R et al (1993) Advanced trauma life support. American College of Surgeons, Chicago, pp 159–190

Bakay L, Crawford JD, White JC (1954) The effects of intravenous fluids on cerebrospinal fluid pressure. Surg Gynec Obstet 99:484

Bakay R, Wood JH (1985) Pathophysiology of cerebral fluid in trauma. In: Beckere DP, Povlishock J (eds) Central nervous system trauma status report. Bethesda, MD. NINCDS, NIH pp 89–122

Battistella ED, Wisner DH (1991) Combined hemorrhagic shock and head injury: Effects of hypertonic saline (7.5%) resuscitation. J Trauma 31:182

Becker DB, Miller JD, Ward JD et al (1977) The outcome from severe head injury with early diagnosis and intensive management. J Neurosurg 47:491

Berger S, Schurer L, Hartl R et al (1995) Reduction of post-traumatic intracranial hypertension by hypertonic/hyperoncotic saline/dextran and hypertonic mannitol. Neurosurgery 37:98

Bouma GJ, Muizelaar JP (1990) Relationship between cardiac output and cerebral blood flow in patients with intact and with impaired autoregulation. J Neurosurg 73:368

Bowser-Wallace BH, Cone JB, Caldwell FT Jr (1985) Hypertonic lactated saline resuscitation of severely burned patients over 60 years of age. J Trauma 25:22

Brown FD, Johns L, Jafar JJ et al (1979) Detailed monitoring of the effects of mannitol following experimental head injury. J Neurosurg 50:243

Brown MM, Marshall J (1982) Effect of plasma exchange on blood viscosity and cerebral blood flow. Br Med J 284:1733

Brown MM, Marshall J (1985) Regulation of cerebral blood flow in response to changes in blood viscosity. Lancet 1:604

Brown MM, Wade JP, Marshall J (1985) Fundamental importance of arterial oxygen content in the regulation of cerebral blood flow in man. Brain 108:81

Bruce DA, Langfitt TW, Miller JE et al (1973) Regional cerebral blood flow, intracranial pressure, and brain metabolism in comatose patients. J Neurosurg 38:131

Bustad LK, Horstman VG, Swindle MM et al (1986) Swing in biomedical research. Plenum, New York, pp 1–6

Carrel M, Moeschler O, Ravussin P et al (1994) Prehospital air ambulance and systemic secondary cerebral damage in severe craniocerebral injuries. Ann Fr Anesth Reanim 13:326

Chappell JE, McBride WJ, Shackford SR (1995) Hemodilution with diaspirin cross linked hemoglobin lowers intracranial pressure, improves cerebral perfusion pressure, and reduces fluid requirement following head injury and shock. Surg Forum 46:569

Chestnut RM, Marshall LS, Klauber M (1993) The role of secondary brain injury in determining outcome from severe head injury. J Trauma 34:216

Civetta JM (1979) A new look at the Starling equation. Crit Care Med 7:84

Clasen RA, Prouty RR, Bingham WG, Martin FA, Hass GM (1957) Treatment of experimental cerebral edema with intravenous hypertonic glucose, albumin and dextran. Surg Gynecol Obstet 104:591

Cole DJ, Schell RM, Drummond JC, Reynolds L (1993) Focal cerebral ischemia in rats. Effect of hypervolemic hemodilution with diaspirin cross-linked hemoglobin versus albumin on brain injury and edema. Anesthesiology 78:335

Cote CJ, Greenhow DE, Marshall BE (1979) The hypotensive response to rapid intravenous administration of hypertonic solutions in man and in the rabbit. Anesthesiology 50:30, 1979

Cruz J (1988) Continuous versus serial global cerebral hemometabolic monitoring: Applications in acute brain trauma. Acta Neurochir Suppl (Wien) 42:35

Davis JW, Shackford SR, Mackersie RC, Hoyt DB (1988) Base deficit as a guide to volume resuscitation. J Trauma 28:1464

DeSalles AA, Muizelaar P, Young HG (1987) Hyperglycemia, cerebrospinal fluid lactic acidosis and cerebral blood flow in severely head-injured patients. Neurosurgery 21:45

DeWitt DS, Jenkins LW, Lutz H (1981) Regional cerebral blood flow following fluid percussion injury. J Cereb Blood Flow Metab 1 [Suppl] 5:579

Dewitt DS, Jenkins LW, Wei EP et al (1986) Effects of fluid-percussion brain injury on regional cerebral blood flow and pial arteriolar diameter. J Neurosurg 64:787

Ducey JP, Mozingo DW, Lamiell JM et al (1989) A comparison of the cerebral and cardiovascular effects of complete resuscitation with isotonic and hypertonic saline, hetastarch, and whole blood following hemorrhage. J Trauma 29:1510

Feldman Z, Zachari S, Reichenthal E, Artru AA, Shapira Y (1995) Brain edema and neurological status with rapid infusion of lactated Ringer's or 5% dextrose solution following head trauma. J Neurosurg 83:1060

Fenstermacher JD (1984) Volume regulation of the central nervous system. In: Staub NC, Taylor AE (eds) Edema. Raven, New York, p 383

Fenstermacher JD, Johnson JA (1966) Filtration and reflection coefficients of rabbit blood-brain barrier. Am J Physiol 211:341

Gazitua S, Scott JB, Swindall B et al (1971) Resistance responses to local changes in plasma osmolality in three vascular beds. Am J Physiol 220:3384

Gennari FJ, Kaissirer JP (1974) Osmotic diuresis. N Engl J Med 291:714

Graham DI, Adams H, Doyle D (1978) Ischemic brain damage in fatal non-missile head injuries. J Neurol Sci 39:213

Graham DI, Ford I, Adams JH et al (1989) Ischemic brain damage is still common in fatal non-missile head injuries. J Neurol Neurosurg Psychiatry 52:346

Graham DI, Adams JH, Nicoll JAR, Maxwell WL, Gennarelli TA (1995) The nature, distribution and causes of traumatic brain injury. Brain Pathol 5:397–406

Greenberg JH, Alavi A, Reivich M et al (1978) Local cerebral blood volume response to carbon dioxide in man. Circ Res 43:325

Greenburg AG, Hayashi R, Siefert BA, Reese H, Peskin GW (1979) Intravascular persistence and oxygen delivery of pyridoxalated, stroma-free hemoglobin during gradiations of hypotension. Surgery 86:13

Gunnar W, Jonasson O, Merlotti G et al (1988) Head injury and hemorrhage shock: studies of the blood brain barrier and intracranial pressure after resuscitation with normal saline solution 3% saline solution, and dextran-40. Surgery 103:398

Hamaguchi S, Ogata (1995) Does hypertonic saline have preventive effects against delayed neuronal death in gerbil hippocampus? Shock 3:280

Hariri RJ, Firlick AD, Shepard SR et al (1993) Traumatic brain injury, hemorrhagic shock, and fluid resuscitation: effects on intracranial pressure and brain compliance. J Neurosurg 79:421

Hartl R, Schurer L, Goetz et al (1995) The effect of hypertonic fluid resuscitation on brain edema in rabbits subjected to brain injury and hemorrhagic shock. Shock 3:274

Heistad DD, Kontos HA (1983) Cerebral circulation. In: Shepard JT, Abboud FM (eds) The cardiovascular system. Williams, Baltimore, pp 137–182 (Handbook of physiology, vol 3)

Hermann HD, Newenfeld HD (1972) Development and regression of a disturbance of the blood brain barrier and of edema in the tissue surrounding a circumscribed cold lesion. Exp Neurol 34:115

Holcroft JW, Vassar MJ, Turner JE et al (1987) 3% NaCl and 7.5% NaCl/dextran 70 in the resuscitation of severely injured patients. Ann Surg 206:279

Ishsige N, Pitts LH, Berry I et al (1988) The effects of hypovolemic hypotension on high-energy phosphate metabolism of traumatized brain in rat. J Neurosurg 68:129

Israel RS, Marx JA, Lowenstein SR (1988) Hemodynamic effect of mannitol in a canine model of concomitant increased intracranial pressure and hemorrhagic shock. Ann Emerg Med 17:560

Jaggi JL, Obrist WD, Gennarelli TA, Langfitt TW (1990) Relationship of early cerebral blood flow and metabolism to outcome in acute head injury. J Neurosurg 72:176

Jenkins LW, Moszynski K, Lyeth BG et al (1989) Increased vulnerability of the mildly traumatized rat brain to cerebral ischemia; the use of controlled secondary ischemia as a research tool to identify common or different mechanisms contributing to mechanical and ischemic brain injury. Brain Res 477:21

Johnson SD, Lucas CD, Gerrick SJ et al (1979) Altered coagulation after albumin supplements for treatment of ligemic shock. Arch Surg 114:370

Kaieda R, Todd MM, Cook LN, Warner DS (1989) Acute effects of changing plasma osmolarity and colloid oncotic pressure on the formation of brain edema after cryogenic injury. Neurosurgery 24:61

Kassell NF, Baumann KW, Hitchon PW et al (1982) The effects of high dose mannitol on cerebral blood flow in dogs with normal intracranial pressure. Stroke 13:59

Kien ND, Kramer GC, White DA (1989) Direct cardiac effect of hypertonic saline in anesthetized dogs. Anesth Analg 68:5147

Kien ND, Reitan JA, White DA et al (1991) Cardiac contractility and blood flow distribution following resuscitation with 7.5% hypertonic saline in anesthetized dogs. Circ Shock 35:109

Klauber MR, Barrett-Connor EB, Marshall LF, Bowers SA (1981) The epidemiology of head injury. Am J Epidemiol 113:500

Klauber MR, Marshall LF, Toole BM, Knowlton SL, Bowers SA (1985) Cause of death in head-injury mortality rate in San Diego County, California. J Neurosurg 62:528

Kontos HA (1981) Regulation of the cerebral circulation. Annu Rev Physiol 43:397

Kraus JF (1993) Epidemiology of head injury. In: Cooper PR (ed) Head injury. Williams, Baltimore, pp 1–25

Kreimeier U, Brueckner UB, Schmidt J, Messmer K (1990) Instantaneous restoration of regional organ blood flow after severe hemorrhage: effect of small-volume resuscitation with hypertonic-hyperoncotic solutions. J Surg Res 49:493

Luh EH, Shackford SR, Shatos MA, Pietropaoli JA (1996) The effects of hyperosmolarity on the viability and function of endothelial cells. J Surg Res 60:122

Manningas PA (1987) Resuscitation with 7.5% NaCl in 6% dextran-70 during hemorrhagic shock in swine: effect on organ blood flow. Crit Care Med 15:1121

Manningas PA, Mattox KL, Pepe RE et al (1989) Hypertonic saline-dextran solutions for the prehospital management of traumatic hypotension. Am J Surg 157:528

Marion DW, Darby J, Yonas H (1991) Acute regional cerebral blood flow changes caused by severe head injuries. J Neurosurg 74:407

Marmarou A, Anderson RL, Ward JD et al (1991) Impact of ICP instability and hypotension on outcome in patients with severe head trauma. J Neurosurg 75:S1591

Marshall LF, Welsh F, Durity F (1975) Experimental cerebral oligemia and ischemia produced by intracranial hypertension: 3. Brain energy metabolism. J Neurosurg 43:323

Marshall LF, Smith RW, Rauscher LA, Shapiro HM (1978) Mannitol dose requirements in brain injured patients. J Neurosurg 48:169

Mattox KL, Manningas PA, Moore EE et al (1991) Prehospital hypertonic saline/dextran infusion for post-traumatic hypotension: The U.S.A. Multicenter Trial. Ann Surg 231:482

Max W, Mackenzie EJ, Rice DP (1991) Head injuries, costs and consequences. J Head Trauma Rehab 6:76

Mazzoni MC, Lundgren E, Arfors KE, Intaglietta M (1989) Volume changes of an endothelial cell monolayer on exposure to anisotonic media. J Cell Physiol 140:272

Mazzoni MC, Borgstrom P, Intaglietta M, Arfors KE (1990) Capillary narrowing in hemorrhagic shock is rectified by hyperosmotic saline-dextran reinfusion. Circ Shock 31:407

McGraw CP, Howard G (1983) Effect of mannitol on increased intracranial pressure. Neurosurgery 13:269

McIntosh TK, Vink R, Noble L et al (1989) Traumatic brain injury in the rat: Characterization of a lateral fluid-percussion model. Neuroscience 28:233

McManus ML, Churchill KB, Straage K (1995) Regulation of cell volume in health and disease. N Engl J Med 333:1260

Mendelow AD, Teasdale GM, Russell T et al (1985) Effect of mannitol on cerebral blood flow and cerebral perfusion pressure in human head injury. J Neurosurg 63:43

Matildi LA, Shackford SR, Virgilio RW, Peters RM (1984) Crystalloid versus colloid in fluid resuscitation of patients with severe pulmonary insufficiency. Surg Gynecol Obstet 158:207

Miller JD, Becker DP, Ward JH et al (1977) Significance of intracranial hypertension in severe head injury. J Neurosurg 54:289

Miller JD, Sweet RC, Narayan R et al (1978) Early insults to the injured brain. JAMA 240:439

Miller JD, Butterworth JF, Gudeman SK et al (1981) Further experience in the management of severe head injury. J Neurosurg 54:289

Monafo WW, Halverson JD, Schectman K (1984) The role of concentrated sodium solutions in the resuscitation of patients with severe burns. Surgery 95:129

Morse ML, Milstein JM, Haas JE, Taylor E (1985) Effect of hydration on experimentally induced cerebral edema. Crit Care Med 113:563

Muizelaar JP, Wei EP, Kontos HA, Becker DP (1983) Mannitol causes compensatory cerebral vasoconstriction and vasodilation in response to blood viscosity changes. J Neurosurg 59:822

Muizelaar JP, Marmarou A, DeSallels AA et al (1989) Cerebral blood flow and metabolism in severely head-injured children. J Neurosurg 71:63

Nakayama S, Sibley L, Gunther RA et al (1984) Small-volume resuscitation with hypertonic saline (2400 mOsm/liter) during hemorrhagic shock. Circ Shock 13:149

Nath F, Galbraith S (1986) The effect of mannitol on cerebral white matter water content. J Neurosurg 65:41

Obrist WD, Langfit TW, Jaggi JL (1984) Cerebral blood flow and metabolism in comatose patients with acute head injury: Relationship to intracranial hypertension. J Neurosurg 61:241

Overgaard J, Mosdal C, Tweed WA (1981) Cerebral circulation after head injury: 3. does reduced regional cerebral blood flow determine recovery of brain function after blunt head injury. J Neurosurg 5:63

Pacult A, Gudeman SK (1989) Medical management of head injuries. In: Becker DP, Gudeman SK (eds) Textbook of head injury. Saunders, Philadelphia, pp 192–220

Pfenninger EG, Reith A, Bretig D et al (1989) Early changes in intracranial pressure, perfusion pressure, and blood flow after acute head injury: I. an experimental study of the underlying pathophysiology. J Neurosurg 70:774

Pietropaoli JA, Rogers FB, Shackford SR (1992) The deleterious effects of intraoperative hypotension on outcome in patients with severe head injuries. J Trauma 33:403

Pitts LH, Kaktis JV, Juster R, Heilbron D (1980) ICP and outcome in patients with severe head injury. In: Shulman K, Marmarou A, Miller JD et al (eds) Intracranial pressure IV. Springer Berlin Heidelberg New York, pp 5–9

Poole GV, Prough AS, Johnson JC et al (1987) Effects of resuscitation from hemorrhagic shock on cerebral hemodynamics in the presence of an intracranial mass. J Trauma 27:18

Prough DS, Rogers AT (1989) Physiology and pharmacology of cerebral blood flow and metabolism. Crit Care Clin 5:713

Prough DS, Johnston JC, Poole GV Jr et al (1985) Effects on intracranial pressure of resuscitation from hemorrhagic shock with hypertonic saline versus lactated Ringer's solution. Crit Care Med 13:407

Prough DS, Johnson JC, Stump DA et al (1986) Effects of hypertonic saline versus lactated Ringer's solution on cerebral oxygen transport during resuscitation from hemorrhagic shock. J Neurosurg 64:627

Przybelski RJ, Kant GJ, Bounds MJ, Slayter MV, Winslow RM (1990) Rat maze performance after resuscitation with cross-linked hemoglobin solution. J Lab Clin Med 115:579

Ramming S, Shackford SR, Zhuang J, Schmoker JD (1994) The relationship of fluid balance and sodium administration to cerebral edema formation and intracranial pressure in a porcine model of brain injury. J Trauma 705

Rango M, Lenkinski RE, Alves WM (1990) Brain pH in head injury: An image-guided P magnetic resonance spectroscopy study. Ann Neurol 28:661

Reed DJ, Woodburg DM (1962) Effect of hypertonic urea on cerebrospinal fluid pressure and brain volume. J Physiol (Lond) 164:252

Reivich M (1965) Arterial PCO_2 and cerebral hemodynamics. Am J Physiol 206:25

Reulan HG (1976) Vasogenic brain edema: new aspects in its formulation, resolution and therapy. Br J Anaesth 48:741

Ring L, Messmer RJ (1977) Incidence and severity of anaphylactoid reactions to colloid volume substitute. Lancet 1:466

Rowe GG, Mckenna DH, Corliss RJ, Sialer S (1972) Hemodynamic effects of hypertonic sodium chloride. J Appl Physiol 32:182

Schmoker JD, Zhuang J, Shackford SR (1991) Hemorrhage hypotension after brain injury causes an early and sustained reduction in cerebral oxygen delivery despite normalization of systemic oxygen delivery. J Trauma 31:1038

Schmoker JD, Shackford SR, Wald SL, Pietropaoli JA (1992) An analysis of the relationship between fluid and sodium administration and intracranial pressure after head injury. J Trauma 33:476

Schmoker JD, Zhuang J, Shackford SR, Pietropaoli J (1993) Effect of lesion volume on cerebral hemodynamics after focal brain injury and shock. J Trauma 35:627

Shackford SR (1987a) Fluid resuscitation of the trauma victim. In: Shackford SR, Perel A (eds) Problems in critical care, vol 1. Lippincott, Philadelphia, p 550

Shackford SR (1990) Fluid resuscitation in head injury. J Intensive Care Med 5:59

Shackford SR, Sise MJ, Fridlund PH, Rowley WR, Peters RM, Virgilio RW, Brimm JE (1983) Hypertonic sodium lactate versus lactated Ringer's solution for intravenous fluid therapy in operations on the abdominal aorta. Surgery 94:41

Shackford SR, Fortlage DA, Peters RM et al (1987b) Serum osmolar and electrolyte changes associated with large infusions of hypertonic sodium lactate for intravascular volume expansion of patients undergoing aortic reconstruction. Surg Gynecol Obstet 164:127

Shackford SR, Norton CK, Todd MM (1988) Renal, cerebral, and pulmonary effects of hypertonic resuscitation in a porcine model of hemorrhagic shock. Surgery 104:553

Shackford SR, Zhuang J, Schmoker J (1992) Intravenous fluid tonicity: effect on intracranial pressure, cerebral blood flow, and cerebral oxygen delivery in focal brain injury. J Neurosurg 6:91

Shackford SR, Mackersie RC, Holbrook TL et al (1993) The epidemiology of traumatic death: a population-based analysis. Arch Surg 128:571

Shackford SR, Schmoker JD, Zhuang J (1994) The effect of hypertonic resuscitation on pial arteriolar tone after brain injury and shock. J Trauma 37:899

Shapira Y, Artru AA, Qassam N et al (1992) Brain edema and neurologic status following head trauma in the rat. No effect from large volumes of isotonic or hypertonic intravenous fluids, with or without glucose. Anesthesiology 77:79

Shenkin HA, Gutterman P (1964) The analysis of body water compartments in postoperative craniotomy patients. J Neurosurg 31:400

Siesjo BK (1984) Cerebral circulation and metabolism. J Neurosurg 60:883

Silva MR, Negraces GA, Soares AM et al (1986) Hypertonic resuscitation from severe hemorrhage shock: Patterns of regional circulation. Circ Shock 19:165

Snyder SR, Welty EV, Walder RY, Williams LA, Walder JA (1987) HbXL99a: A hemoglobin derivative that is cross-linked between the a subunits is useful as a blood substitute. Proc Natl Acad Sci USA 84:7280

Sood SC, Gulati SC, Kidman M, Kak VK (1980) Cerebral metabolism following brain injury: II. Lactic acid changes. Acta Neurochir (Wien) 53:47

Sosin DM, Sniezek JE, Waxweiler RJ (1995) Trends in death associated with traumatic brain injury, 1979 through 1992-Success and Failure. JAMA 273:1778

Stahl WM (1965) Effect of mannitol on the kidney-Changes intrarenal hemodynamics. N Engl J Med 272:381

Starling EH (1896) On the absorption of fluids from the connective tissue spaces. J Physiol (Lond) 19:312

Staverman AJ (1952) Non-equilibrium thermodynamics of membrane processes. Trans Faraday Soc 48:176

Todd M, Tommasino C, Moore S (1985) Cerebral effects of isovolemic hemodilution with a hypertonic saline solution. J Neurosurg 63:944

Tranmer BI, Lacobacci RI, Kindt GW (1989) Effects of crystalloid and colloid infusions on intracranial pressure and computerized electroencephalographic data in dogs with vasogenic brain edema. Neurosurgery 25:173

Vassar MJ, Perry CA, Holcroft JW (1991) Analysis of potential risks associated with 7.5% NaCl dextran for resuscitation of trauma patients undergoing helicopter transport. Arch Surg 126:43

Velasco IT, Pontieri V, Rochae-Silva M Jr, Lopes OU (1980) Hyperosmotic NaCl and severe hemorrhagic shock. Am J Physiol 239:H664

Virgilio RW, Metilddi LA, Peters RM, Shackford SR (1979) Crystalloid vs colloid in fluid resuscitation of patients with severe pulmonary insufficiency. Surg Forum 30:166

Wagner EM, Traystman RJ (1983) Cerebral venous outflow and arterial microsphere flow with elevated venous pressure. Am J Physiol 244:H505

Wahl M, Kuschinsky W, Bosse O (1973) Dependency of pial arterial and arteriolar diameter on perivascular osmolarity in the cat: A microapplication study. Circ Res 32:162

Wald SL, Shackford SR, Fenwick J (1993) The effect of secondary insults on mortality and long-term disability after severe had injury in a rural region without a trauma system. J Trauma 34:377

Walsh J, Zhuang J, Shackford SR (1990) Fluid resuscitation of focal brain injury and shock. Surg Forum 41:46

Walsh JC, Zhuang J, Shackford SR (1991) A comparison of hypertonic to isotonic fluid in the resuscitation of brain injury and hemorrhagic shock. J Surg Res 50:248–292

Warner DS, Boehland LA (1988) effects of iso-osmolar intravenous fluid therapy on post-ischemic brain water content in the rat. Anesthesiology 68:86

Waters DC, Hoff JT, Black KL (1986) Effect of parenteral nutrition on cold-induced vasogenic edema in cats. J Neurosurg 64:460

Wei EP, Dietrich WD, Provlishock JT et al (1980) Functional, morphological, and metabolic abnormalities of the cerebral microcirculation after concussive brain injury in cats. Circ Res 46:37

Wildenthal K, Shelton CL, Coleman HN (1969) Cardiac muscle mechanics in hyperosmotic solutions. Am J Physiol 217:302

Wilkinson HA, Rosenfeld SR (1983) Furosemide and mannitol in the treatment of acute experimental intracranial hypertension. Neurosurgery 12:405

Wisner D, Busche F, Sturm J et al (1989) Traumatic shock and head injury: Effects of fluid resuscitation on the brain. J Surg Res 46:49

Wisner DH, Schuster L, Quinn C (1990) Hypertonic saline resuscitation of head injury: Effects on cerebral water content. J Trauma 30:75

Yuan XQ, Wade CE (1992) Traumatic brain injury attenuates the effectiveness of lactated ringer's solution resuscitation of hemorrhagic shock in rats. Surg Gynecol Obstet 174:305

Yuan XQ, Wade CE (1993) Influences of traumatic brain injury on the outcomes of delayed and repeated hemorrhages. Circ Shock 35:231

Yuan XQ, Prough DS, Smith T, Dewitt DS (1988) The effects of traumatic brain injury on regional cerebral blood flow in rats. J Neurotrauma 5:289

Zarins CK, Rice CL, Peters RM, Virgilio RW (1978) Lymph and pulmonary response to isobaric reduction in plasma oncotic pressure in baboons. Circ Res 43:925

Zhuang J, Shackford SR, Schmoker JD, Pietropaoli JA (1995) Colloid infusion after brain injury. Crit Care Med 23:140

Zornow MH, Prough DS (1995) Fluid management in patients with traumatic brain injury. New Horiz 3:488

Zornow MH, Scheller MS, Todd MM, Moore SS (1988) Acute cerebral effects of isotonic cystalloid and colloid solutions following cryogenic brain injury in the rabbit. Anaesthesiology 69:180

Zornow MH, Scheller MS, Shackford SR (1989) Effect of a hypertonic lactated ringers lactate solution on intracranial pressure and cerebral water content in a model of traumatic brain injury. J Trauma 29:484

Discussion

Traber:

I have a number of questions about the hemoglobin study. When we gave hemoglobin to our animal models they produced a relatively marked increase of pulmonary artery pressure. I was wondering whether you saw that. And the other thing I was wondering, did you measure cerebral blood flow in the animals that were given the hemoglobin?

Shackford:

We saw an increase in both the mean and the systolic pulmonary artery pressure when we gave the animals diaspirin crosslinked hemoglobin. We are now analyzing its effect on stroke work, because head injury, as you know, is thought to impair cardiac function and the combination of increased afterload produced by the hemoglobin and the cardiac "dysfunction" produced by head injury may be devastating.

We did measure cerebral blood flow, and cerebral blood flow was increased in these animals that got the hemoglobin.

Traber:

The other question I was going to ask was related to the colloid that you used with the hypertonic solution, was that albumin?

Shackford:

We did two studies. The study I showed you today was albumin.

Traber:

Have you looked at dextran? I think they are getting ready to come out of or go into clinical trials with hypertonic solution with dextran now.

Shackford:

We used dextran and virtually every animal had an element of intracerebral hemorrhage. We are very concerned about this effect. The use of dextran in this model appeared to increase bleeding associated with the cryogenic agent and was very disconcerting to us.

Traber:

And that was at a concentration that the hypovolemia people are using?

Shackford:

It was 7.5% hypertonic saline with 6% dextran 70.

Young:

There are a number of interesting positive aspects that you brought up, Dr. Shackford, in particular for patients with shock and neurological injuries. I was wondering, though, about a couple of issues that might be worth exploring just to make sure the crystalloid resuscitation is safe as far as the brain is concerned. One would be central pontine myelinolysis. I do not know if that was something that was looked for. Raising the plasma osmolarity, even if it is initially normoosmolar (a setting that was found in a published series of burn patients) in which a number of patients developed osmotic demyelination syndrome. It may not apply to trauma, but it might be worth looking at. The second issue is increased subfalcine herniation. Did you find there was any increase in the shift from one side to the other, when you use this? If fluid is being taken from the relatively normal hemisphere, there may be more side-to-side brain shift.

Shackford:

We did not look at shift. That is a good point. Your point about pontine myelinolysis is also a good one. I think that most of that work, however, dealt with chronic states and the rapid correction of a chronic state. We have not looked specifically at it, although most of the animals do undergo histologic evaluation, and we had not seen any evidence of it.

Baethmann:

Dr. Shackford, I enjoyed your presentation very much as we also studied hypertonic-hyperoncotic fluid resuscitation. You mentioned that colloids do not confer additional benefit to hypertonic fluid resuscitation. I wonder whether this is valid for the "small volume resuscitation fluid"?

Shackford:

Dr. Baethmann, I apologize for the confusion. From both my reading of the literature and my experience looking at surrogates for secondary injury, such as cortical water content and ICP at 24h, the use of a colloid resuscitation appeared to have no benefit on either of those two surrogates. Clearly, however, the animals that get the small volume hypertonic saline and dextran required less fluid to restore their physiology, i.e., get their cardiac output back to baseline or actually exceed baseline, and get their blood pressure back to baseline. The dextran, as I am sure you know and your work would suggest it, sustains the hemodynamic stability, whereas when just hypertonic sodium chloride is given, without dextran, there is a later attenuation of the initial beneficial effect.

Should the Hypotensive, Brain-Injured Patient Be Resuscitated with Hypertonic Solutions?

D.S. Prough, M.H. Zornow, and D.S. DeWitt

Summary

Hypertonic solutions appear promising for acute resuscitation of hypotensive, brain-injured patients. If the blood–brain barrier (BBB) is intact, movement of water between the brain and the intravascular space is highly dependent on osmotic gradients, which may be established by the administration of either hyper- or hypo-osmolar solutions. Acute bolus administration of hypertonic saline solutions decreases brain water in uninjured brain and decreases intracranial pressure (ICP) while temporarily increasing blood pressure and cardiac output. However, if the BBB is damaged, hypertonic saline will not decrease brain water or ICP. In head-injured children, 3% saline reduces ICP. In humans, acute resuscitation from hemorrhagic shock with hypertonic solutions (7.5% saline) is associated with improved outcome in multiply traumatized head-injured patients. However, some experimental studies fail to demonstrate benefit from hypertonic solutions. Insufficient data are currently available to justify the routine use of hypertonic fluids in hypotensive, brain-injured patients.

Effects of Hypertonic Solutions on Brain Water

Despite years of clinical and laboratory research, controversy still exists over the optimal fluid management for patients with traumatic brain injury (TBI). This article will review some of the important characteristics of hypertonic fluids, both experimentally and as applied to patients with TBI, with special attention to the influence of hypertonic fluids on intracranial hypertension.

Much of the confusion regarding fluid management of patients with intracranial hypertension arises from a failure to clearly distinguish intravascular volume from osmolality and tonicity. The osmolality of a solution is a measure of the number of solute particles per kilogram of solvent, reported as milliosmoles/kg (mOsm/kg). Serum osmolality is estimated by the equation:

$$\text{Osmolality} = \left(\left[\text{Na}^+\right] \times 2\right) + \left(\text{glucose} \div 18\right) + \left(\text{BUN} \div 2.8\right) \tag{1}$$

where sodium concentration ($[\text{Na}^+]$) is expressed in mEq/l, serum glucose is expressed in mg/dl, and blood urea nitrogen (BUN) is expressed in mg/dl. Osmolarity differs from osmolality in that it quantifies the number of particles per liter of sodium.

Table 1. Composition of commercially available intravenous fluids

Solution	Dextrose (g/l)	Na^+ (mEq/l)	Cl^- (mEq/l)	Osmolarity (mOsm/l)
5% Dextrose in water	50	–	–	253
5% Dextrose in 0.45% saline	50	77	77	505
Lactated Ringer's solution[a]	–	130	109	273
0.9% ("normal") saline	–	154	154	308[b]
3.0% saline	–	513	513	1026[b]
6% dextran 70 in 0.9% saline	–	154	154	310
6% HES in 0.9% saline	–	154	154	310
5% albumin	–	~154	~154	~310

HES, hydroxyethylstarch.
[a] Lactated Ringer's Solution also contains (per liter) 4 mEq K^+, 3 mEq Ca^{++}, 28 mEq lactate.
[b] Calculated osmolarity.

These solute particles may be small charged ions, e.g., sodium or chloride, or much larger protein molecules, e.g., albumin or globulins. In determining osmolality, only the number of molecules is important; the sizes of the particles are immaterial.

Osmolality provides no information, however, about whether particles can penetrate cell membranes or are retained intracellularly. The tonicity of a solution is a measure of the number of osmotically active particles. Osmotically active solutes cannot freely cross semipermeable cell membranes; therefore, such solutes can produce an osmotic pressure gradient. Although a concentrated solution of urea will be hyperosmolar to plasma, it cannot establish a sustained osmotic gradient because urea crosses most cell membranes. In contrast, 20% mannitol solutions or saline solutions containing more than physiologic concentrations of sodium are both hyperosmolar and hypertonic since mannitol and sodium do not readily pass through cell membranes. Moreover, sodium that does enter cells is actively pumped out.

The term "tonicity" also is used colloquially to compare the osmotic pressure of a solution to that of plasma. A fluid in which the osmotic pressure is similar to that of plasma is termed "isotonic". Hypotonic solutions exert lower osmotic pressures than plasma; hypertonic solutions exert higher osmotic pressures (Table 1). Note that in this colloquial usage an isotonic fluid may produce serum hypotonicity if glucose rather than sodium salts represents a substantial proportion of osmoles and if, as a consequence, infusion reduces serum sodium.

The brain, unlike peripheral tissues, is isolated from the intravascular space by the BBB. Anatomically, this barrier consists of endothelial tight junctions that effectively preclude the movement not only of plasma proteins, but also of low molecular weight ions, including sodium, potassium, and chloride. In effect, the BBB functions as a semipermeable membrane that allows only water to move between the brain's interstitial space and the vasculature, i.e., the brain acts as an osmometer. Administration of hypertonic solutions will increase plasma osmolality and cause water to move from the brain into the vascular space. These effects of hypertonic solutions on the central nervous system were demonstrated in studies conducted as long ago as 1919 by Weed and McKibben [1]. These early experiments examined the effects of intravenous administration of hypo- and hypertonic saline solutions on brain bulk and protrusion through a craniotomy. As would be predicted, hypotonic solutions visibly increased brain volume and worsened herniation through the craniotomy site, whereas hypertonic saline shrank the brain.

The osmotic effects exerted by low molecular weight ions are potent. The change (Δ) in osmotic pressure produced by a change in osmolality is approximated by the equation:

$$\Delta \text{ Osmotic pressure (mmHg)} = 19.3 \times \Delta \text{ osmolality (mOsm/kg)} \qquad (2)$$

This effect far exceeds the hydrostatic pressure gradient that can be generated by changes in plasma oncotic pressure. Because the BBB is highly impermeable to protein, clinicians have assumed that administration of colloid-containing solutions should increase ICP less than crystalloid solutions. However, because the BBB also is highly impermeable to sodium, small changes in serum sodium generate greater osmotic pressure gradients across the cerebral capillary bed than do relatively large changes in serum protein concentrations. For instance, an increase of 5 mEq/l in serum sodium would increase osmolality by 10 mOsm/kg, or 193 mm Hg of osmotic pressure (Table 2), more than sevenfold greater than the osmotic pressure exerted by all serum proteins. However, after acute head injury, especially compounded by shock, it is impossible to predict the integrity of the BBB. Tanno et al. studied rats subjected either to lateral fluid-percussion injury alone or lateral fluid-percussion injury accompanied by hypoxia (10% inspired oxygen) [2]. Although BBB function was similar 1 h after injury, it was significantly worse in the combined injury group 6 h after injury and remained more permeable to protein in the injured hemisphere for at least 72 h.

TBI produces a heterogeneous lesion, presumably consisting of regions with varying degrees of BBB integrity. Clearly, in some regions, there is a complete breakdown of the BBB with extravasation of blood into the brain tissue. Other regions of the traumatized brain may function similarly to peripheral tissues, in that the capillaries

Table 2. Acute effects of changes in plasma sodium and proteins on osmotic pressure in the cerebral capillaries

Physiologic state	Site (cerebral capillary plasma or cerebral interstitium)	Osmolality (mOsm/kg)	Osmotic pressure difference (mm Hg)	Net change (mm Hg)
Baseline, sodium,	Plasma	280	5404	
protein and non-	Cerebral interstitium	280	5404	
protein osmoles				
Plasma [Na$^+$] acutely	Plasma	290	5597	
increased by 5 mEq/l	Cerebral interstitium	280	5404	193
Baseline protein	Plasma	1.2	23	
	Cerebral interstitium	0	0	
Plasma protein	Plasma	2.4	46	
acutely doubled	Cerebral interstitium	0	0	23

[Na$^+$] = sodium concentration; mEq/l = milliequivalents per liter.

leak water and low molecular weight compounds into the parenchyma, but remain capable of retaining macromolecules. Demonstration of such areas has been difficult both in clinical and experimental studies. Finally, there is usually a significant portion of the brain with an intact, functional BBB. Indeed, presence of normal brain is essential if osmotherapy is to be successful.

Intravenous Solutions

A variety of solutions are commonly administered to patients with brain injury. For the purposes of this discussion, they can be conveniently divided into crystalloids and colloids. Crystalloid solutions can be further subdivided into hypotonic, isotonic and hypertonic solutions.

Crystalloids

Crystalloids are solutions composed solely of low molecular weight (MW) solutes (MW < 30000). These solutes may be either ionic (e.g., Na^+,Cl^-) or nonionic (e.g., mannitol, dextrose). Although the osmolarity of crystalloid solutions may range from near zero into the thousands, by definition they have a colloid osmotic (i.e., oncotic) pressure of zero.

Hypertonic Crystalloids

For many years, mannitol has been the primary agent used for osmotherapy. Mannitol, a six-carbon sugar with a molecular weight of 182 daltons, cannot be metabolized by the body and is excreted unchanged in the urine. Available as 20% and 25% solutions (osmolarities of 1098 and 1372 mOsm/l), mannitol is often given in 0.5–1.0 g/kg doses. Mannitol does not pass through the intact BBB; hence, intravenous administration increases plasma osmolality and generates an osmotic gradient favoring the movement of water from the brain's interstitial space into the vasculature. Rapid administration of large doses of mannitol may have a biphasic effect on ICP. Initially, ICP may increase due to an increase in cerebral blood volume. Subsequently, ICP will decrease, owing to the movement of water from the brain interstitial space into the vasculature [3].

Hypertonic solutions, by creating osmotic gradients, can recruit water from the intracellular space. The effects of hypertonic solutions can be approximated by calculating the amount of water that will move from the intracellular to the extracellular space, based upon the change in total osmolality, and then estimating what fraction will remain in the intravascular compartment. Table 3 displays the volumes of various fluids required to increase plasma volume (PV) by 1 l. For example, for each liter of 3% hypertonic saline infused, PV will increase by about 500 ml after equilibration. The immediate effects will be greater because of transient movement of interstitial fluid into the PV.

Table 3. Fluid volumes necessary to expand plasma volume by 1 L

Fluid	ΔPV (ml)	ΔIFV (ml)	ΔICV (ml)	Infused volume (ml)
D5W	1000	3700	9300	14000
LRS	1000	3700	0	4700
5% Albumin	1000	0	0	1000
25% Albumin	1000	(–)750	0	250
7.5% Saline				
Immediate	1000	(–)285	(–)575	140
At equilibrium	170	630	(–)800	140

PV, plasma volume; IFV, interstitial fluid volume; ICV, intracellular volume; D5W, 5% dextrose in water; LRS, lactated Ringer's solution; "immediate" assumes rapid bolus infusion; "at equilibrium" assumes distribution as proposed by Spital [9].

Recently, there has been considerable interest in the use of hypertonic saline solutions for control of intracranial hypertension and treatment of hemorrhagic shock. Intravenous infusions of small volumes of hypertonic saline solutions have been reported to rapidly restore intravascular volume, improve myocardial contractility, and decrease ICP [4–7]. The primary mechanism by which hyperosmotic saline increases venous return is plasma volume expansion [8]. Hypernatremic fluids acutely increase plasma volume both by osmotic attraction of water from the intracellular volume into the extracellular volume and by transient translocation of interstitial fluid volume into the plasma volume. Immediately after infusion, the combination of 7.5% saline and 6% dextran 70 increases plasma volume by a volume approximately seven times the original infused volume [8]. The immediate effect is attributable in part to the fact that permeability of the systemic capillaries to sodium is not complete; therefore, interstitial fluid volume is translocated into the plasma volume until equilibration occurs.

The effects after equilibration on extracellular volume and intracellular volume of adding hyperosmotic saline can be calculated as follows [9] (Table 3):

$$\frac{\text{new total extracellular solute}}{\text{new ECV}} = \frac{\text{total intracellular solute}}{\text{new ICV}} \tag{3}$$

For instance, assume that a healthy 70-kg patient ($[\text{Na}^+] = 140\,\text{mEq/l}$) were to receive 2.0 ml/kg of 7.5% saline. A total of 173 mEq of sodium would be added as new extracellular solute. Before infusion, total extracellular sodium would be 1960 mEq (140 mEq/l × 14 l) and total intracellular potassium, the predominant intracellular solute, would be 3920 mEq (140 mEq/l × 28 l). The equation would then be calculated:

$$\frac{1960\,\text{mEq} + 173\,\text{mEq}}{14\,\text{l} + x} = \frac{3920\,\text{mEq}}{28\,\text{l} - x} \tag{4}$$

where x = the added extracellular volume. The new total extracellular volume would equal 14.8 l (14 l + 0.8 l), and the new total intracellular volume would equal 27.2 l (28 l – 0.8 l). Assuming that the increase in extracellular volume were equal to 0.8 l, the increase in plasma volume would be approximately 170 ml.

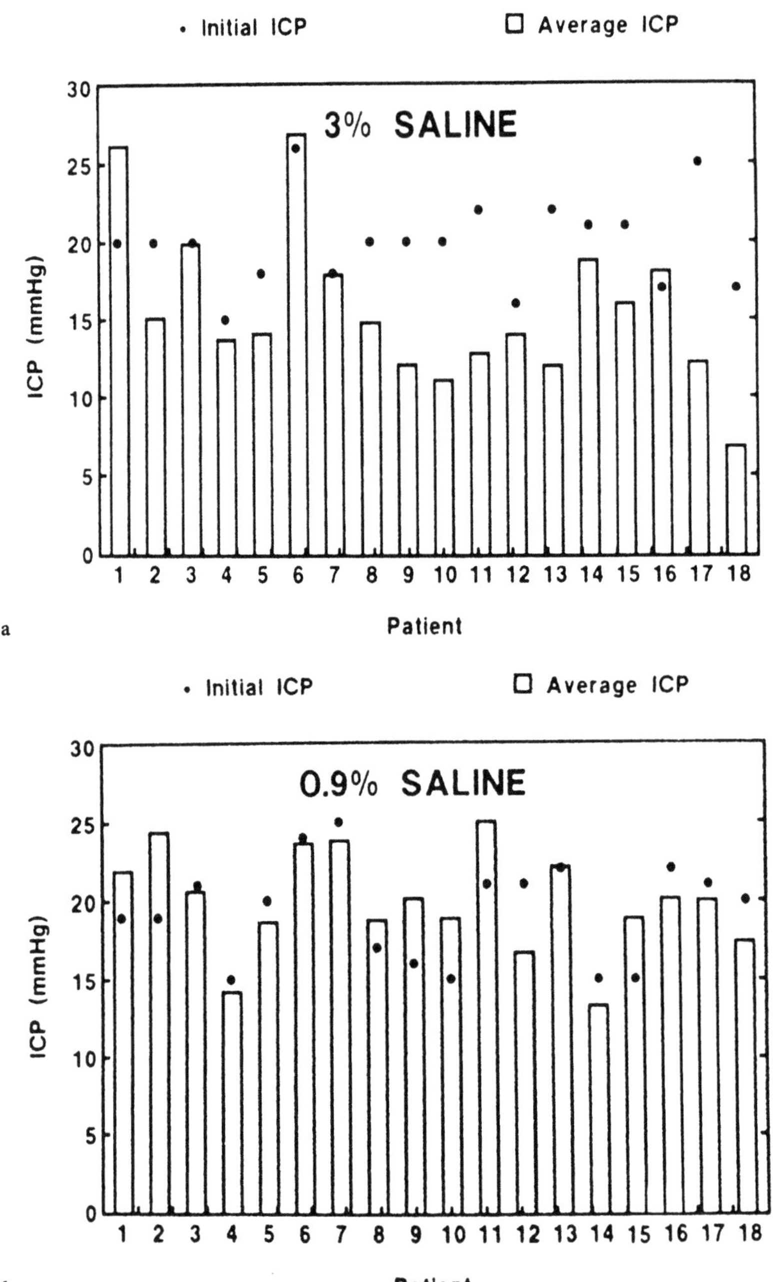

Fig. 1a,b. Intracranial pressure (*ICP*; *vertical axis*) in 18 head-injured children (*horizontal axis*) receiving 3.0% (**a**) or 0.9% (**b**) saline (10 ml/kg) over 120 min. The initial ICP is represented by the *dots*. Average ICP after infusion is displayed by the *open bars*. (From [11])

There have been anecdotal reports of successful treatment of intracranial hypertension with hypertonic saline in patients who have failed to respond to large doses of mannitol [10]. In a randomized, crossover study of hypertonic saline (3%) vs 0.9% saline, Fisher and colleagues reported significant reductions in ICP in 18 pediatric head-trauma patients [11]. Patients received a 10 ml/kg bolus of either 0.9% saline or 3% saline and ICP was monitored for the ensuing 2 h. The administration of 3% saline was associated with a 4 mm Hg decline in ICP as compared to a 0.7 mm Hg increase in patients receiving normal saline (Fig. 1).

In animal studies using a cryogenic lesion as a model of TBI, hypertonic saline solutions are effective for control of ICP [12,13]. In one study, equiosmolar doses of either mannitol or hypertonic saline were administered to animals with intracranial hypertension secondary to cryogenic injury [13]. The effects of these two agents were compared to those of a third group that received an identical volume of normal saline. ICP decreased in both of the groups receiving hypertonic solutions and remained significantly less than that in the saline group for the ensuing 90 min. However, there were no differences at any time point between the mannitol and hypertonic saline groups.

Concerns that increased serum sodium may be detrimental have not been substantiated when hypertonic saline has been used for acute resuscitation from hemorrhage; however, seizures and a decreased level of consciousness may occur with serum sodium levels >170 mEq/l [14]. Thus, these solutions should be administered in judicious amounts and with frequent monitoring of plasma osmolarity and sodium concentrations. A theoretical concern is the production by rapid increases in serum sodium of central pontine myelinolysis, a syndrome that is characterized pathologically by demyelination, primarily of the pons, and clinically by the onset of lethargy and quadriparesis. Most frequently reported after the rapid correction of chronic hyponatremia [15–17], similar lesions have not been reported as a result of the increase in serum sodium associated with the rapid infusion of large volumes of hypertonic saline in patients who initially had normal serum sodium levels [18].

The least encouraging observations regarding hyperosmotic resuscitation involve experimental models of uncontrolled hemorrhage [19], in which hyperosmotic solutions increase bleeding and may adversely affect mortality. In urban trauma patients, Bickell et al. reported that immediate, prehospital resuscitation did not improve mortality in comparison to resuscitation initiated only after arrival at the hospital [20].

Experimental Effects of Hypertonic Fluid Administration

Investigation of the effects of fluid infusion on ICP and cerebral edema has generally been carried out in animals, although a few studies have been performed in humans. The studies vary in several critical details. Osmolality, colloid osmotic pressure, and hemoglobin concentration have been altered in several ways: by simple fluid infusion; fluid infusion as blood is removed (isovolemic hemodilution); or a sequence of hemorrhage followed by fluid infusion (analogous to hemodilution during resuscitation after trauma). Some investigators have studied acute, single-bolus resuscitation (similar to prehospital treatment), while others have studied more prolonged infusions (comparable to management in the emergency department, operating room, or intensive care unit). In attempting to replicate the features of clinical lesions, studies have been performed both in animals without intracranial pathology and in those with a variety of brain injuries, including focal cryogenic injury (which causes vasogenic brain edema), space-occupying lesions, cerebral ischemia, and concussive brain injury.

Cerebral Effects of Hypertonic Fluid Infusion (No Hemorrhagic Shock)

The simplest models are those in which fluid or blood is infused in the absence of hemorrhage or shock (Table 4). In such a model, Weed and McKibben [1] showed in cats that hypertonic solutions shrank while hypotonic solutions expanded the brain. They also demonstrated that 0.9% saline had little effect on intracranial volume. These observations were expanded by Wilson [21], who demonstrated in dogs that hypertonic salt solutions decreased ICP but that hypertonic glucose solutions actually increased ICP after a transient decrease, presumably reflecting equilibration of glucose across the BBB. In head-injured children, Fisher et al. showed, in a double blind, crossover study, that 3.0% saline significantly reduced ICP while 0.9% saline exerted no effect (Fig. 1) [11]. It is necessary to note, however, that hypertonic fluids may reduce brain interstitial fluid while only transiently influencing intracellular fluid volume. In cultures of brain glioma cells, after hypertonic challenge cellular volume was quickly restored by a mechanism that was inhibited by loop diuretics [22] (Fig. 2).

Cerebral Effects of Acute Isovolemic Hemodilution with Hypertonic Solutions (No Brain Lesion)

Perhaps the most appropriate model of perioperative fluid administration is isovolemic hemodilution (Table 5), since that technique mimics the intraoperative sequence of blood loss and concurrent fluid replacement, without intervening

Table 4. Cerebral effects of hypertonic fluid infusion (no hemorrhage or shock)

First author	Reference	Species (lesion(s))	Interventions	Observations
Weed	[1]	Cats	30% saline; distilled water; 0.9% saline	30% saline shrank brain; distilled water expanded brain; 0.9% saline had little effect
Wilson	[41]	Dogs	$1.0\,M$ sodium lactate or saline; $0.67\,M$ sodium succinate; $2\,M$ glucose	$1.0\,M$ salts decreased ICP; after initial decrease, $2.0\,M$ glucose increased ICP
Fisher	[11]	Children (head injury)	3% saline vs. 0.9% saline (crossover design)	3.0% saline decreased ICP; 0.9% did not

ICP, intracranial pressure.

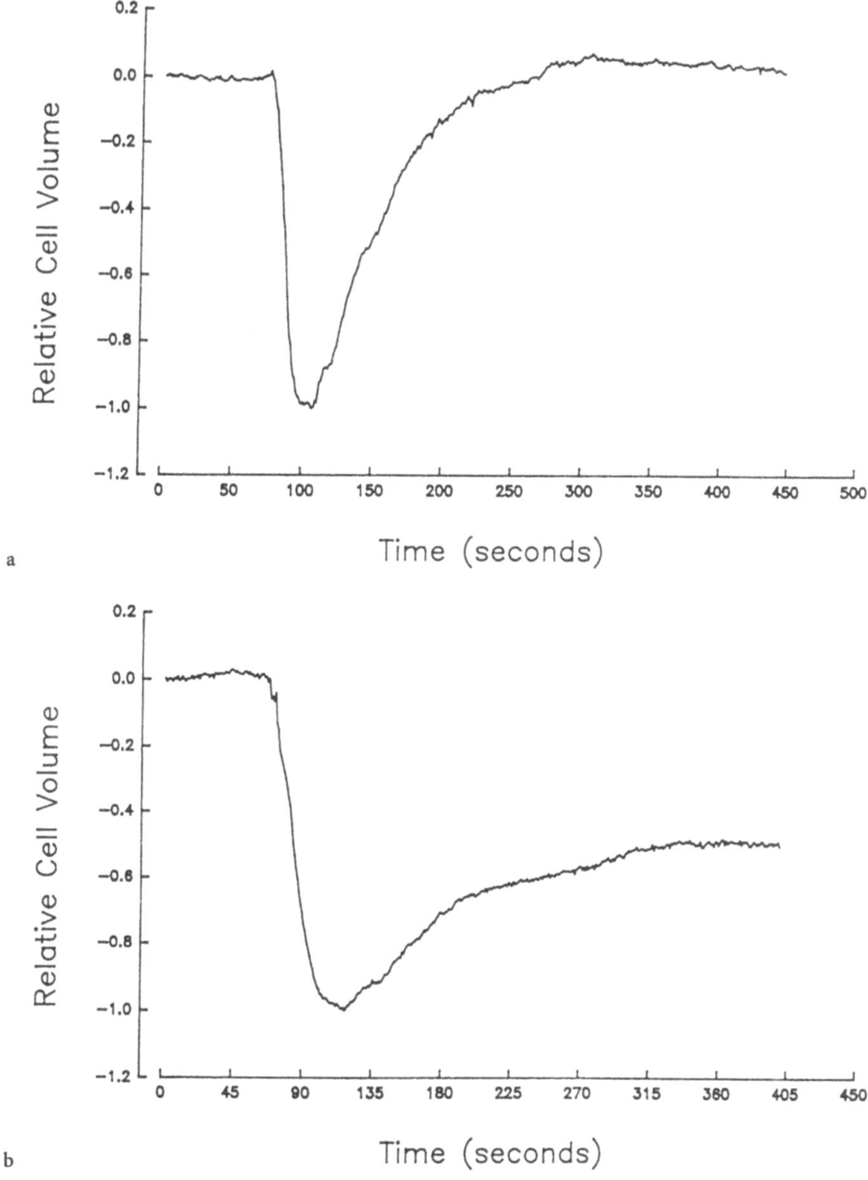

Fig. 2a,b. Volume behavior of cultured glioma cells exposed to hypertonic saline. **a** Cells were equilibrated in an isotonic solution until the voltage signal remained stable for 15–30 min, then were abruptly exposed to the hypertonic solution. Light-scattering voltages are normalized to the maximal voltage change and presented as relative changes in cell volume. Note the rapid and complete recovery of cell volume despite maintenance of the hypertonic environment. **b** Cells exposed to hypertonic saline in the presence of $10^{-4}\,M$ bumetanide. The experimental protocol is the same as in **a**. (From McManus [22])

Table 5. Cerebral effect of acute isovolemic hemodilution with hypertonic solutions (with or without brain lesion)

First author	Reference	Species	Interventions	Observations
Todd	[4]	Rabbits (no lesion)	0.9% saline; hypertonic LRS (Na$^+$ 252 mEq/l); Hct 40% → 20%	Hypertonic LRS decreased brain water and ICP; 0.9% saline slightly increased ICP; increased CBF > 60%
Zornow	[12]	Rabbits (cryogenic lesion)	Hemodilution with hypotonic or hypertonic LRS to decrease Hct to 23%	ICP increased more in the hypotonic LRS group. Brain water similar in lesioned, more in nonlesioned hemisphere in hypotonic LRS group

LRS, lactated Ringer's solution; Hct, hematocrit; ICP, intracranial pressure; CBF, cerebral blood flow.

hypovolemia. Isovolemic hemodilution produces several effects. First, in the absence of shock, a reduction in hematocrit increases cerebral blood flow (CBF) in animals [4] and humans [23]. The acute effects on ICP depend upon the tonicity of the infused fluid. Hypertonic fluids decreased brain water and ICP (4) in rabbits; 0.9% saline increased ICP slightly, but did not change brain water.

Cerebral Effects of Acute Isovolemic Hemodilution with Hypertonic Solutions (Brain Injury Present)

In the presence of cryogenic or ischemic brain injury, damage to the BBB tends to reduce the differences in CBF, ICP and brain water produced by acute hemodilution with different solutions (Table 5). In rabbits with cryogenic brain lesions, hemodilution to reduce hematocrit to approximately 23% using hypotonic lactated Ringer's solution or hypertonic lactated Ringer's solution resulted in a greater increase in ICP in the hypotonic group [12]. Brain water was similar in the lesioned hemispheres but less in the nonlesioned hemisphere in rabbits given the hypertonic solution.

Cerebral Effects of Hemorrhage and Resuscitation with Hypertonic Solutions (No Brain Lesion)

In the absence of brain lesions, the sequence of hemorrhage followed by resuscitation with crystalloid or colloid produces changes in ICP similar to those seen in animals subjected to isovolemic hemodilution (Table 6). However, CBF, which usually is increased after isovolemic hemodilution, often is not increased in the sequence of hemorrhage followed by fluid resuscitation. Hypertonic solutions, whether given as

Table 6. Cerebral effects of hemorrhage and resuscitation with hypertonic solutions (no brain lesion)

First author	Reference	Species	Interventions	Observations
Prough	[24]	Dogs	LRS; 7.5% saline	ICP lower with 7.5% saline; CBF no different
Prough	[25]	Dogs	7.5% saline (4 ml/kg); LRS (45 ml/kg)	ICP lower after 7.5% saline
Gunnar	[6]	Dogs	Resuscitation with shed blood plus 0.9% saline; 3% saline; 10% dextran 40	ICP lower with 3% saline
Schmoker	[26]	Swine	4 ml/kg of HSL or LRS as bolus, then HSL or LRS to restore MAP to baseline for 24 h	ICP lower; brain water lower; CDO_2 greater in HSL animals
Whitley	[27]	Dogs	Small volume resuscitation with 7.2% saline; 20% HES	Regional CBF no different; ICP no different
Prough	[28]	Dogs	Small volume resuscitation with 7.2% saline; 20% HES; 20% HES in 7.2% saline	CBF transiently increased with 7.2% saline; no other important differences
Smith	[42]	Rats	HLS vs. LRS (volume = blood loss)	Shock increased brain water; fluid had little additional effect

HES, hydroxyethylstarch; CBF, cerebral blood flow; ICP, intracranial pressure; LRS, lactated Ringer's solution; HSL, hypertonic sodium lactate; CDO_2, cerebral oxygen delivery; MAP, mean arterial pressure; HLS, hypertonic lactated saline.

boluses or as boluses followed by continued infusions, have been associated with considerably lower ICP [6,24–28] and brain water. In general, hypertonic solutions did not improve CBF, although CBF improved in some experimental models [26,29]. Perhaps the most striking observation about the sequence of hemorrhage followed by single-bolus resuscitation is that CBF may not recover well, despite substantial improvements in mean arterial pressure and cardiac output [24,25,27,28].

Cerebral Effects of Hemorrhage and Resuscitation with Hypertonic Solutions (Intracranial Mass Lesion)

Addition of a mass lesion to the sequence of hemorrhage and resuscitation produces similar, but exaggerated effects (Table 7). However, if the experimental model produces cerebral ischemia, it is likely that the resulting changes in BBB function reduce the differences between fluids in the affected brain. In dogs after hemorrhagic shock for 30 min accompanied by inflation of a subdural balloon, 7.2% saline (6 ml/kg) decreased ICP and increased CBF in the hemisphere adjacent to the balloon in comparison to 0.8% saline (54 ml/kg) (Table 8) [29]. Gunnar et al. [5,30] resuscitated

Table 7. Cerebral effects of hemorrhage and resuscitation with hypertonic solutions (mass lesion)

First author	Reference	Species (lesion)	Interventions	Observations
Prough	[29]	Dogs (subdural balloon)	0.8% saline (54 ml/kg); 7.2% saline (6 ml/kg)	7.2% saline decreased ICP, increased CBF in the lesioned hemisphere
Whitley	[32]	Dogs (subdural balloon)	0.73% saline, with and without 10% pentastarch; 1.46% saline, with and without 10% pentastarch to maintain cardiac output	No effect of fluid choice on ICP or CBF
Gunnar	[30]	Dogs (epidural balloon)	0.9% saline; 3% saline; 10% dextran 40 for 2 h after resuscitation	ICP lower with 3% saline; CBF similar in all groups
Gunnar	[5]	Dogs (epidural balloon)	0.9% saline; 3% saline; 10% dextran 40 for 2 h after resuscitation	ICP lower; cerebral edema less with 3.0% saline; no difference in blood–brain barrier function
Ducey	[31]	Swine (epidural balloon)	Blood; 0.9% saline; 6.0% saline; 6.0% HES to normalize DO_2	6.0% saline decreased ICP, improved intracranial elastance

ICP, intracranial pressure; CBF, cerebral blood flow; LRS, lactated Ringer's solution; HES, hydroxyethylstarch; DO_2, systemic oxygen delivery.

Table 8. Cerebral oxygen delivery (means ± SEM)

	Group	Baseline	T15	T35	T95	T155
Right frontoparietal cortex (ml/100 g per minute)	1 HS	9.4 ± 1.3	6.5 ± 0.9	9.1 ± 1.9	6.5 ± 0.7	5.1 ± 0.5
	1 SAL	7.7 ± 0.5	5.2 ± 0.3	5.0 ± 0.4	5.0 ± 0.2	5.6 ± 0.5[a]
	2 HS	9.9 ± 1.7	4.1 ± 1.6	4.8 ± 1.1	6.2 ± 2.0	3.9 ± 1.3
	2 SAL[b]	9.8 ± 1.7	2.0 ± 0.4	1.6 ± 0.8[c]	1.2 ± 0.6[c]	1.0 ± 0.6[d]
Right cerebral hemisphere (ml/100 g per minute)	1 HS	9.8 ± 1.1	6.7 ± 0.9	9.2 ± 1.8	7.2 ± 1.0	5.7 ± 0.7
	1 SAL	8.2 ± 0.6	5.6 ± 0.3	5.3 ± 0.4	5.5 ± 0.3	6.1 ± 0.5[a]
	2 HS	9.6 ± 1.6	4.5 ± 1.5	5.4 ± 1.1	5.8 ± 1.6	3.9 ± 1.2
	2 SAL[e]	8.8 ± 1.3	2.5 ± 0.5	2.1 ± 0.8[c,f]	1.5 ± 0.7[c,f]	1.2 ± 0.7[d,f]

Cerebral oxygen delivery in the right frontoparietal cortex and right cerebral hemisphere. Group 1 animals were subjected to hemorrhagic shock alone; group 2 animals were subjected to hemorrhagic shock after inflation of a right hemispheric subdural balloon to 20 mm Hg. All animals were resuscitated with 7.2% saline (HS) or 0.8% saline (SAL). [a]$p < 0.001$ T155 versus baseline; [b]$p < 0.05$ by ANOVA, group 2-SAL versus group 2-HS; [c]$p < 0.05$ group 2-SAL versus group 2-HS at specific interval; [d]$p = 0.0001$ T155 versus baseline; [e]$p < 0.01$ by ANOVA, group 2-SAL versus group 2-HS; [f]$p < 0.01$ group 1-SAL versus group 2-SAL. *$p = 0.05$ by ANOVA, group 2-SAL versus group 2-HS. Data from [29] with permission.

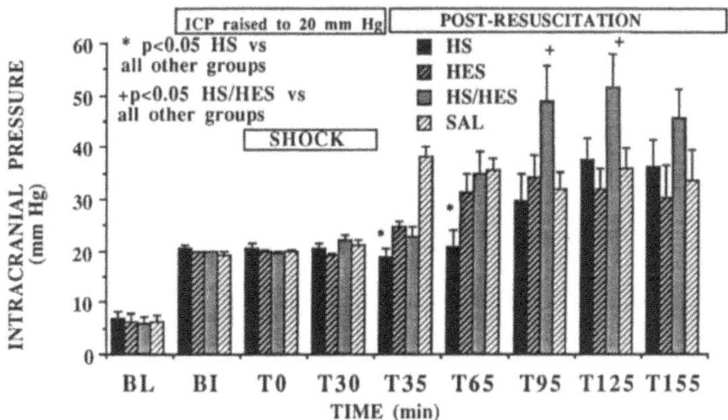

INTRACRANIAL PRESSURE (mm Hg)
ICP raised to 20 mm Hg
POST-RESUSCITATION
* p<0.05 HS vs all other groups
+p<0.05 HS/HES vs all other groups
SHOCK
HS
HES
HS/HES
SAL
60
50
40
30
20
10
0
BL
BI
T0
T30
T35
T65
T95
T125
T155
TIME (min)

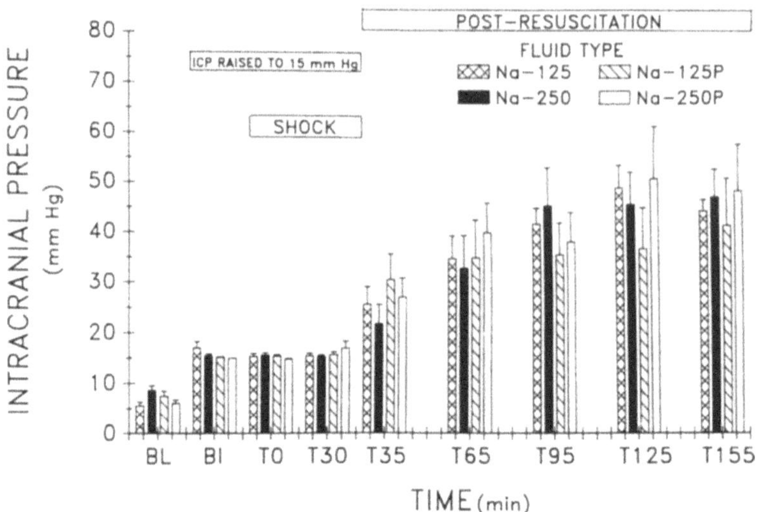

INTRACRANIAL PRESSURE (mm Hg)
80
70
60
50
40
30
20
10
0
ICP RAISED TO 15 mm Hg
SHOCK
POST-RESUSCITATION
FLUID TYPE
Na-125
Na-125P
Na-250
Na-250P
BL
BI
TO
T30
T35
T65
T95
T125
T155
TIME (min)

Table 9. Cerebral effects of hemorrhage and resuscitation with hypertonic solutions (brain injury)

First author	Reference	Species (lesions(s))	Interventions	Observations
Warner	[33]	Rats (forebrain ischemia)	40% hemorrhage replaced by blood; HES; 0.9% saline (vol = shed blood)	No difference in edema at 6 or 24h
Walsh	[34]	Swine (cryogenic injury)	4 ml/kg bolus of LRS or 7.5% saline in 6.5% dextran 70, then LRS or HSL	7.5% saline/6.5% dextran 70 increased CBF, decreased ICP
Battistella	[35]	Sheep (cryogenic injury)	LRS or 7.5% saline after shock to keep MAP $\geq$ 80 mm Hg for 1h	7.5% saline decreased ICP, brain water (uninjured hemisphere)
Wisner	[36]	Sheep (fracture/ crush injury plus cryogenic injury)	LRS or 4% albumin for 2h	ICP increased in both groups
Wisner	[37]	Rats (fluid percussion injury)	LRS vs. 6.5% saline	6.5% saline decreased brain water in uninjured, not injured brain
Prough	[38]	Cats (fluid percussion injury)	Resuscitation with 3.0% saline or 10% HES	3.0% saline increased ICP, did not increase CBF

HES, hydroxyethylstarch; LRS, lactated Ringer's solution; HSL, hypertonic sodium lactate; CBF, cerebral blood flow; ICP, intracranial pressure; MAP, mean arterial pressure.

unit. Physicians caring for these patients must balance adequate volume resuscitation against the need to minimize exacerbation of cerebral edema and swelling. Although not yet considered a standard of care, hypertonic saline solutions may be useful in certain situations. In the presence of hypovolemia accompanied by intracranial hypertension or when large volumes of isotonic crystalloid solutions are not available or cannot be rapidly infused, the use of hypertonic saline appears to be an attractive option. Extensive animal experience supports the efficacy of hypertonic solutions in reversing shock and, usually, decreasing ICP. In those few studies in which hypertonic saline did not reduce ICP [32,38], it is likely that the BBB was diffusely damaged by ischemia or trauma. The value of small-volume hypertonic resuscitation may be greatest when dealing with mass or combat casualties; however, hypertonic saline solutions have been extensively studied for prehospital resuscitation in the USA and are currently being used in the prehospital transport of hypovolemic, TBI patients in Europe. Whether this approach will gain popularity in the United States remains to be seen.

Clinical trials have evaluated whether rapid infusion of hypertonic solutions might improve outcome when used for prehospital resuscitation. In a multicenter

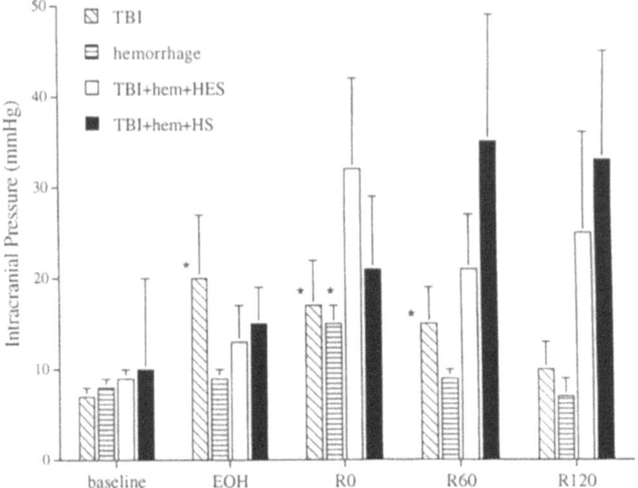

Fig. 5. Intracranial pressure (ICP) in four groups of cats. One group received only traumatic brain injury (*TBI*), one underwent hemorrhage to a mean arterial pressure of 90 mm Hg (no *TBI*), and two received a combination of *TBI*, hemorrhage and single-bolus fluid resuscitation with either 18 ml/kg of 10% hydroxyethylstarch or 3% saline. $*p < 0.05$ compared to baseline within groups. (From DeWitt [38])

Table 10. Predicted (from TRISS scores) versus acutal survival

	LRS	HS	HSD-6%	HSD-12%
Entire cohort (*n*)	45	50	50	49
Predicted (%)	47	48	52	40
Actual (5)	49	60	56	45
GCS $\leq$ 8 (*n*)	25	29	26	30
Predicted (%)	14	13	16	14
Actual (%)	12	34	27	30

Patients randomized to immediate resuscitation with 250 ml of lactated Ringer's solution (LRS) or 250 ml of 7.5% saline (HS), 7.5% saline with 6% dextran 70 (HSD-6%), or 7.5% saline with 12% dextran 70 (HSD-12%). GCS, Glasgow Coma Scale score. (Data from [40] with permission.)

trial in which trauma patients were randomly assigned to receive 250 ml of either a balanced salt solution or 7.5% saline in 6.0% dextran 70 (HSD) [39], HSD improved blood pressure but did not improve overall survival; however, in the patients who required surgery, survival was improved in those who received HSD [39]. Vassar et al. compared 250 ml of lactated Ringer's solution to 7.5% saline in 6.0% dextran 70 for prehospital resuscitation of trauma patients in whom systolic blood pressure was $\leq$100 mm Hg [18]. Although there was no overall difference in mortality, in the subset of patients with severe head injury (53 of 186 patients), 32% of those who received HSD survived, versus only 16% of the patients who received lactated Ringer's solution

($p = 0.04$). In a subsequent randomized multicenter study, Vassar et al. (Table 10) evaluated the effects of 250 ml of sodium chloride with and without 6% and 12% dextran 70 for the prehospital resuscitation of hypotensive trauma patients [40]. A small subgroup of patients with Glasgow Coma Scale scores <8 but without severe anatomic injury seemed to benefit most from resuscitation with 7.5% saline [40].

Conclusion

In summary, hypertonic saline solutions exert advantageous effects if the BBB is intact. Clinical studies suggest that hypertonic solutions may be better in hypotensive, brain-injured patients during transport to the hospital. Further data are necessary to clarify the physiologic effects of hypertonic solutions and to determine their application after admission to the hospital.

References

1. Weed LH, McKibben PS (1919) Experimental alteration of brain bulk. Am J Physiol 48:531–558
2. Tanno H, Nockels RP, Pitts LH, Noble LJ (1992) Breakdown of the blood-brain barrier after fluid percussive brain injury in the rat. Part 1: distribution and time course of protein extravasation. J Neurotrauma 9:335–347
3. Shenkin HA, Goluboff B, Haft H (1964) Further observations on the effects of abruptly increased osmotic pressure of plasma on cerebrospinal-fluid pressure in man. J Neurosurg 22:563–568
4. Todd MM, Tommasino C, Moore S (1985) Cerebral effects of isovolemic hemodilution with a hypertonic saline solution. J Neurosurg 63:944–948
5. Gunnar W, Jonasson O, Merlotti G, Stone J, Barrett J (1988) Head injury and hemorrhagic shock: studies of the blood brain barrier and intracranial pressure after resuscitation with normal saline solution, 3% saline solution, and dextran-40. Surgery 103:398–407
6. Gunner WP, Merlotti GJ, Jonasson O, Barrett J (1986) Resuscitation from hemorrhagic shock: alterations of the intracranial pressure after normal saline, 3% saline and dextran-40. Ann Surg 204:686–692
7. Shackford SR, Zhuang J, Schmoker J (1992) Intravenous fluid tonicity: effect on intracranial pressure, cerebral blood flow, and cerebral oxygen delivery in focal brain injury. J Neurosurg 76:91–98
8. Schertel ER, Valentine AK, Rademakers AM, Muir WW (1990) Influence of 7% NaCl on the mechanical properties of the systemic circulation in the hypovolemic dog. Circ Shock 31:203–214
9. Spital A, Sterns RD (1989) The paradox of sodium's volume of distribution. Why an extracellular solute appears to distribute over total body water. Arch Intern Med 149:1255–1257
10. Worthley LIG, Cooper DJ, Jones N (1988) Treatment of resistant intracranial hypertension with hypertonic saline. Report of two cases. J Neurosurg 68:478–481
11. Fisher B, Thomas D, Peterson B (1992) Hypertonic saline lowers raised intracranial pressure in children after head trauma. J Neurosurg Anesthesiol 4:4–10
12. Zornow MH, Scheller MS, Shackford SR (1989) Effect of a hypertonic lactated Ringer's solution on intracranial pressure and cerebral water content in a model of traumatic brain injury. J Trauma 29:484–488
13. Scheller MS, Zornow MH, Oh YS (1991) A comparison of the cerebral and hemodynamic effects of mannitol and hypertonic saline in a rabbit model of acute cryogenic brain injury. J Neurosurg Anesthesiol 3:291–296

14. Sotos JF, Dodge PR, Meara P, Talbot NB (1960) Studies in experimental hypertonicity. I: Pathogenesis of the clinical syndrome, biochemical abnormalities and cause of death. Pediatrics 26:925–938
15. Sterns RH, Riggs JE, Schochet SS Jr (1986) Osmotic demyelination syndrome following correction of hyponatremia. N Engl J Med 314:1535–1542
16. Kleinschmidt-DeMasters K, Norenberg MD (1981) Rapid correction of hyponatremia causes demyelination: relation to central pontine myelinolysis. Science 211:1068–1070
17. Arieff AI (1986) Hyponatremia, convulsions, respiratory arrest, and permanent brain damage after elective surgery in healthy women. N Engl J Med 314:1529–1535
18. Vassar MJ, Perry CA, Gannaway WL, Holcroft JW (1991) 7.5% sodium chloride/dextran for resuscitation of trauma patients undergoing helicopter transport. Arch Surg 126:1065–1072
19. Gross D, Landau EH, Klin B, Krausz MM (1990) Treatment of uncontrolled hemorrhagic shock with hypertonic saline solution. Surg Gynecol Obstet 170:106–112
20. Bickell WH, Wall MJ, Jr., Pepe PE, Martin RR, Ginger VF, Allen MK, Mattox KL (1994) Immediate versus delayed fluid resuscitation for hypotensive patients with penetrating torso injuries. N Engl J Med 331:1105–1109
21. Wilson BJ, Jones RF, Coleman ST, Moyer CA (1951) The effects of various hypertonic sodium salt solutions on cisternal pressure. Surgery 30:361–366
22. McManus ML, Strange K (1993) Acute volume regulation of brain cells in response to hypertonic challenge. Anesthesiology 78:1132–1137
23. Hino A, Ueda S, Mizukawa N, Imahori Y, Tenjin H (1992) Effect of hemodilution on cerebral hemodynamics and oxygen metabolism. Stroke 23:423–426
24. Prough DS, Johnson JC, Stump DA, Stullken EH, Poole GV Jr, Howard G (1986) Effects of hypertonic saline versus lactated Ringer's solution on cerebral oxygen transport during resuscitation from hemorrhagic shock. J Neurosurg 64:627–632
25. Prough DS, Johnson JC, Poole GV, Jr., Stullken EH, Johnston WE, Royster R (1985) Effects on intracranial pressure of resuscitation from hemorrhagic shock with hypertonic saline versus lactated Ringer's solution. Crit Care Med 13:407–411
26. Schmoker JD, Zhuang J, Shackford SR (1991) Hypertonic fluid resuscitation improves cerebral oxygen delivery and reduces intracranial pressure after hemorrhagic shock. J Trauma 31:1607–1613
27. Whitley JM, Prough DS, Taylor CL, Deal DD, DeWitt DS (1991) Cerebrovascular effects of small volume resuscitation from hemorrhagic shock: comparison of hypertonic saline and concentrated hydroxethyl starch in dogs. J Neurosurg Anesthesiol 3:(1):47–55
28. Prough DS, Whitley JM, Olympio MA, Taylor CL, DeWitt DS (1991) Hypertonic hyperoncotic fluid resuscitation after hemorrhagic shock in dogs. Anesth Analg 73:738–744
29. Prough DS, Whitley JM, Taylor CL, Deal DD, DeWitt DS (1991) Regional cerebral blood flow following resuscitation from hemorrhagic shock with hypertonic saline: Influence of a subdural mass. Anesthesiology 75:319–327
30. Gunnar W, Kane J, Barrett J (1989) Cerebral blood flow following hypertonic saline resuscitation in an experimental model of hemorrhagic shock and head injury. Braz J Med Biol Res 22:287–289
31. Ducey JP, Mozingo DW, Lamiell JM, Okerburg C, Gueller GE (1989) A comparison of the cerebral and cardiovascular effects of complete resuscitation with isotonic and hypertonic saline, hetastarch, and whole blood following hemorrhage. J Trauma 29:1510–1518
32. Whitley JM, Prough DS, Brockschmidt JK, Vines SM, DeWitt DS (1991) Cerebral hemodynamic effects of fluid resuscitation in the presence of an experimental intracranial mass. Surgery 110:514–522
33. Warner DS, Boehland LA (1988) Effects of iso-osmolal intravenous fluid therapy on post-ischemic brain water content in the rat. Anesthesiology 68:86–91
34. Walsh JC, Zhuang J, Shackford SR (1991) A comparison of hypertonic to isotonic fluid in the resuscitation of brain injury and hemorrhagic shock. J Surg Res 50:284–292
35. Battistella FD, Wisner DH (1991) Combined hemorrhagic shock and head injury: effects of hypertonic saline (7.5%) resuscitation. J Trauma 31:182–188
36. Wisner DH, Busche F, Sturm J, Gaab M, Meyer H (1989) Traumatic shock and head injury: effects of fluid resuscitation on the brain. J Surg Res 46:49–59

37. Wisner DH, Schuster L, Quinn C (1990) Hypertonic saline resuscitation of head injury: effects on cerebral water content. J Trauma 30:75–78
38. DeWitt DS, Prough DS, Taylor CL, Deal DD, Vines SM (1996) Hypertonic saline does not improve cerebral oxygen delivery after head injury and mild hemorrhage in cats. Crit Care Med 24:109–117
39. Mattox KL, Maningas PA, Moore EE, Mateer JR, Marx JA, Aprahamian C, Burch JM, Pepe PE (1991) Prehospital hypertonic saline/dextran infusion for post-traumatic hypotension. The U.S.A. Multicenter Trial. Ann Surg 213:482–491
40. Vassar MJ, Fischer RP, O'Brien PE, Bachulis BL, Chambers JA, Hoyt DB, Holcroft JW (1993) A multicenter trial for resuscitation of injured patients with 7.5% sodium chloride: The effect of added dextran 70. Arch Surg 128:1003–1013
41. Wilson BJ, Jones RF, Coleman ST, Moyer CA (1958) The effects of various hypertonic sodium salt solutions on cisternal pressure. Surgery 30:361
42. Smith SD, Cone JB, Bowser BH, Caldwell FT (1982) Cerebral edema following acute hemorrhage in a murine model: the role of crystalloid resuscitation. J Trauma 22:(7):588–590

Discussion

Baethmann:
I am addressing the point of Dr. Prough that, in the situation where the blood–brain barrier is broken, hypertonic fluid does not work. It depends, of course, on the extent of blood–brain barrier disruption, and I think there is a variety of data available on the experimental and also clinical part, where there is a barrier disruption and still hypertonic solutions work to lower intracranial pressure. So I would not say it generally that hypertonic fluid should not be given in a situation of open blood–brain barrier. I think one should try it, anyway, and in your situation I think the benefit of hypertonic fluid is really the resuscitation of the general circulatory system, which then would benefit the brain and I would not worry too much about whether the blood–brain barrier is open or not.

Traber:
I would like to comment on the studies that were brought up about resuscitation of burned patients with hypertonic solutions. First of all, that hypertonic solution was the formula of monofo; these data are about 20–30 years old. The hypertonicity was only 50% more than normal hypertonicity. Secondly, there are a lot of data showing demyelination of burned children's brains during that time period whether or not they received hypertonic saline solution, so I think perhaps that demyelination is a wild card, and that perhaps we should look at demyelination more closely as hypertonic solutions are used more in a clinical situation.

Prough:
I agree. The question is relevant. Although burned patients have received hypertonic fluids, most clinicians have used solutions containing 250–300 mEq/l of sodium. Although they gave much less concentrated sodium solutions, they gave much larger volumes. So the patients' final serum sodium concentrations were typically in the range of 155–160 mEq/l, which is analogous to the hypernatremia that you see with acute resuscitation with small volumes of 7.5% saline.

Traber:
That is sort of like comparing apples and oranges, because the patients who received the hypertonic saline for resuscitation were mostly getting silver nitrate for their burned coverage instead of the sulphur compounds. This is a very hypertonic solution that really was pulling a lot of fluid out of the burned wounds.

Sprung:
I would just like to toss in some more apples and oranges concerning the question of acute pontine myelinolysis. When we looked at our septic shock patients in the early 1980s, a large number of those patients at autopsy had acute pontine myelinolysis. These were medical patients who typically received large amounts of normal saline. Therefore, prior to using a new therapeutic modality for patients that indeed may be helpful, I believe we really ought to make sure that it is not harmful.

Prough:
That also is an important point. Mildly hypertonic solutions given in enormous volumes may produce changes in serum sodium that are similar to the changes produced by small volumes of very hypertonic solutions. So patients that receive large volumes of normal saline (0.9%) solutions will begin to approximate a serum sodium concentration of 154 mEq/l. The difficulty in interpreting pontine myelinolysis in septic patients might be, though, that they often were hospitalized before they became septic for other illnesses, including surgery, and hospitalized patients tend to become hyponatremic. So that is not a population quite like the acute trauma patients; it might be oranges and grapefruits, rather than apples and oranges.

Kochanek:
A very nice talk. I was just wondering if you are aware of anyone studying the combination of uncontrolled hemorrhagic shock plus traumatic brain injury in any animal model.

Prough:
No, I think they would be short-duration studies.

Kochanek:
Not necessarily. I think it would just depend on how you produced your uncontrolled hemorrhage. I think that is relatively controllable. Peter Safer has been, for the last several years, studying uncontrolled hemorrhagic shock plus hypothermia using a tail-cut model in rats.

Prough:
There are rat models of uncontrolled hemorrhage that would be easy enough to combine with traumatic brain injury. It is an intriguing concept because you would really want to combine established models.

Shackford:
Don, this was a very nice presentation. We have used a pressure-driven hemorrhage model, because the aortotomy wire model is so uncontrollable that you cannot get an equal lesion in every animal. So we have used a pressure-driven hemorrhage model in a pig with an uninjured brain. We are now about to add the injury part of it.

Using the pressure-driven model, you cannot get the blood pressure low enough to produce cerebral ischemia. That is, cerebral blood flow really is unaffected even when we get blood pressures down around 40. But I have a hunch that when we add the brain injury we are going to see a problem, and like you I am very concerned that a lot of clinical resuscitalogists will take the Bickell data and will apply it to brain-injured patients. I think that would be a great step backwards. The question I have for you is: As a clinical anesthesiologist who takes care of patients every day, where would you get concerned about a patient that you have treated, given an anesthetic to, who might have a head injury and a fractured femur and then post-operative day 1 in the ICU has received some mannitol, where do you get concerned about the serum osmolarity? At what serum sodium or serum osmolarity would you add in some free water?

Prough:
I am really afraid to answer that question, given the breadth and depth of expertise in this room. So I am really sticking my neck out. I frankly do not worry much, even up into the range of 350 mOsm/kg, assuming that the patient is normovolemic. A great deal of our concern about clinical hypertonicity is related to experience with patients who come to the hospital both hypovolemic and hypertonic. I think it is very difficult to separate the adverse effects of the two lesions. What our models produce and what most models of hypertonic resuscitation produce, after additional fluid is given to stabilize the circulation, is a good cardiac index, good oxygen delivery, and hyperosmolality. I am not sure that is the same as the hypertonicity that we have learned to fear. I think the safety of moderate hypertonicity is reasonably consistent with data in burned children and in burned adults, in whom hypertonic solutions have been used, and in the trauma studies. But that is certainly not a majority viewpoint. A lot of clinicians do not like to see osmolality greater than 320 mOsm/kg.

Gennarelli:
You mention that hyperosmotics tend to lose their effectiveness if there is a large amount of blood–brain barrier disruption. There has been clinical concern in the use of other hyperosmotics that small areas of intense blood–brain barrier disruption such as around hemorrhages will cause localized problems with reversals of osmotic gradients. Is this a concern at all in the resuscitative phase?

Prough:
One set of data that I decided not to show has not yet gone through the peer-review process. (It is not because they are fresh, it is because they were misplaced about the time I moved from North Carolina to Galveston.) We did not specifically study blood–brain barrier function, but did look at intracranial pressure. It actually appears to me as if we were seeing "rebound", perhaps the same kind of phemonemon that was seen with urea and perhaps with mannitol. I think you could speculate that there may be some subset of patients who have an injury that is severe enough to change blood–brain barrier permeability to small molecules such as sodium, but not necessarily change permeability to larger molecules. But I am just not comfortable enough about those data to present them in this context. I think you might see "rebound" and I think you also might see local brain swelling and brain distortion if the possibility of sodium were clearly increased.

Brain Dysfunction Secondary to Sepsis

Brain Dysfunction Secondary to Sepsis

A. OPPENHEIM, L.A. EIDELMAN, and C.L. SPRUNG

Septic encephalopathy is a reversible dysfunction of the central nervous system (CNS) that develops in seriously ill patients with sepsis. Conditions in which altered mental status results from localized infections of the CNS, such as meningitis, encephalitis and brain abscess, are not considered septic encephalopathy, and so are beyond the scope of this chapter. We will review the manifestations, incidence, etiology, and treatment of septic encephalopathy. In addition, we will review the spectrum of the systemic inflammatory response syndrome (SIRS) and sepsis, based on the American College of Chest Physicians and the Society of Critical Care Medicine (ACCP/SCCM) Consensus Conference Committee statement [1]. This statement came in response to the need for guidelines for sepsis studies and the knowledge that as long as definitions remained ambiguous and controversial, it would be impossible to compare incidence of sepsis, outcome and effect of new therapies in different studies [1–3].

Systemic Inflammatory Response Syndrome

Infection is a continuum which starts locally and which may progress with a systematic inflammatory response. This response is not distinguishable from the inflammatory response to non-infectious etiologies, such as trauma, burns, or pancreatitis, and patients with these disorders are also said to be "septic". Because the term "sepsis" relates only to patients who have an infection, the Consensus Conference Committee decided that a new term was required to describe patients with a systemic inflammatory response who may or may not have an infection. The term chosen was the systemic inflammatory response syndrome. Patients with SIRS include patients who are septic, i.e., who have a systemic response to infection, and those who do not have an infection (Fig. 1) [1].

The criteria for SIRS selected by the committee were deliberately broad, so as to include as many patients suffering from an inflammatory response as possible, and therefore all patients with sepsis. SIRS is defined as the presence of two or more of the following signs: tachycardia, tachypnea, alteration in body temperature, and alteration in white blood cell count. Sepsis is the systemic inflammatory response to infection. Severe sepsis occurs when hypoperfusion or hypotension occurs and septic shock is associated with hypotension that does not respond to adequate fluid replacement, together with hypoperfusion. The definitions agreed upon by the committee are detailed in Table 1.

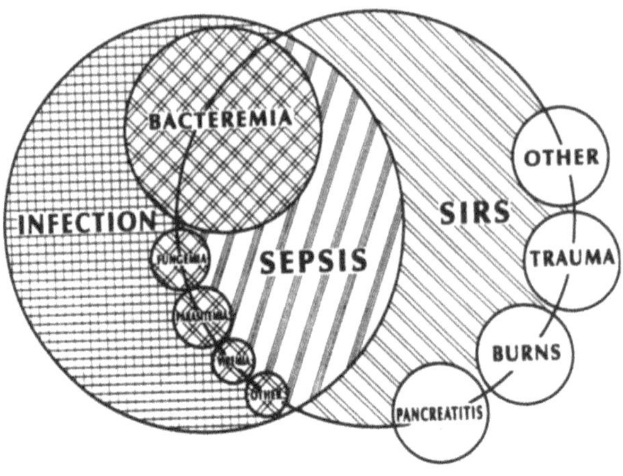

INFECTION
BACTEREMIA
FUNGEMIA
PARASITEMIA
VIREMIA
OTHERS
SEPSIS
SIRS
OTHER
TRAUMA
BURNS
PANCREATITIS
BLOOD BORNE INFECTION

Two recent studies examined the incidence of SIRS and found it to be extremely high [4,5]. In a prospective study by Pittet et al. [4], 93% of 158 patients hospitalized in a surgical intensive care unit (ICU) were found to have SIRS. Of these, 49% developed sepsis, 16% severe sepsis, and 7% septic shock. The 28-day mortality was 6% for patients with SIRS, 35% for those with severe sepsis, and 58% for those with septic shock. Patients with sepsis and severe sepsis had a longer mean length of ICU stay (2.1 ± 0.2 and 7.5 ± 1.5 days, respectively) and of hospital stay (24 ± 2 and 35 ± 9 days, respectively) than patients with SIRS (ICU stay 1.5 ± 0.1 days, hospital stay 11 ± 0.8 days) or control patients (ICU stay 1.2 ± 0.1 days, hospital stay 9 ± 0.1 days) ($p < 0.01$) [4].

In a prospective survey of 3708 patients hospitalized in three ICUs and three wards, Rangel-Frausto et al. found that 68% of the patients met the criteria for SIRS. Among the patients with SIRS, 26% developed sepsis, 18% severe sepsis, and 4% septic shock [5]. The median interval from SIRS to sepsis was inversely correlated with the number of SIRS criteria (two, three, or all four) met by the patient. As patients progressed from SIRS to septic shock, an increasing proportion of them developed adult respiratory distress syndrome, disseminated intravascular coagulation, acute renal failure, and shock. There was also a stepwise increase in the mortality rate from SIRS (7%), sepsis (16%), and severe sepsis (20%) to septic shock (46%) [5].

These studies demonstrate that sepsis is a continuum and that patients may deteriorate from SIRS to sepsis, severe sepsis and, finally, septic shock [4,5]. Moreover, they suggest that mortality is related to the severity of the inflammatory response [4,5].

Acute alteration in mental status is a sign of hypoperfusion which is a component of severe sepsis and septic shock. Septic encephalopathy is thus clinically relevant to management of these conditions. In addition, growing recognition of the importance of a universally accepted definition for the SIRS continuum has highlighted the need for an accepted definition for septic encephalopathy. To date, there is no such definition. A review of the literature reveals a number of different definitions for septic encephalopathy (Table 2). The diversity of definitions means that the results of different studies cannot easily be compared. Moreover, many of the definitions used are subjective rather than objective, and thus not easily reproducible.

Manifestations

The manifestations of encephalopathy range from agitation, irritability, lethargy, disorientation and confusion, to obtundation, stupor and coma [6]. There may be associated fluctuating focal signs, seizures and myoclonic jerks [7]. Milder cases manifest confusion and disorientation along with inappropriate behavior, inattention and writing errors [8]. Altered mental status often appears early in sepsis and resolves as the patient's condition improves.

Electroencephalography (EEG) in patients with septic encephalopathy demonstrates abnormalities reflecting the clinical severity of sepsis. In Young et al.'s study [8], EEG was more sensitive than clinical testing. Dr. Young's chapter discusses the EEG findings in depth.

Table 2. Definitions of septic encephalopathy (SE)

Source	Grade SE	Criteria
Wijdicks [7]		Decreased level of consciousness + seizures, myoclonus, gaze palsy or hemiparesis
Young [8]	Mild	Deficit of two of the following: memory, attention, orientation
	Severe	Mild + impaired consciousness
Pine [9]		Coma
Sprung [10]		Acute cognitive or behavioral changes
Eidelman [11]	1. Altered mental status	Acute cognitive or behavioral changes
	2. Clinical grading	
	1	1 = clouding of consciousness
	2	2 = obtundation
	3	3 = stupor
	4	4 = coma
	3. Glasgow Coma Score	
	Mild	13–14
	Moderate	9–12
	Severe	3–8

Incidence

The incidence of septic encephalopathy has not been extensively studied. In the studies referred to in Tables 2 and 3, the incidence appears to be related to the definitions of sepsis and septic encephalopathy used. In a series of 106 patients with intra-abdominal sepsis, Pine et al. [9] reported a 9% incidence of encephalopathy when coma was the criterion employed. In a study of 84 patients, Wijdicks and Stevens [7] found 17% to be encephalopathic using a definition of decreased level of consciousness accompanied by seizures, myoclonus, gaze palsy, or hemiparesis. Sprung et al. [10] found an incidence of encephalopathy of 23% in 1333 patients when the criterion was an acute behavioral or cognitive abnormality which developed concomitantly with the onset of infection. In a study of 69 infected patients, Young et al. [8] found that 25% had mild encephalopathy (memory, attention, or orientation deficit) while 46% had severe encephalopathy (impaired consciousness in addition to memory, attention, or orientation deficit).

Eidelman et al. [11] recently reported the incidence of septic encephalopathy in 50 septic patients. The incidence varied from 48% to 62% according to the criteria used to define septic encephalopathy (Table 3). When only the presence or absence of altered mental status was recorded, 54% of the patients were found to be encephalopathic. When a clinical grade of encephalopathy was used, 36% of the patients were found to have mild septic encephalopathy and 12% to have severe septic encephalopathy. Using the Glasgow Coma Score (GCS), 30% of the patients had mild

Table 3. Incidence and mortality of septic encephalopathy (SE)

Source	Grade SE	Patients (*n*)	Incidence (%)	Mortality SE (%)	Mortality non-SE (%)
Pine [9]		106	9	100	11
Sprung [10]		1333	23	49	26
Young [8]	Total	69	71	47	0
	Mild		25	35	
	Severe		46	53	
Widjicks [7]		84	17	79	51
Eidelman [11]	Total	50	48–62	33–39	16–27
1. Altered mental status			54	33	26
2. Clinical grading	Total		48	33	27
	1–2		36	28	
	3–4		12	50	
3. Glasgow Coma Score	Total		62	39	16
	13–14		30	20	
	9–12		16	50	
	3–8		16	63	

septic encephalopathy (GCS 13–14), 16% had moderate septic encephalopathy (GCS 9–12), while 16% had severe septic encephalopathy (GCS $\leq$ 8). Eidelman et al. [11] thus demonstrated that considerable variation in the incidence of septic encephalopathy may be found if different criteria are used, even in the same group of patients. In addition, the authors employed the GCS – an objective, widely recognized and easy-to-use scale – to study the spectrum of septic encephalopathy. Use of the GCS is especially attractive because it does not require special training. It is used extensively in ICUs around the world, and has proven beneficial for evaluating patients with brain dysfunction from various causes [12,13]. Another advantage of the GCS is that it is a graded score and different grades of septic encephalopathy have been shown to correlate with APACHE II, metabolic abnormalities and mortality [11].

Etiology

The etiology of septic encephalopathy has yet to be satisfactorily elucidated. Many possible causes have been suggested, including:

- Systemic metabolic derangements
- Microabscesses in the brain
- Endotoxin effect on the brain
- Inadequate or altered cerebral perfusion
- Altered amino acid profiles and brain metabolism
- Thrombocytopenia
- Complications of medical therapy [6,14].

Septic encephalopathy is probably not due to any one factor, but rather to a combination of mechanisms.

Systemic metabolic derangements can result from failure of an organ system due to sepsis, e.g., hepatic failure, renal failure, respiratory failure or pancreatic failure. Other types of metabolic derangements or electrolyte disturbances that may cause mental disturbances are abnormal levels of sodium, calcium, phosphorus and magnesium, hypo- or hyperglycemia, acid-base disturbances, hypo- or hyperthermia, nutritional deficiencies, endocrine abnormalities and exogenous drugs – all widely prevalent in the critical care patient population. Of all these variables, the only ones to have correlated with septic encephalopathy are elevated serum urea nitrogen [8,11], creatinine [8], and bilirubin levels [8,11] and an increased incidence of renal failure [11].

Sepsis is a major catabolic insult which leads to muscle breakdown and nitrogen loss. This is due in part to insulin resistance along with inability to utilize fat. Hepatic failure, an extensively investigated metabolic state, also involves a high catabolic state with decreased glycogen stores, insulin resistance, decreased ketogenesis, decreased fatty acid utilization and increased muscle protein breakdown. It has been postulated that septic encephalopathy is due in part to hepatic failure [15].

A characteristic pattern of amino acids in the plasma develops in hepatic failure. There is an increase in the level of aromatic amino acids (phenylalanine, tyrosine, and tryptophan) and sulphur-containing amino acids, and a decrease in the level of branched-chain amino acids (valine, leucine, and isoleucine) [16–18]. This pattern develops because of the combination of insulin resistance – which prevents utilization of glucose as a source of energy – and inability to utilize fat as a source of energy during hepatic failure. The main source of energy is thus amino acids, specifically branched-chain amino acids. Under normal conditions, aromatic amino acids are metabolized by the liver, while in hepatic failure, they persist in the circulation.

An altered pattern of plasma amino acids affects the pattern of brain amino acids. Both branched-chain amino acids and aromatic amino acids competitively share a transport system for crossing the blood–brain barrier. When the ratio of aromatic amino acids to branched-chain amino acids is high, more aromatic amino acids are transported into the brain. The end result of the altered amino acid pattern is inhibition of dopamine and norepinephrine synthesis along with increased levels of serotonin and 5-hydroxyindolacetic acid (5-HIAA). The enhancement of the serotoninergic pathway may explain the inhibited behavioral and motor activity in septic patients. Altered brain amino acids lead to changes in brain neurotransmitters. Jellinger et al. [19] showed an alteration in brain neurotransmitters occurring in hepatic encephalopathy, with a decrease in dopamine and an increase in serotonin and 5-HIAA.

Hepatic failure occurs early in sepsis [20]. Several investigators believe that the above described alterations in plasma amino acid profiles in sepsis are secondary to the hepatic dysfunction [15]. In sepsis, higher aromatic amino acid levels have been found to correlate with increased mortality [18]. In a comparison of 15 septic shock patients with altered sensorium and 17 infected patients without encephalopathy, Sprung et al. [18] found that the patients with altered sensorium had higher circulating concentrations of ammonia, phenylalanine and tryptophan (the latter two being aromatic amino acids) and lower levels of isoleucine (a branched-chain amino acid).

The encephalopathic patients had a mortality rate of 71% compared to 12% among the non-encephalopathic septic patients.

Another proposed mechanism for septic encephalopathy is that of multiple brain microabscesses. Further discussion of this can be found in Young (this volume).

As to the role of endotoxin in the pathogenesis of septic encephalopathy, many studies have examined the various effects of endotoxin on organ systems. Several mitochondrial functions have been found to be inhibited by endotoxin [21]. The levels of endotoxin in vitro, however, required to produce this effect are several hundred times the concentrations measured in the brains of experimental animals [21]. An interesting finding of the study by Sprung et al. [10] was the relationship between the incidence of altered sensorium and the inciting pathogen. Contrary to accepted clinical belief, patients with gram-negative bacteremia and sepsis were not found to be more likely to develop an acutely altered mental status. The prevalence of encephalopathy was similar in patients with negative blood cultures (23%) and patients with either gram-positive or gram-negative bacteremia (25% and 28%, respectively). Wijdicks and Stevens [7] also found no correlation between gram-negative bacteremia and mortality using the same criteria as the Sprung study. By contrast, Eidelman et al. [11], albeit in a much smaller study group, found a strong correlation between bacteremia (gram-positive or gram-negative) and septic encephalopathy (Table 4). The difference in these findings may be related to the criteria used to define sepsis in the three studies, the patients in the Eidelman et al. study being more severely ill.

Another proposed etiology for septic encephalopathy is inadequate or altered cerebral perfusion. Although cardiac output early in sepsis usually increases, the manifestations of septic encephalopathy may appear at this time. This suggests the possibility of flow maldistribution in sepsis. Studies in animal models of sepsis have been contradictory, possibly a result of interspecies variability: some demonstrate increased cerebral blood flow and others no change [22]. In Wijdicks and Stevens'

Table 4. Septic encephalopathy and presence of bacteremia. (Adapted from [11])

	Bacteremia (%)	p value	Gram-negative bacteremia	p value
Altered mental status		$p < 0.01$		$p < 0.01$
No	13		9	
Yes	59		48	
Clinical grade of encephalopathy		$p < 0.01$		$p < 0.01$
0	15		12	
1–2	78		61	
3–4	17		17	
Glasgow Coma Score		$p = 0.09$		$p = 0.06$
15	21		21	
13–14	60		40	
9–12	25		25	
3–8	50		38	

study [7], the most significant variable associated with septic encephalopathy was severe hypotension, suggesting an ischemic rather than a metabolic pathogenesis of encephalopathy. Similar findings were reported by Sprung et al. [10] and Young et al. [8]. Eidelman et al., however, found no correlation between hypotension and septic encephalopathy, a fact they attributed to aggressive initial treatment [11]. Bowton et al. [22] studied the effects of sepsis on cerebral blood flow and cerebrovascular reactivity to changes in PCO_2 in nine patients meeting criteria for sepsis with acute encephalopathy. Both cerebral blood flow and cerebral oxygen consumption were reduced in these patients, while the cerebrovascular response to PCO_2 remained intact. Maekawa et al. [23] studied cerebral blood flow, cerebral metabolic rate for oxygen ($CMRO_2$) and EEG in six septic patients with encephalopathy. In this study, septic encephalopathy was accompanied by decreases both in cerebral blood flow and in $CMRO_2$, along with EEG slowing. These studies strongly suggest that altered cerebral blood flow in sepsis may participate in the pathogenesis of encephalopathy.

The acute inflammatory response to sepsis entails an inappropriate and at times uncontrolled release of multiple potent mediators, including kinins, prostaglandins, proteases, and cytokines, among others [24]. Some of these mediators have a direct cytotoxic effect, as well as an effect on the distribution of blood flow. The result is inappropriate vasoconstriction, endothelial cell damage, microembolism, thrombosis and interstitial edema. These can affect brain metabolism and lead directly to hypoxia-related cell dysfunction and death.

Thrombocytopenia has also been found to correlate with the development of septic encephalopathy. Sprung et al. [10] found the prevalence of thrombocytopenia to be significantly higher in patients with altered mental status (32%) than in those with normal mental status (18%) ($p < 0.001$). Whether this is an indicator of a more severe illness or a contributing etiological factor has yet to be determined.

Prognosis

The prognosis, like the incidence, of septic encephalopathy reported in the literature (Table 3) is related to the definitions used (Table 2). In Pine et al.'s study [9] the mortality rate among the encephalopathic patients was 100%, while in the series reported by Wijdicks and Stevens [7], the mortality rate was 79% among the encephalopathic patients compared to 51% among the non-encephalopathic ones. Eidelman et al. [11] reported a mortality rate of 16%–27% in the non-encephalopathic septic group, according to the criteria used for diagnosis. The mortality rate among the mildly encephalopathic patients was similar (20%–28%), but in the moderate to severe encephalopathic patients it was significantly higher (50%–63%) ($p < 0.05$ when GCS <12 was used as the criterion for moderate or severe encephalopathy). Young et al. [8] observed a mortality rate of 53% in severely encephalopathic patients, 35% in mildly encephalopathic patients and 0% in non-encephalopathic patients. Sprung et al. [10] reported a mortality rate of 49% for encephalopathic patients and 26% for patients with normal sensorium.

Marshall et al. [25] have devised a scoring system for multiple organ dysfunction in the ICU. The Multiple Organ Dysfunction Score (MODS) is composed of the sum of the scores given to six systems (respiratory, renal, hepatic, cardiovascular, hematologic and central nervous system) (Table 5). Of the six systems reviewed, CNS dysfunction was found to be the strongest predictor of death [25]. While it may be argued that encephalopathy is simply a marker of more severe sepsis and hence associated with an increased mortality, the presence of encephalopathy is still of considerable use to the clinician in identifying a more severely ill subset of patients requiring intensive monitoring and treatment.

Treatment

Mental confusion and obtundation are considered to be early signs of the sepsis syndrome [26]. Survival from sepsis is greatly enhanced by early diagnosis and treatment [27], before the onset of multiple organ dysfunction. Hence, early recognition of septic encephalopathy may lead to improved outcome in sepsis. Prompt diagnosis of septic encephalopathy is also important because of its influence on mortality.

The cardinal treatment of septic encephalopathy is of course eradication of the septic focus, accompanied by aggressive supportive therapies in accordance with the

Table 5. The multiple organ dysfunction score. (From [25])

Organ system	Score				
	0	1	2	3	4
Respiratory[a] (PO_2/ FIO_2 ratio)	>300	226–300	151–225	76–150	≤75
Renal[b] (serum creatinine)	≤100	101–200	201–350	351–500	<500
Hepatic[c] (serum bilirubin)	≤20	21–60	61–120	121–240	>240
Cardio-vascular[d] (PAR)	≤10.0	10.1–15	15.1–20.0	20.1–30	>30.0
Hematologic[e] (platelet count)	>120	81–120	51–80	21–50	≤20
Neurologic[f] (Glasgow Coma Score)	15	13–14	10–12	7–9	≤6

[a] The PO_2/FIO_2 ratio is calculated without reference to the use or mode of mechanical ventilation, and without reference to the use or level of positive end-expiratory pressure.
[b] The serum creatinine concentration is measured in µmol/L, without reference to the use of dialysis.
[c] The serum bilirubin concentration is measured in µmol/L.
[d] The pressure-adjusted heart rate (PAR) is calculated as the product of the heart rate (HR) multiplied by the ratio of the right atrial (central venous) pressure (RAP) to the mean arterial pressure (MAP): PAR = HR × RAP/mean BP.
[e] The platelet count is measured in platelets/ml 10^{-3}.
[f] The Glasgow Coma Score is preferably calculated by the patient's nurse, and is scored conservatively (for the patient receiving sedation or muscle relaxants, normal function is assumed, unless there is evidence of intrinsically altered mentation).

patient's condition. Prompt control of infection is of the utmost importance for reversing the septic encephalopathy and preventing increased mortality. Data on specific treatment modalities for septic encephalopathy are currently scarce. However, as understanding of the various mechanisms involved in sepsis and septic encephalopathy increases, specific therapies for individual derangements may prove helpful. These include infusion of branched-chain amino acids to correct the plasma and ultimately the brain ratio of aromatic to branched amino acids [17], manipulation of cerebral blood flow to improve regional oxygen supply, and of course modulation of the immune response that causes systemic inflammatory response.

References

1. Bone RC, Balk RA, Cerra FB, Delinger RP, Fein AM, Knaus WA, Schein RMH, Sibbald WJ (1992) ACCP/SCCM consensus conference: definitions for sepsis and organ failure and guidelines for the use of innovative therapies in sepsis. Chest 101:1644–1655
2. Zeigler EJ, Fisher CJ, Sprung CL et al for the HA-1A Sepsis Study Group (1991) Treatment of gram-negative bacteremia and septic shock with HA-1A human monoclonal antibody against endotoxin. N Engl J Med 324:429–436
3. Greenman RL, Schein RMH, Martin MA et al (1991) A controlled trial of ES murine monoclonal IGM antibody to endotoxin in the treatment of gram negative sepsis. JAMA 266:1097–1102
4. Pittet D, Rangel-Frausto S, Li N, Tarara D, Costigan M, Rempe L, Jebson P, Wenzel RP (1995) Systemic inflammatory response syndrome, sepsis, severe sepsis and septic shock: incidence, morbidities and outcomes in surgical ICU patients. Intensive Care Med 21:302–309
5. Rangel-Frausto MS, Pittet D, Costigan M, Hwang T, Davis CS, Wenzel RP (1995) The natural history of the systemic inflammatory response syndrome. JAMA 273:117–123
6. Bolton CF, Young GB (1986) In: Sibbald WJ, Sprung CL (eds) Perspectives on Sepsis and Septic Shock. Society of Critical Care Medicine, Fullerton, pp 157–171
7. Wijdicks EFM, Stevens M (1992) The role of hypotension in septic encephalopathy following surgical procedures. Arch Neurol 49:653–656
8. Young GB, Bolton CF, Austin TW, Archibald YM, Gonder J, Wells GA (1990) The encephalopathy associated with septic illness. Clin Invest Med 13:297–304
9. Pine RW, Wertz MJ, Lennard ES, Dellinger EP, Carrico CJ, Minshew BH (1983) Determinants of organ malfunction or death in patients with intra-abdominal sepsis: a discriminate analysis. Arch Surg 118:242–249
10. Sprung CL, Peduzzi PN, Shatney CH, Schein RMH, Wilson MF, Sheagren JN, Hinshaw LB (1990) Impact of encephalopathy on mortality in the sepsis syndrome. Crit Care Med 18:801–806
11. Eidelman LA, Putterman D, Putterman C, Sprung CL (1996) The spectrum of septic encephalopathy. JAMA 275:470–473
12. Teasdale F, Jennet B (1974) Assessment of coma and impaired consciousness. Lancet 81–84
13. Mullie A, Verstinge P, Buylaert W et al (1988) Predictive value of Glasgow Coma Score for awakening after out of hospital cardiac arrest. Lancet 137–140
14. Bowton DL (1989) Central nervous system effects of sepsis. Crit Care Clin 5:785–792
15. Hasselgren PO, Fischer JE (1986) Septic encephalopathy. Etiology and management. Intensive Care Med 12:13–16
16. Fischer JE, Funovics JM, Aguirre A et al (1975) The role of plasma amino acids in hepatic encephalopathy. Surgery 78:276–290
17. Freund HR, Ryan JA, Fischer JE (1978) Amino acid derangements in patients with sepsis: treatment with branched chain amino acid rich infusion. Ann Surg 188:423–429
18. Sprung CL, Cerra FB, Freund HR, Schein RMH, Konstantinides FN, Marcial EH, Pena M (1991) Amino acid alteration and encephalopathy in the sepsis syndrome. Crit Care Med 19:753–757

19. Jellinger K (1978) Brain mono-amines in human hepatic encephalopathy. Acta Neuropathol (Berl) 43:63–68
20. Chaudry IH, Clemens MG, Baue AE (1986) In: Sibbald WJ, Sprung CL (eds) Perspectives on Sepsis and Septic Shock. Society of Critical Care Medicine, Fullerton, pp 61–76
21. Mela L (1981) Direct and indirect effects of endotoxin on mitochondrial function. Prog Clin Biol Res 62:15–21
22. Bowton DL, Bertels NH, Prough DS, Stump DA (1989) Cerebral blood flow is reduced in patients with sepsis syndrome. Crit Care Med 17:399–403
23. Maekawa T, Fujii Y, Sadamitsu D et al (1991) Cerebral circulation and metabolism in patients with septic encephalopathy. Am J Emerg Med 9:139–143
24. Movat HZ, Cybulsky MI, Colditz IG, Chan MKW, Dinarello CA (1987) Acute inflammation in gram-negative infection: endotoxin, interleukin-1, tumor necrosis factor, and neutrophils. Fed Proc 46:97–104
25. Marshall JC, Cook DJ, Christou NV, Bernard GR, Sprung CL, Sibbald WJ (1995) Multiple organ dysfunction score: a reliable descriptor of a complex clinical outcome. Crit Care Med 23:1638–1652
26. Shatney CH, Lillehei RC (1978) Septic shock in patients with surgical disease of the colon and rectum. Dis Colon Rectum 21:480–486
27. Sprung CL, Caralis PV, Marcial EH et al (1984) The effects of high-dose corticosteroids in patients with septic shock. A prospective controlled study. N Engl J Med 311:1137–1143

Discussion

Traber:
That was a very elegant presentation. There are two questions that I want to ask: The first is, there have been a large number of studies that have looked at negative nitrogen balance in many different patient groups, and of those patient groups there have been a large number of septic patients. Mainly they have been looking at the administration of growth hormone in double-blinded close-labeled studies. And growth hormone, at least in some of the data that I have seen, reverses negative nitrogen balance, and I assume that if the elevation in aromatic amino acids was due to the breakdown of protein and gluconeogenesis that aromatic amino acids would have been reduced in those groups. Has anybody looked at a subpopulation of septic patients in those studies to see if there was a lower instance of encephalopathy in the growth hormone-treated individuals? And then the second question I want to ask: Has anyone given aromatic amino acids to volunteers to achieve plasma levels similar to what is seen in sepsis? And in those cases, have they seen encephalopathy?

Sprung:
As far as the first question is concerned, I am not aware of any data looking at subgroups of septic patients in those studies. Frank Cerra did a multicenter trial in hepatic encephalopathy looking at the use of branched-chain amino acids and found a decrease in encephalopathy and, in fact, mortality. But it is still not used routinely in that patient group and the use of branched-chain amino acids in hepatic encephalopathy remains controversial. There are also studies showing no differences. As for the second question, I am not aware of any patient data. There are data in animals with portocaval shunts in whom aromatic amino acids were injected and encephalopathy was induced in those animals.

Zornow:
I really appreciated this lecture. I do not have to take care of intensive care unit patients, so I may be naive about some of these issues. Has anybody done a study to compare the incidence of encephalopathy, of whatever definition, in patients with sepsis versus a matched control group of patients with similar degrees of illness? This would help to determine whether or not the encephalopathy is associated with sepsis or just a sort of an ICU psychosis. Has this been done?

Sprung:
Not really. Mizock looked at CSF amino acids in patients who had septic encephalopathy or hepatic encephalopathy and showed some similarities but also differences; but looking prospectively at different groups – no. There are not a lot of data related to septic encephalopathy. The Pine study was not looking at septic encephalopathy but rather at organ system failure in patients with abdominal infections. There are other studies that look at it peripherally, but septic encephalopathy has been a neglected field.

Shackford:
Charlie, that was a very nice presentation about a very important problem. I may have missed it, but I was wondering if anybody has done any comprehensive or compulsive histologic sections of patients dying of multiple organ failure looking specifically at the brain. I think all of us around the table recognize the incredible contribution that Graham made years ago looking at patients who had died following head injury, and discovered this incidence of secondary ischemic brain injury occurring in areas remote from the primary injury. Has there been any kind of a similarly compulsive postmortem histologic examination of brains of patients dying of sepsis who had septic encephalopathy?

Young:
We have studied a group of twelve sequential patients who died of sepsis, and we have continued to examine cases since, and found somewhat similar findings. The problem is that you have to see things at the end of the road. Some findings are possibly merely agonal phenomena. At least the early part of the encephalopathy is almost certainly a metabolic and fully reversible phenomenon, but things happen with protracted sepsis that structurally damage the brain. We find neurological problems in some of the follow-ups of survivors who nearly died. So, I think septic encephalopathy has a mixed pathogenesis; sometimes there can be structural damage in protracted sepsis.

Shackford:
Knowing that, or realizing that you are looking at an end-stage phenomenon, perhaps, there are techniques now, microdialysis being one, for example, that is being used in head-injured patients and has advanced significantly our understanding of what is going on on a continuing basis. Has anybody put in microdialysis catheters in patients with septic encephalopathy that you are aware of?

Young:
I am not aware of that, but it is a good idea.

Sprung:

I am not aware of that either. Just a further comment on your first question. At least in the ICU patient there are so many variables that are involved besides sepsis and encephalopathy, so at the end of the road, when you have a finding, to say that it was related to the sepsis is very, very difficult. Looking for septic encephalopathy in patients in our units is very difficult, because most of our patients are sedated and we must exclude these patients from analysis, so it is a real problem.

Baethmann:

Are there sepsis-specific neuropathological changes in the brain? You were mentioning that some findings suggest formation of microthrombosis and of microabscesses. The similarity of the septic encephalopathy with the encephalopathy from hepatic failure is striking, raising the question whether the pathophysiology observed in the brain could be attributed to secondary effects of hepatic failure from sepsis.

Sprung:

I agree with you and it is clear that in the early stages of sepsis there is hepatic dysfunction. We may not even see it with enzymes, but Chaudry had data that early in sepsis there is hepatic dysfunction. Our hypothesis was that the amino acid changes are related to hepatic dysfunction. The increased bilirubin that we found in our patients might go along with that hypothesis.

Bolton:

I enjoyed that excellent review. Just a comment, without getting into too much controversy, about the Glasgow Coma Score. It was not originally designed to classify encephalopathies in the intensive care unit, but classify encephalopathies before intensive care treatment was started. Among the problems is the endotracheal tube which eliminates assessment of the verbal response. The assessment of the best motor response may be done poorly in the unit. Charlie, in your own study it was obviously done very well, but in many units they just do not know how to interpret it. So you have two of the three categories that are suspect. I would recommend that if we are going to do a study, we probably should do something other than the Glasgow Coma Scale. Brian Young has looked into some of the other scaling mechanisms.

Sprung:

I would agree that there are problems with the Glasgow Coma Score. Obviously, in patients who are intubated we do not have a reliable verbal component. In addition, there are agitated patients who have a change in their mental status and the Glasgow Coma Score will not pick that up either. I do not think the score is perfect. Yet it is something that is used routinely throughout the world and there are other areas, patients after cardiac arrest where the Glasgow Coma Score has been found to be helpful. Many other tests of cerebral function are just too complex and too difficult to perform.

Young:

I agree with your comments. The Glasgow Coma Score is standardized, has the advantage of being universal, and is incorporated into the APACHE scoring system. But there are a number of problems, as Dr. Bolton has mentioned, in that the different subsets are added and you can derive the same total score with very different subset values, which is a disadvantage. I think the best scoring system that has been published is one called the Reaction Level Score-85, which was published, I believe, in a Scandinavian journal. In that scoring system moving up one point is very significant. The score is a continuous ordinal scale that is not divided into subsets that are then added on to each other. It suffers the problem of not being universal and not being as familiar. But it is quite easy to apply and to grade severity. I think it might have some advantages looking at encephalopathies over other scoring systems. I would also argue that electrophysiological tests could be used in an objective way to check the brain function, but this needs to be better standardized.

Traber:
I can understand your point relative to the interpretation of the Glasgow Coma Score in ICU patients. I was on the other end of the line. I was in a bad automobile accident and they were trying to get a Glasgow Coma Score on me. An ophthalmologist in the trauma room of the ER had noticed that I had some eye pathology and put atropine in my eye that was really causing a lot of excitement. They were using the Glasgow Coma Score on me. I fully appreciate the idea about brains from patients who died of sepsis. You know, when you look at the residents who tried to resuscitate some of these septic patients for 3 h and then the body goes to autopsy, and the pathology does not get around to preserving the brain until 12 h later, there is a lot of variation. But I think you can look at the chart and get brains from patients who died at different moments of sepsis. I think that this microthrombosis might be a very interesting thing to evaluate in these brains. There are some new data that might tie microthrombosis together with some of the metabolic changes that are seen. It appears that platelets deliver interleukin-1 to the tissues and, therefore, can definitely affect the metabolism of that. So it might be of interest in looking at the pathology of some of these brains from septic individuals, to look for the microthrombosis and see if there is any correlation with metabolic changes.

Morganti:
I have another comment concerning the inflammatory response, which we also see in head trauma patients. It is known that cytokines can increase the permeability of the blood–brain barrier. This may play a very important role, because once a breakdown of this barrier occurs, there is penetration of serum components plus bacteria, which may penetrate the brain. And locally, the alteration of the homeostasis of the nervous environment certainly may lead to brain dysfunction. And the second thing is that when we look at it the other way round, head trauma patients very often show an acute phase response characterized by an increase of acute phase proteins which correlate with increased serum interleukin-6. We suppose that interleukin-6 may come from the brain since the levels we measure in CSF are higher compared to the levels we find in serum. This represents another approach to study these events, showing again that when the barrier is dysfunctional there is a change which can either come from the brain or come from the septical environment, the periphery.

Traber:
May I ask you a question: there are a large number of patients that receive interleukin-2 administration for treatment of cancer. These patients develop many of the same side effects as septic patients. Do those patients show an encephalopathy?

Young:
I think they can and there is an increased permeability of the blood–brain barrier with interleukin-2 administration; it has been used in cancer. I do not know if it is universal, though.

Morganti:
It is known that injection of cytokines in the ventricles can increase the permeability of the blood–brain barrier, and this increase has been correlated to recruitment of neutrophils and increased synthesis or expression of adhesion molecules. But I am not aware of the study on interleukin-2.

The Encephalopathy Associated with Septic Illness: Clinical Neurological Features

G.B. YOUNG

Summary

Septic encephalopathy resembles many metabolic encephalopathies and is largely reversible, although some survivors of severe septic illness may have residual cognitive problems. These deficits may relate to microscopic abnormalities in the brain that we have found at autopsy. Biochemical abnormalities are directly related to the severity of the encephalopathy. It is unlikely that organ failure accounts for the early encephalopathy, but multi-organ failure probably contributes to brain dysfunction in advanced sepsis.

Electroencephalographic (EEG) changes run parallel to the clinical severity of the brain dysfunction, biochemical derangements and the failure of other organ systems. Each of these stages is potentially reversible, although mortality rises proportionally with the severity of the EEG abnormality. Deaths are usually due to multi-organ, rather than brain, failure.

Introduction

The following discussion is concerned with the clinical neurological features of septic encephalopathy, including relevant investigative tests. We have gained some further insights from pathological studies and a preliminary study on the follow-up of survivors.

Clinical Features

The acute encephalopathy associated with sepsis is similar to most metabolic encephalopathies (Plum and Posner 1980; Young et al. 1990). Impairment in alertness can range from delirium or acute confusional state to coma. There is often considerable fluctuation in the early stages. The principal or universal mental status abnormality is impairment of attention. A test for impaired attention is counting backwards from 20 to one. The patient should make no more than one error and should be able to do this within 15 s, assuming a previously normal mental status. Impaired orientation and poor writing ability are common early accompaniments.

Cranial nerve functions, including pupillary size and reactivity and extra-ocular movements, are spared. This is essential in differentiating an encephalopathy from impaired consciousness from a single structural lesion in either the supratentorial or infratentorial compartment. We have found that gegenhalten, or paratonic rigidity, is the most common motor abnormality (Young et al. 1990). The essential feature is a resistance to the passive movement of a limb that is velocity-dependent. With movements at normal or rapid rate the resistance is felt by the examiner, but the resistance disappears when the limb is moved more slowly. This differentiates gegenhalten from Parkinsonian rigidity. Other motor abnormalities, including tremor, asterixis, multifocal myoclonus and seizures, occur infrequently in our experience. A sometimes helpful clue on general examination is the presence of hyperventilation. This may be due to respiratory alkalosis in the early phase of sepsis, but it may later relate to metabolic acidosis with failure of organ perfusion and increased lactic acid production. Other clinical features of septic illness, including fever and tachycardia, are common but not universal. Patients who are elderly or seriously debilitated may not show these features.

The diagnosis of septic encephalopathy is one of exclusion. Table 1 lists other conditions that may produce an acute confusional state and fever. These should be considered in the differential diagnosis when seeing such a patient. Clinical and laboratory features will help to make the necessary exclusions. Sometimes it is necessary to perform a lumbar puncture to exclude a central nervous system infection, especially bacterial meningitis. Herpes simplex encephalitis, the main treatable viral encephalitis, is diagnosed by clinical features, electroencephalography (EEG), showing abnormalities, especially periodic sharp waves, localized to one or both temporal lobes, magnetic resonance imaging (MRI), showing altered signal in the mesial temporal and insular cortex, and CSF analysis, especially the polymerase chain reaction, confirming the presence of DNA from herpes simplex.

In severely affected patients in the intensive care unit (ICU), 70% in our experience develop a critical illness polyneuropathy (CIP) (Young et al. 1990; Zochodne et al. 1987). This is usually noted after the encephalopathy has peaked or after the patient has regained consciousness in the ICU (Bolton et al. 1993). Such patients do not move their limbs, and only grimace when a limb is given a noxious stimulus. Deep tendon reflexes are lost. Critical illness polyneuropathy is one of the principal reasons for the failure to wean septic patients from the ventilator. It is often noted after the septic illness and adult respiratory distress syndrome (ARDS) have resolved (Bolton et al. 1993).

Laboratory Features

The EEG is more sensitive to the encephalopathic effects of sepsis than our bedside screening tests for attentional deficits (Young et al. 1992). The severity of the encephalopathy and the mortality are directly related to the EEG abnormalities. The latter can be broadly categorized into four groups: mild slowing in the theta (>4 but <8 Hz frequencies), excessive delta (less than 4 Hz), triphasic waves, and burst-suppression, in ascending order of severity (Figs. 1–5). Rarely, patients may have

Table 1. Causes of encephalopathy in febrile patients

Infections
  Central nervous system
    Bacterial: meningitis, cerebritis, brain abscess, subdural–epidural empyema
    Viral: encephalitis (herpes simplex)
    Other: spirochetal, rickettisial, protozoal, helminthic
  Septic intracranial thrombophlebitis
  Bacterial endocarditis: produces multiple emboli, meningitis, or mycotic aneurysm, or
    arteritis
  Systemic inflammation: sepsis or SIRS with "septic encephalopathy" picture, direct organ
    damage, and secondary encephalopathy
Vascular Accidents
  Pulmonary emboli
  CNS: vertebrobasilar stroke, intracranial hemorrhage
Trauma
  Cerebral injury
  Fat embolism with fractures of long bones
  SIRS
Immunological conditions
  Drug fever
  Acetylsalicylic acid toxicity
  Connective tissue disease
Metabolic conditions
  Acute adrenal failure
  Thyroid storm
  Porphyria
Reye's syndrome (children)
Neoplasms
  Systemic malignancy with multiple organ failure
  Brain tumors, primary or secondary, affecting thermoregulation
Hematological causes
  Hemolytic episodes, e.g., sickle cell disease
  Leukemia
Increased muscular activity
  Seizures
  Malignant hyperthermia
  Malignant neuroleptic syndrome

SIRS, systemic inflammatory response syndrome.

focal or generalized or focal epileptiform discharges. These often correlate with cortical lesions discovered later at autopsy. CSF is usually normal, although some severely encephalopathic patients have a slight elevation of protein concentration (Young et al. 1990). This is also helpful in differentiating CIP from Guillain-Barré syndrome. In the latter the CSF shows a marked rise in protein concentration, while it is normal or only mildly elevated in CIP.

Neuro-imaging of the brain with computed tomography (CT) is negative. Our limited experience with standard MRI has also been unremarkable. Functional MRI would be expected to show abnormalities, in keeping with previous blood flow and metabolic studies. Leukocytosis, hyperglycemia, increased lactate, hyperuricemia, hypertriglyceridemia, hypocalcemia, and hypoxemia are common. Serum concentrations of urea, creatinine, phosphate, potassium, alkaline phosphatase, and bilirubin

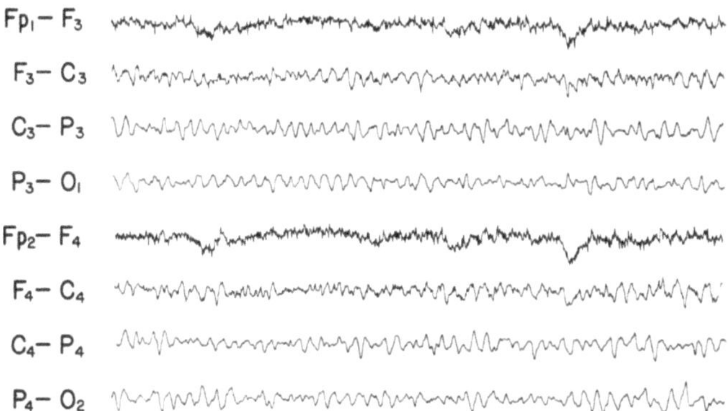

THETA
AWAKE
67 yrs
Fp₁– F₃
F₃– C₃
C₃– P₃
P₃– O₁
Fp₂– F₄
F₄– C₄
C₄– P₄
P₄– O₂
50μV
1 SEC

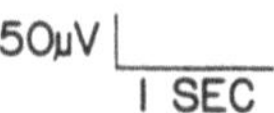

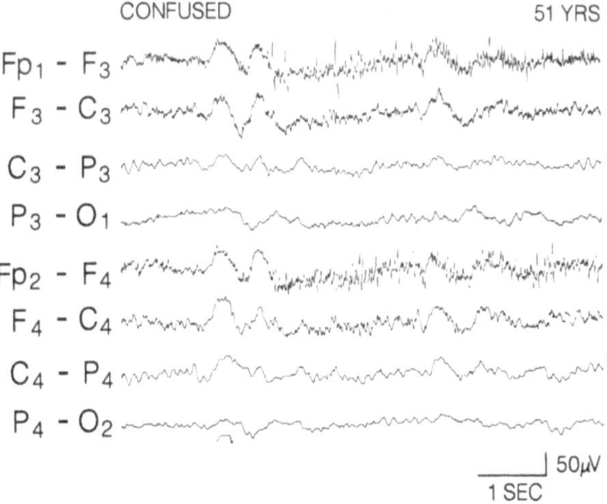

CONFUSED
51 YRS
Fp₁ - F₃
F₃ - C₃
C₃ - P₃
P₃ - O₁
Fp₂ - F₄
F₄ - C₄
C₄ - P₄
P₄ - O₂
50μV
1 SEC

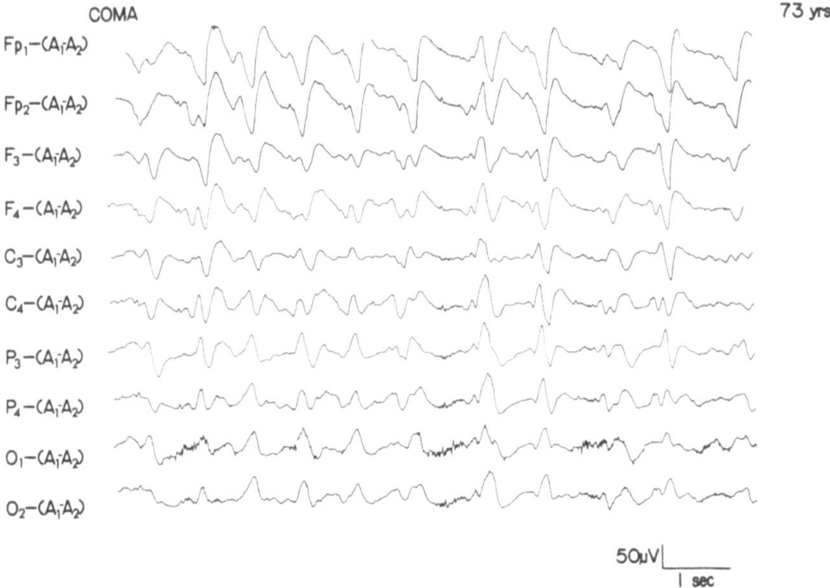

Fig. 3. The third stage in the progression of electroencephalography abnormality in septic encephalopathy is triphasic waves. These are bilateral, frontally predominant phenomena that are sharply contoured and occur in trains

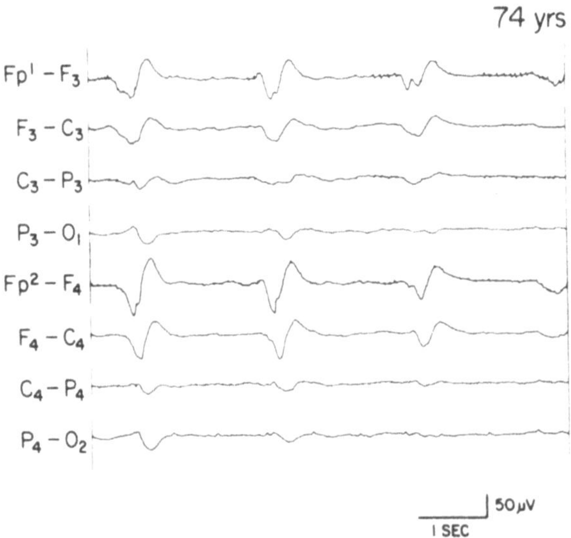

Fig. 4. A burst-suppression pattern in which periods of generalized attenuation of voltage alternate with bursts of activity, or incomplete generalized suppression is the most marked electroencephalography abnormality

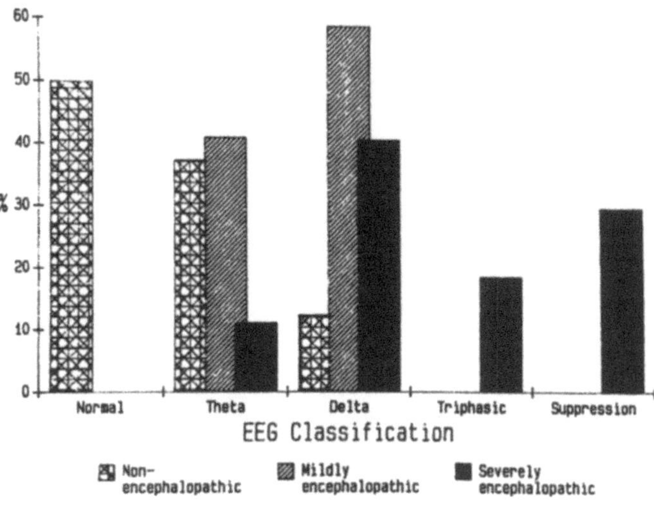
60
50
40
%
30
20
10
0
Normal
Theta
Delta
Triphasic
Suppression
EEG Classification
Non-encephalopathic
Mildly encephalopathic
Severely encephalopathic

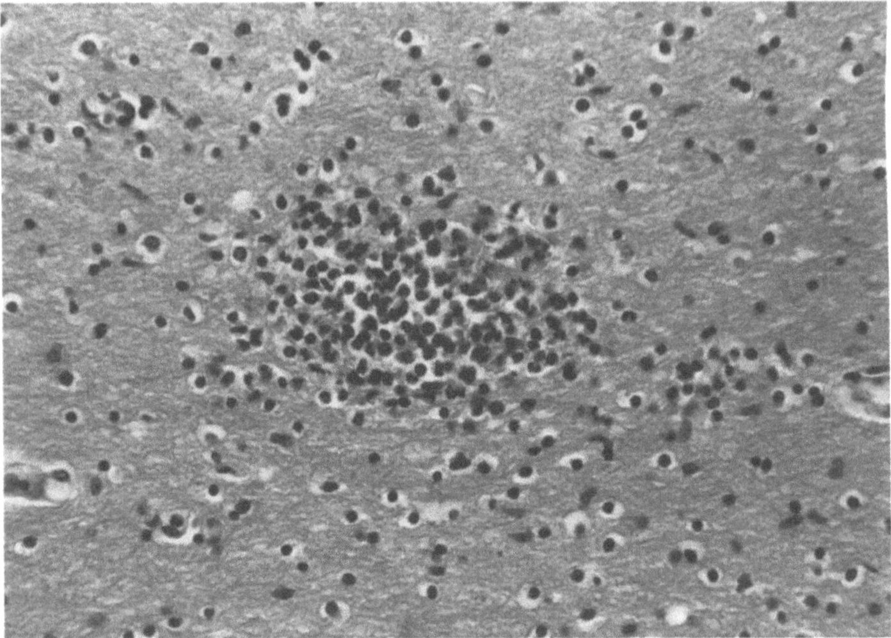

Fig. 6. A photomicrograph of a microabscess in the cerebral cortex of a patient who died after a protracted septic illness. There is an inflammatory infiltrate of polymorphonuclear leukocytes, macrophages, and lymphocytes. The surrounding brain shows microglial proliferation (×627). (Reproduced with permission from Jackson et al. 1985)

essential for the development of encephalopathy, however, which is likely on a reversible (metabolic) basis in the early phases of the condition.

Neurological Outcome of Survivors of Septic Encephalopathy

Patients who survive septic illness recover consciousness and awareness (Young et al. 1990). During their hospital stay the main neurological abnormalities often lie in the peripheral nervous system: Recovery from critical illness polyneuropathy may take many months (Bolton et al. 1993).

We are conducting a questionnaire study on survivors of coma-producing septic encephalopathy at 6 months and 1 year after discharge from the intensive care units (Lazosky et al. 1995). A significant number, probably more than half of these survivors, have behavioral and cognitive problems, especially memory and the speed of cognitive processing. The study is not completed; we plan to follow this with a more detailed neuropsychological, clinical neurological and electroencephalographic follow-up. Some survivors do very well and appear to recover completely, but it is likely that some are left with cognitive problems that persist at least for several months.

References

Bolton CF, Young GB, Zochodne DW (1993) The neurological complications of sepsis. Ann Neurol 33:297–304

Jackson AC, Gilbert JJ, Young GB, Bolton CF (1985) The encephalopathy of sepsis. Can J Neurol Sci 12:303–307

Lazosky A, Young GB, Archibald YM (1995) Cognitive deficits in survivors of severe septic encephalopathy. Presented at Conference of the Canadian Trauma Society, London, Ontario, Canada

Norenberg MD (1983) A hypothesis of osmotic endothelial injury. Arch Neurol 40:66–69

Plum F, Posner JB (1980) The Diagnosis of Stupor and Coma. FA Davis, Philadelphia

Young GB, Bolton CF, Archibald YM, Gonder J, Wells GA (1990) The encephalopathy associated with septic illness. Clin Invest Med 13:297–304

Young GB, Bolton CF, Austin TW, Archibald YM, Gonder J, Wells GA (1992) The electroencephalogram in sepsis-associated encephalopathy. J Clin Neurophysiol 9:145–152

Discussion

Prough:

Two questions: First, have you done any neuropsychologic testing during the confusional state that occurs early in sepsis? Is there a way to quantify that stage? Second, have you done any neuropsychologic testing in the survivors of sepsis? I may have missed some detail about whether they show any specific changes. Our group at Brurnan Gray School of Medicine had a lot of experience with cognitive dysfunction after cardiac surgery. One of the striking observations was that the subjective complaints and objective evidence of neuropsychologic dysfunction often occurred in totally different sets of patients.

Young:

Those are good questions. We have found it difficult to test patients with the confusional state, as adequate testing of memory and other higher functions is precluded if the person has problems with attention and concentration. These are universal in the acute confusional state that these patients show earlier in sepsis. I am not sure if a grading of acute confusion exists, perhaps a neuropsychologist could develop a system. With regards to the second question about follow-up, no, we have not yet done detailed neuropsychological testing on these patients. That is planned, though, as a later phase. We are just doing a questionnaire so far, which seems to be picking up a fair degree of psychosocial and cognitive dysfunction in survivors, and we need to have them back and really do a proper neuropsychological evaluation on those patients (and probably neurological and psychological as well).

I do not want to imply that this cognitive dysfunction is universal, as the patients we have surveyed so far have all been in coma with sepsis. I think if they survived acute reversible sepsis they probably would fully recover. In the very severely ill patients with protracted sepsis, I think there will be a significant morbidity.

N. Zarkovic:
I was wondering, how much is the red blood cell count?

Young:
I do not think we found any significant changes in hemoglobin or red cell counts in the blood.

N. Zarkovic:
Namely, as Dr. Morganti mentioned, the data you said, and what she said already, fit into a general, I would say acute phase reaction, which absolutely has to be associated with cytokine release on one side and on the other due to the activity of the granulocytes and monocytes one has to expect an enormous oxidative burst within the blood. That should, of course, induce lipid peroxydation of the erythrocytes as well. They should be damaged, and afterwards eliminated and this should cause an increase of bilirubin. All the data that you have are rather in favor of the acute phase response than of the liver malfunction. I would say the liver is functioning pretty well, but this is a general systemic response to bacteremia.

Young:
Maybe so, but we have not found that when we looked at all our variables as a phenomenon and changes in the red cells. Do you suggest any particular, more sophisticated testing of red cells?

N. Zarkovic:
Yes, I think, for example, one should follow the content of glutathione, for example, particularly liver glutathion, which could indicate the scavenger activity of the liver to defend the organism against the systemic oxidative stress, which is a normal thing to happen in case of really severe trauma, and I expect sepsis as well.

Young:
That is a good suggestion.

Regel:
You were mentioning organ failure in your set up with encephalopathy and my question is: We are looking mostly at multiple trauma patients that are *ventilated* and develop multiple organ failure, so how would you monitor these patients in relation to the severity of encephalopathy? You were just mentioning most of them are awake, what do you do with the ventilated patients? Most of the multiple organ failure scores include encephalopathy but nobody knows how to handle this factor in intubated ventilated patients.

Young:
It is really harder to monitor the brain dysfunction in those severely ill patients. I think the best way is electrophysiologically. One problem is of course the drugs, which have a profound effect on the EEG. It is difficult to get around that; sometimes you can reverse this with naloxone or flumazenil if you want. However, I think it is a rather brutal thing to be doing. Perhaps some types of evoked responses might be useful. The N20 response, following median nerve stimulation, is too robust to detect subtle changes. The person has to practically lose his cortex to lose that response.

I think if we can try to hold off as much as possible on the use of sedative drugs, we use continuous EEG monitoring at the bedside. The nurses are trained to recognize patterns, doses of drugs can be titrated, so patients are not overly sedated. One can follow those patients electrophysiologically in a much more sensitive clinical method.

Regel:
Just one more question in this concern: Would you consider maybe using a biochemical monitoring? Both of you mentioned a lot of factors and parameters you could look at that are disturbed during the encephalopathy. Is there any advice for this aspect?

Young:
I think that of commonly available laboratory tests it is true that there certainly are strong parallels of these various tests in the encephalopathy, but you really are looking at a general or systemic phenomenon rather than the brain. You could probably use these blood tests to get an index of the severity of the illness. What you want to do I suppose is trending to see if the patient is improving or worsening. That is certainly possible with EEG or quantitative EEG analysis. Additionally, you could trend systemically with biochemical data.

Schlag:
Maybe I have an answer, we are monitoring in our septic baboons the neuronic specific amylase and in the baboons which die we see this increase in neuronic specific amylase; but the problem is always to do it in the right way and to do it several times, not only once. But you will see this tomorrow in our presentation. I have another question: I was wondering: Do you still believe in a sepsis syndrome without infection?

Young:
I know, we discussed this and from a theoretical point of view I think SIRS could occur with the cytokine release alone. But I must say that in our experience there has usually been the presence of an underlying infection in our patients. When we did our prospective study, the presence of infection was in our operational definition, so they had to have it. But in other patients we have seen in the intensive care unit, usually there is an infection underlying the encephalopathy. Charles might have some comments about more pure cases of SIRS without infection.

Sprung:
I have seen patients who had pancreatitis, burns, multiple trauma patients, who appeared to be encephalopathic. The biggest problem in the ICU is the problem that you mentioned, of sedation. The best place to find these patients is not in the ICU, it is on the wards and in the emergency department, and that's where we have been looking for these patients. We have not objectively studied the problem and my bias is that it exists. I would bet that we would find a lot of encephalopathic patients in the SIRS group of patients who are non-infected, if we used sophisticated ways to test CNS functioning, but I am not aware of any data in the literature.

Schlag:
You see, I know I am in contrast to these consensus conferences, because I believe there is no multiorgan failure without infection. Also in pancreatitis you see translocation, which can cause an infection. I do not believe there is multi-organ failure without infection.

Sprung:
I do not think we have enough data on that subject. We have been looking for SIRS patients without sepsis, without infections in the ICU.

Schlag:
It depends on the time.

Sprung:
The problem is, SIRS patients, if they spend enough time in the ICU become infected and septic. You can follow up SIRS patients for a long period of time in terms of mortality, organ system dysfunction and failure, but most of them become infected sooner or later.

Schlag:
But to speak of organ failure without infection is not right. We could show this very nicely in a study with femur fractures in baboons which were nailed. These baboons showed inflammatory mediators in the reamed group. I am sure during the first hour there is no infection, but the translocation starts very early, which we could show in our shock animals. You cannot detect this translocation in patients, because if you wait till you get the mesenteric lymph node it is already too late. Positive blood cultures are only observed in 40% or 50% because the clearance rate is very high.

Sprung:
But in orthopedic patients with fat embolization, you will see patients who become encephalopathic or who develop ARDS, but who are not infected.

Schlag:
Of course.

Sprung:
So you will see multi-organ failure without infection.

Schlag:
Maybe during the first hours, but not later, they are infected. I am sure, because they have the translocation, they have an endotoxemia and they have a bacteremia, but it is always the time where you detect this, because, as you know, the clearance rate is very fast, and so is the binding rate of endotoxin. You do not detect endotoxin, and you say "This patient is not septic" but he has already been septic, or he is going to be septic again, if he has a hypoperfusion of his gut tract. So I do not think that that is not infectious.

Regel:
I just have to confirm your opinion, I think it is only a matter of definition. As far as the discussion is concerned, at least in multiple trauma patients we do not see bacteremia. You see endotoxemia, and this is also a result of bacterial translocation,

as far as we believe. But endotoxemia is also a systemic infection. So, I think it is just a matter of definition.

Sprung:
I just have a comment for Dr. Regel in terms of what we should be using to follow these patients: It is a real problem. I was part of the Marshall study using a multiple organ dysfunction syndrome scoring system. In reviewing the literature of different studies that have used different scores for various organ dysfunction and failure, looking at the brain, there have not been real good scoring systems. The best we could come up with was the Glasgow Coma Scale. The European Society for Intensive Care Medicine's Working Group on Sepsis has used a "SOFA" Score that has also used the Glasgow Coma Scale for assessing brain dysfunction. We talked about the deficiencies of the Glasgow Coma Scale, particularly when patients are sedated or are intubated. But the bottom line is to date there is just nothing better. I just have a question for Dr. Young: Is there any typical EEG finding in patients who are agitated?

Young:
It is often hard to do an EEG if patients are in a delirious–agitated state. When we do the EEG of course they tend to be just mildly abnormal. They can have decreased voltage if they are really agitated, the voltage goes down, But we usually found some excessive theta (5–7 Hz rythmus), slight slowing and flattening of voltage.

Gennarelli:
The high oxidative metabolism of macrophages in some instances, particularly in stroke, allows them to be imaged with single photon emission computed tomography (SPECT) or position emission tomography (PET) scanning. I wonder with regard to the diagnosis of the microabscesses whether either of these has been used?

Young:
I am not aware if that has been examined, but probably it would be worthwhile looking at. You are suggesting, I believe, the microabscesses show up as an increased metabolic activity.

Gennarelli:
In the areas around stroke and some cases of abscess and infarct, the periphery of those necrotic areas where a large number of macrophages have high oxidative metabolism, have shown metabolic areas using fluorodeoxy glucose.

Regel:
I am not satisfied yet. I think from our opinion, maybe also from the Vienna group, it would be very nice if you could maybe categorize these three severity levels: You mentioned the stages "no" encephalopathy and "mild" as well as "severe". Could you quantify these EEG phenomena in these patients, that would allow a grading: Let us say grade 0 to 2, as is suggested in the MOF-score of Goris?

Young:
With power spectral analysis you could quantify early rythmic changes, but with greater severity of encephalopathy there are qualitative changes in EEG that appear,

particularly triphasic waves, which would not really be recognizable with this quantitative method. Quantitative methods could probably separate out the non-encephalopathic from mild encephalopathic patients if you control for normal drowsiness. Severe encephalopathy requires, I think, the raw EEG for adequate classification. Quantitative EEG may still help, however, in showing suppression and lack of variability in very severe septic encephalopathy.

Baethmann:
I have two points: One is, to call your attention to specific components of the bacterial cell membranes, the so-called muramyl peptides, which are released to my knowledge when bacteria are destroyed. These muramyl peptides have been reported to have powerful sedating benzodiazepine-like properties in the brain. Thus, accumulation of this material in septic patients may in part play a role in the clinical encephalopathy syndrome. Further you were mentioning the so-called triphasic waves observed in your EEG analysis and I wonder whether you have some explanation as to their origin and significance.

Young:
The answer to the first question is that we have not addressed the issue of bacterial biochemical components. The triphasic waves, I think, are a marker for fairly severe encephalopathy. We have seen them in only three instances in our intensive care unit patients: in sepsis, in renal failure and in hepatic failure. The mechanism for the production of triphasic waves is a traveling wave usually delayed from the front to the back of the head or the reverse, so that the wave appears to travel across the cortex, and we see approximately a 150 ms delay from the front to the back of the head. This is probably due to a series of interconnected oscillating neuronal systems. Triphasic waves are always a very pathological phenomenon, implying a very abnormal type of physiological oscillation that occurs to cause this slow traveling wave over the cortex. Looking at the reversible nature of most of those cases it has to be something that reversibly affects the synaptic function in the cortex, but that is speculation on my part.

The Investigation of Respiratory Insufficiency in Nervous System Trauma and Sepsis

C.F. BOLTON

Introduction

Many disorders of the nervous system affect respiration. The reasons involve either lack of central drive or weakness of the muscles of respiration. The former are induced by a wide variety of encephalopathies and the latter by diseases of anterior horn cells, peripheral nerve, neuromuscular junction, or muscles of the chest wall or diaphragm (Bolton 1993a).

The lack of central drive may be due to disturbances of voluntary or automatic respiration. The former, served by the corticospinal tract, can be tested by asking the patient to cough or "voluntarily" breathe for a short time at a faster rate. Automatic respiration, served by centers in the brainstem, occurs when a person is completely relaxed and not undertaking voluntary respiration, and is influenced by metabolic changes, particularly blood pH. A lack of central drive due to encephalopathy can often be discerned by observing specific patterns of respiration which are of localizing value (Fig. 1) (Plum and Posner 1980). These clinical signs, however, are often absent or are interfered with by ventilatory assistance. In many instances, it is not possible to determine whether there is a lack of central drive or a neuromuscular problem. The early clinical signs of neuromuscular respiratory dysfunction are rapid, shallow breathing and a rise in blood carbon dioxide levels. In later stages, hypoventilation, hypoxia, and potential apnea prompt assisted ventilation. The observation of "respiratory alternans" (alternation of rib cage and abdominal movement) or "abdominal paradox" (inward movement of the abdominal wall during inspiration), which may suggest neuromuscular respiratory failure, are often absent or are overlooked. More sophisticated measurements such as vital capacity, high airway occlusion pressure, the peak-negative pressure on maximal inspiration from full expiration, breathing frequency and tidal volume (Munro 1987) may also provide inconclusive results. Even unilateral damage to the phrenic nerve due to operative trauma (Abd et al. 1989) is often undiagnosed, despite chest X-rays and fluoroscopy.

In trauma the initial onset may induce immediate dysfunction of respiratory pathways, soon to be augmented by edema, hemorrhage and other pathophysiological changes. After the patient has been stablized and on a ventilator for more than a week, sepsis or the systemic inflammatory response syndrome (SIRS)(American College of Chest Physicians) which arises from severe trauma (Roumen et al. 1995) or infections of any type, may further impair these respiratory pathways.

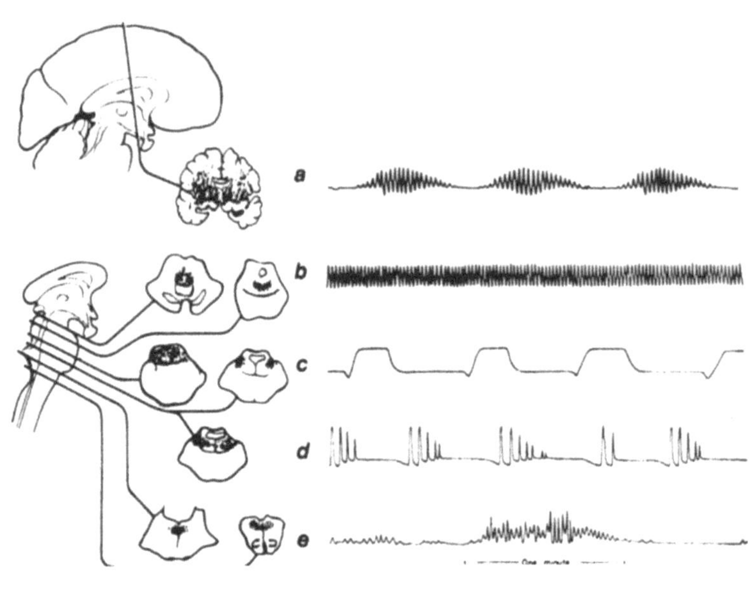

a
b
c
d
e
One minute

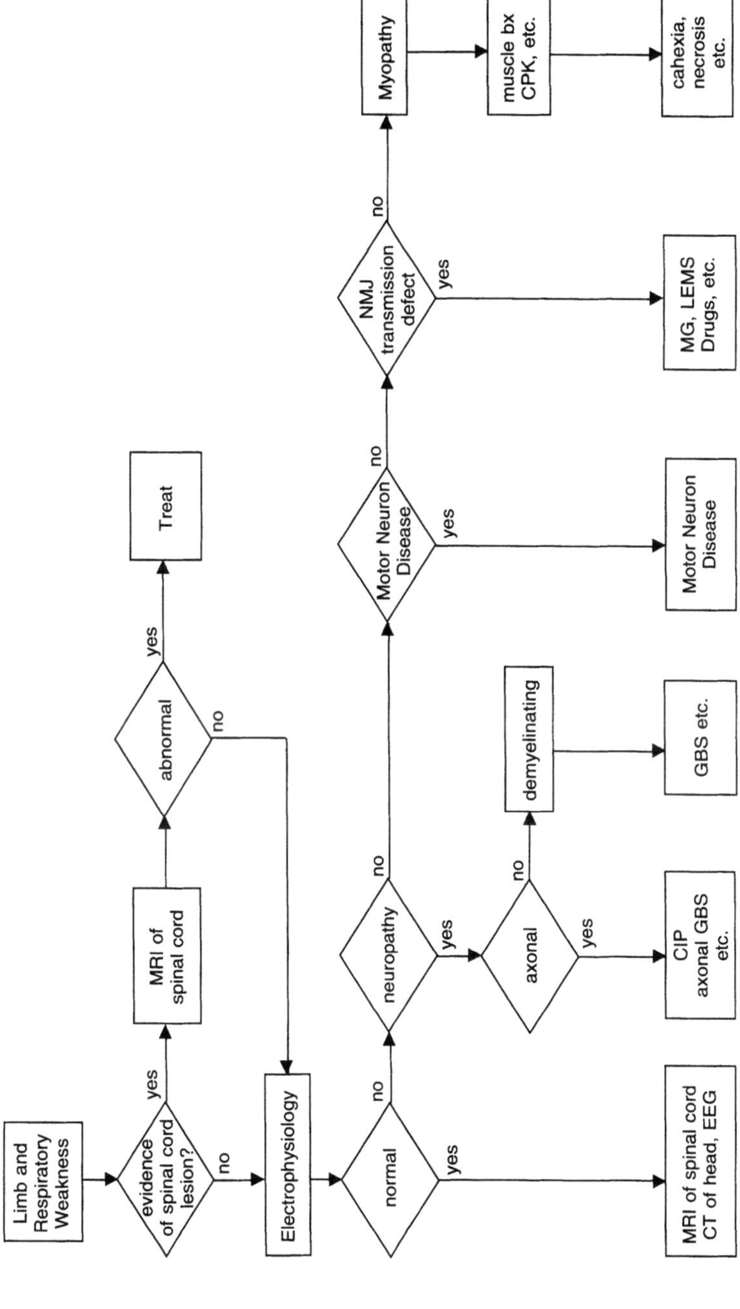

Fig. 2. Electrophysiological resting, measurements of creatine phosphokinace (*CPK*) and at times muscle biopsy are necessary for a thorough investigation. *MRI*, magnetic resonance imaging; *NMJ*, neuromuscular junction; *bx*, biopsy; *CT*, computed tomography; *CIP*, critical illness polyneuropathy; *GBS*, Guillain–Barre syndrome; *MG*, myasthenia gravis; *LEMS*, Lambert–Eaton myasthenia syndrome. *Note:* Positive serology or stool culture for *C. jejuni* may be the earliest warning of the axonal form of GBS

Table 1. Neuromuscular conditions presenting in the intensive care unit often associated with sepsis (SIRS)

Conditions	Incidence	Clinical features	Electrophysiology	Creatine phosphokinase	Muscle biopsy
A Polyneuropathy					
Critical illness polyneuropathy	Common in septic patients	Flaccid limbs and respiratory weakness	Axonal degeneration of motor and sensory fibers	Near normal	Denervation atrophy, mild necrosis
Motor neuropathy	Common with N-M blocking agents	Flaccid limbs and respiratory weakness	Axonal degeneration of motor fibers	Near normal	Denervation atrophy, mild necrosis
B Neuromuscular Transmission Defects					
Use of N-M blocking agents	?	Transient weakness	Neuromuscular transmission block	Normal	Normal
C Myopathy					
The necrotizing myopathy of critical care	Rare	Flaccid weakness, myoglobinuria	Abnormal spontaneous activity in muscle	Markedly elevated	Panfascicular muscle fiber necrosis
Thick filment myopathy	Common with steroids, N-M blocking agents and asthma	Flaccid limbs and respiratory weakness	Abnormal spontaneous activity in muscle	Elevated	Central loss of thick filaments
Polymyositis	Common in tropical countries	Severe generalized weakness	?	Elevated	Multiple microabcesses
Disuse (cachectic myopathy)	Common (?)	Muscle wasting	Normal	Normal	Normal or type 2 fiber atrophy

N-M, neuromuscular.

Critical Illness Polyneuropathy

Polyneuropathy occurs in 70% of patients with SIRS (Witt et al. 1991). However, clinical signs are often absent and it remains an occult condition in many ICUs throughout the world (Bolton 1996; Leijten and de Weerd 1994). Nonetheless, it is important to establish the diagnosis since it is an important cause of difficulty in weaning from the ventilator (Spitzer et al. 1989) and problems in rehabilitation after the acute illness has been treated. Only in more severe critical illness polyneuropathy will there be obvious limb weakness and reduced deep tendon reflexes. Signs of sensory impairment are difficult to test in the ICU. Electrophysiological studies are essential to establish the diagnosis. These will reveal a primary axonal degeneration of first motor and then sensory fibers. Phrenic nerve conduction and needle electromyography (EMG) of the diaphragm will disclose that the difficulty in weaning from the ventilator is due to involvement of the nerves and muscles of respiration (Maher et al. 1995). The CPK is either normal or mildly elevated. Muscle biopsy will reveal the presence of both acute and chronic denervation of muscle. Often the muscle is involved directly to varying degrees by the sepsis; this causes muscle necrosis, the severity being reflected in the degree of elevation of the CPK.

If the sepsis and multiple organ failure can be successfully treated (the mortality rate remains as high as 50%) one can expect a recovery from the critical illness polyneuropathy. This will occur in a matter of weeks in mild cases and in months in more severe cases. Electrophysiological studies will provide valuable information as to the time it may take for successful weaning from the ventilator (Maher et al. 1995).

Axonal Motor Neuropathy Associated with the Use of Neuromuscular Blocking Agents

A number of reports in the literature (Gooch et al. 1991; Giostra et al. 1994) have associated the use of neuromuscular blocking agents, particularly vecuronium or pancuronium bromide, with the development of polyneuropathy. These drugs are used to ease mechanical ventilation. The clinical features are similar to critical illness polyneuropathy. In my opinion, this is simply a variant of that condition, with sepsis as an important underlying factor. The practical implications are that these neuromuscular blocking agents should be used as sparingly as possible, and of course, in the event of signs of a polyneuropathy, be promptly discontinued. Like critical illness polyneuropathy, the prognosis for recovery is good.

Neuromuscular Transmission Defects

Non-competitive neuromuscular blocking agents such as succinylcholine are rarely used in the ICU setting because they may induce prolonged blockade, circulatory collapse and hyperkalemia. Sepsis and multiorgan failure in themselves will not cause a defect in neuromuscular transmission (Bolton, Laverty et al. 1986). However, whenever competitive neuromuscular blocking agents are used to ease mechanical ventilation, there is a risk of muscle weakness as a complication. As noted, this may occur through the induction of a pure axonal motor neuropathy. A second mechanism is a defect in neuromuscular transmission, which occurs when neuromuscular blocking agents such as vecuronium or pancuronium bromide are given in the presence of renal failure. The action of these drugs are prolonged beyond hours to a number of days after they been discontinued (Segredo et al. 1992). Nerve stimulation studies show a typical postsynaptic defect. There is a decrement of the compound muscle action potential at slow rates of stimulation (Fig. 3). The prognosis for recovery of muscle strength is quite good, although, an accompanying critical illness polyneuropathy is often present and may further prolong recovery (Fig. 3).

The third situation results in the induction of a thick filament myopathy (see below).

Myopathies Presenting After Admission to the ICU

Myopathies presenting in this situation are most often associated with sepsis, and share theoretical pathophysiological mechanisms with neuropathy (see "Pathophysiology" below).

Thick Filament Myopathy

A distinctive syndrome (Barohn et al. 1994; Lacomis et al. 1993; Danon and Carpenter 1991; Douglass et al. 1991; Hirano et al. 1992) occurs in children or adults in the setting of sudden, severe asthma. Endotracheal intubation and placement on a ventilator is necessary. High dose steroids to treat the asthma and neuromuscular blocking agents to ease ventilation are given, often for a number of days. Again, on attempted weaning from the ventilator, it will be noted that the patient has severe neuromuscular respiratory insufficiency and limb weakness. Ophthalmoplegia may be present (Sitwell et al. 1991). CPK levels are often considerably elevated. Repetitive nerve stimulation studies are usually normal. Sensory conduction is normal, as is motor conduction, except for a low amplitude compound muscle action potential. On needle EMG, motor unit potentials tend to be low amplitude, short duration and polyphasic, indicating a primary myopathy. The muscle may be electrically inexcitable on direct stimulation, suggesting inactivation of sodium, chloride or potassium channels (Rich et al. 1996). Muscle biopsy shows a loss of structure centrally in muscle fibers. Under the electron microscope, this has been shown to be due to destruction of the thick myosin filaments (Danon and Carpenter 1991). Denervation of muscle, secondary to either critical illness polyneuropathy or the neuromuscular blocking agent, likely predisposes to this distinctive pathological change (Bolton, editorial, 1994; Karpati et al. 1972). This type of myopathy may also occur in patients who are critically ill following organ transplantation, and receive high dose steroids to prevent rejection (Faragher et al. 1996).

Recovery occurs quite rapidly. The clinical and electrophysiological features are usually so distinctive in this syndrome that muscle biopsy is often not necessary, a worthwhile consideration in children because of the disfiguring scar.

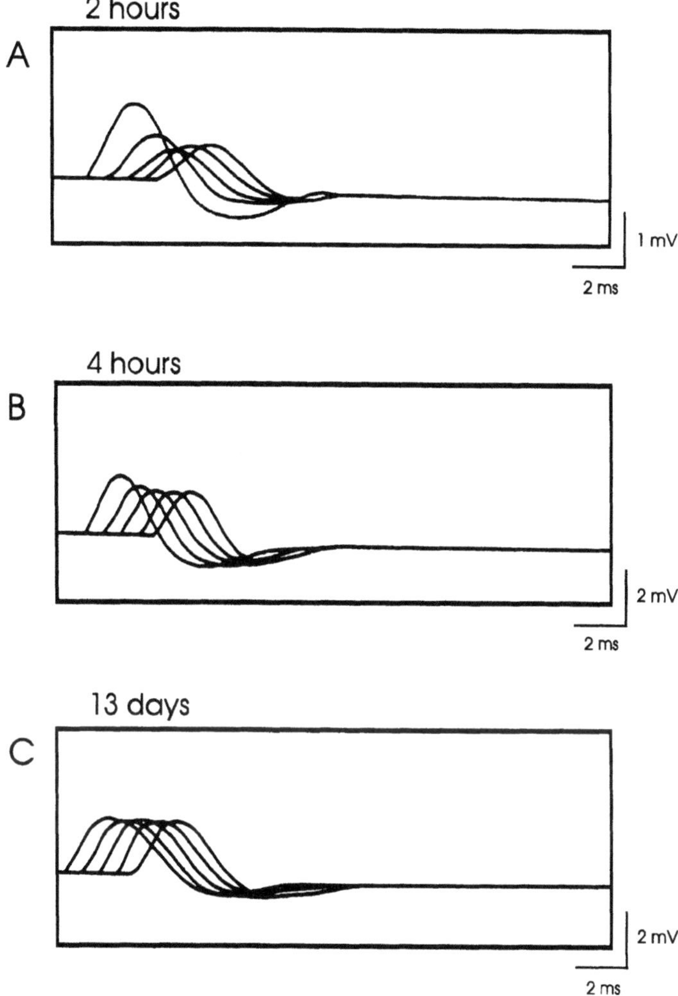

Fig. 3A–C. Critical illness polyneuropathy plus neuromuscular blockade (vecuronium 10 mg i.v.). The patient had had the septic syndrome for 6 weeks, and weakness after a single injection of vecuronium seemed more severe and prolonged than expected. Repetitive median nerve stimulation with recordings from the thenar muscle showed a decremental response, typical of vecuronium-induced block, except in the initial action potential which was quite low. Needle electromyography (EMG) at 2 and 4h (**A,B**) showed EMG signs of denervation which had become more severe at 13 days (**C**), when the neuromuscular block had disappeared. We suspect critical illness polyneuropathy was the main cause of weakness in this patient and was probably present before vecuronium was used

While the subject is still controversial, I believe that neuromuscular blocking agents should be used to ease ventilation in asthmatics only when there are clearcut indications, and in as low a dosage and for as short a period as possible. The use of steroids should also be limited as much as possible.

Cachectic Myopathy

Cachectic myopathy, disuse atrophy and catabolic myopathy (Clowes et al. 1983) are often cited as complications of critical illness. However, even though they cause muscle weakness and wasting, all are ill-defined in clinical terms (Bolton, editorial, 1994). Motor and sensory nerve conduction studies, needle EMG of muscle and creatine kinase levels are all normal. Muscle biopsy may be normal or show Type 2 muscle fiber atrophy, a nonspecific finding.

Acute Necrotizing Myopathy of Intensive Care

Rarer, but more well-defined, is "acute necrotizing myopathy of intensive care" (Zochodne et al. 1994; Ramsay et al. 1993). It may be precipitated by a wide variety of infective, chemical and other insults, basically involving the differential diagnosis of acute myoglobinuria (Penn 1986). It would be expected to occur with increased frequency in critical care units, in which there is a high incidence of trauma, infection and the use of various medications. Thus, Ramsay et al. (1993) and Zochodne et al. (1994) reported 11 cases in critical care units in which there was severe weakness with high levels of CPK and often myoglobinuria. Electrophysiological studies were consistent with a severe myopathy, and muscle biopsy showed widepsread necrosis of muscle fibers. Rapid and spontaneous recovery is expected to occur in milder cases, but in more severe cases, notably the ones reported by Ramsay et al. (1993), the prognosis may be poor.

We have observed mild elevations of creatine kinase and scattered necrosis of muscle fibers on muscle biopsy in some critically ill patients, suggesting primary involvement of muscle, as well as denervation atrophy. This may be due to a reduction in bioenergetic reserves as measured by ^{31}P magnetic resonance spectroscopy, since two of our patients had very low ratios of phosphocreatine to inorganic phosphate, more than would be expected from denervation of muscle alone (Bolton et al. 1994). These abnormalities returned towards normal as the patients recovered from the critical illness and from the polyneuropathy. Nonetheless, biopsy performed in 11 of our patients in the critical care unit, because of uncertainties about the nature of the neuromuscular condition, were all dominated by denervation atrophy, presumably secondary to a critical illness polyneuropathy (Pringle et al. 1992).

The Pathophysiology of the Neuromuscular Complications of SIRS (Sepsis)

Retrospective (Zochodne et al. 1987) and prospective (Witt et al. 1991) studies have failed to incriminate a variety of potential causes of critical illness polyneuropathy, including types of primary illness or injury, Guillain–Barre syndrome, medications including aminoglycoside antibiotics and neuromuscular blocking agents and specific nutritional deficiencies. We have speculated that sepsis is the cause (Zochodne et al. 1987; Witt et al. 1991). The severity of the polyneuropathy can be quantified from

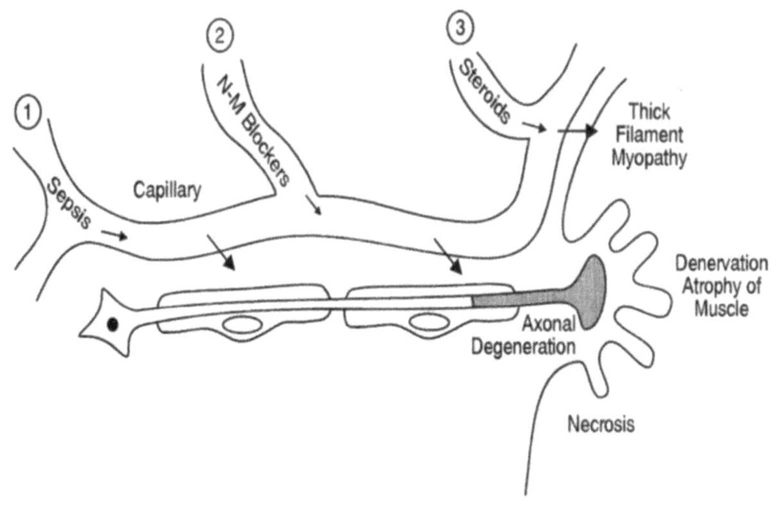

1
2
3
Sepsis
Capillary
N-M Blockers
Steroids
Thick
Filament
Myopathy
Denervation
Atrophy of
Muscle
Axonal
Degeneration
Necrosis

permeability induced by the sepsis, neuromuscular blocking agents, notably vecuronium or its metabolite, 3-desacetyl-vecuronium (Segredo et al. 1992), could have a direct toxic effect on peripheral nerve axons. These neuromuscular blocking agents may also cause functional denervation through their prolonged neuromuscular blocking action (Wernig et al. 1980). The result would be denervation atrophy of muscle and a relatively pure motor neuropathy.

We have always been concerned that antibiotics, particularly aminoglycosides with their known neural toxicity, might cause critical illness polyneuropathy. They might gain access to peripheral nerve as a result of increased capillary permeability. However, there has been no statistical proof that antibiotics cause peripheral nerve dysfunction in sepsis (Witt et al. 1991). Nonetheless, this possibility should be explored by basic experiments.

This schema (Fig. 4) also explains the acute myopathy which develops when asthmatic patients or post transplant patients are treated with neuromuscular blocking agents and steroids. We suspect that many of these patients suffer from SIRS, since infection is often a precipitating event in acute, severe asthma. Animal experiments by Karpati et al. (1972) have shown that if the muscle is first denervated by nerve transsection and then steroids are given, a thick filament myopathy similar to that seen in humans can be induced. Thus, in the human condition, critical illness polyneuropathy and the additional effects of neuromuscular blocking agents would first denervate muscle and then steroids would induce the typical myopathic changes. The rapidly evolving myopathy reported recently by Al-Lozi et al. (1994), characterized by destruction of thick filaments throughout the muscle fibers, and the acute, necrotizing myopathy of intensive care (Zochodne et al. 1994; Clowes et al. 1983) may simply represent further stages of this process.

Electrophysiological Studies of the Respiratory System

The various sites of stimulation and recording that test the motor and sensory pathways of respiration are shown in Fig. 5.

The Central Pathways of Respiration

Observations During Needle Electromography

The central drive to phrenic neurons during inspiration can be accurately tested by observations with a recording needle in the diaphragm (see below). If firing of motor unit potentials does occur with inspiration, the pattern may suggest dysfunction of specific areas in the brain (see Fig. 1).

Magnetic Stimulation of the Cerebral Cortex and Cervical Spinal Cord with Recording from the Diaphragm

Gandevia and Rothwell (1987) performed percutaneous stimulation of the motor cortex with electric shocks and demonstrated that conduction in oligosynaptic path-

SENSORY PATHWAYS **MOTOR PATHWAYS**

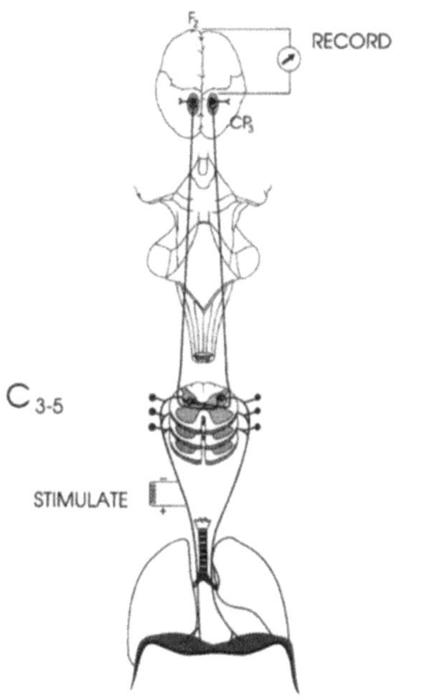

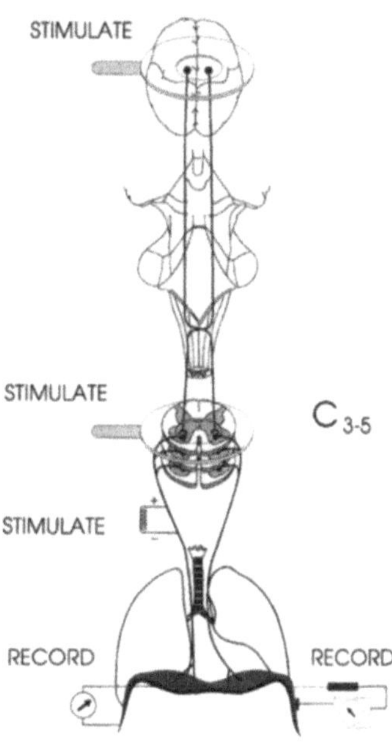

Motor Magnetic Transcranial Stimulation with Recording from Abdominal Muscles

This technique, developed by Lissens et al. (1995), consists of stimulating with a 90-mm diameter coil at C7, as well as the T10 roots, both during inspiration and expiration. Normal values were as follows: motor provoked potential (MEP) latency time and MEP amplitude were found to be 20.28 ± 0.51 ms and 0.91 ± 0.49 mV at inspiration, and 17.55 ± 0.81 ms and 2.01 ± 0.59 mV at expiration. The central motor conduction time was 13.18 ± 1.64 ms and 11.01 ± 1.51 ms at inspiration and at expiration, respectively. This study confirms a direct projection from the motor cortex to the human abdominal muscles through rapidly conducting mono- or oligosynaptic pathways. The rectus abdominus muscle is mainly an expiratory muscle.

Somatosensory Evoked Potentials of the Phrenic Nerve

The phrenic nerve is generally regarded as the motor nerve to the diaphragm but it contains about half as many sensory fibers as motor fibers. These fibers mediate sensory input from the costal and mediastinal pleura over the apex of the lung, the upper part of the pericardium and the serosa of liver, gall bladder, and pancreas. Physiological assessment of the sensory fibers in the phrenic nerve can now be tested according to the somatosensory evoked potential technique developed by Zifko et al. (1995). The nerve is stimulated just above the clavicle, percutaneously or with needle electrodes in the neck, and recordings made with subcutaneous needles at various sites over the scalp determined by the modified 10–20 electroencephalography (EEG) system. Sites with active scalp electrodes (G1) over C3, P3, CP1 and CP3 gave the best responses with the reference electrode G2 positioned over Fz. The normal values are for latency, P1–12 ms ± 0.8 ms and N1–17 ms ± 1.3 ms. For P2 the values were 20–26 ms and N2 31–45 ms. Peak to peak amplitudes ranged from 0.3 to 0.6 uV. This method allows evaluation of sensory fibers of the phrenic nerve and its central nervous system projections. The practical implications of this have yet to be determined.

Testing the Peripheral Pathways of Respiration

Phrenic Nerve Conduction Studies

This is a method of assessing the function of phrenic motor neurons which supply the diaphragm. A number of different methods have been adopted, which include percutaneous stimulation at the posterior border of the sternomastoid muscle, needle stimulation behind the sternomastoid muscle at the level of the thyroid cartilage and magnetic stimulation. The various recording sites used include esophageal electrodes, surface electrodes on the anterior or lateral chest wall or needle electrode in the diaphragm. Both monopolar and bipolar recordings have been used (Chen et al. 1995a; Lagueny et al. 1992; Markand et al. 1984; Mier et al. 1992; Newsom-Davis 1967; Swenson and Rubenstein 1992). Each laboratory will decide its own preferences in technique. We (Chen et al. 1995a) have used a modification of the technique by Markand et al. (1984) and Newsom-Davis (1967). Briefly, the phrenic nerve is stimulated percutaneously in the neck just above the clavicle and the compound muscle action potential from the diaphragm recorded at the lower costal margin with surface electrodes. Either phrenic nerve can be stimulated in this way and a well-defined compound muscle action potential obtained. It is important not to inadvertently stimulate the brachial plexus, which will spuriously shorten the latency and distort the waveform. With this recording technique, the amplitude of the response will vary with the phase of respiration, being of higher amplitude during inspiration and of lower amplitude during expiration. In practical terms, this problem can be overcome by repeating the supramaximal stimulus several times during the various phases of respiration and choosing the two highest amplitude responses. An electrocardiography (ECG) artifact may interfere with the waveform and then the response is simply rejected and the stimulus repeated when an artifact-free response can be obtained. With this technique, repeatability and comparison of right to left differences indicate that the technique is valuable in serial recordings and in identifying unilateral dysfunction of the diaphragm (Chen et al. 1995a). Disturbances of anterior horn cells, involvement of the phrenic nerve in axonal or demyelinating polyneuropathies, and traumatic damage to the phrenic nerve can now be identified.

Repetitive Phrenic Nerve Stimulation

This technique can be used to study neuromuscular transmission failure involving the phrenic nerve and diaphragm in patients who have a variety of neuromuscular transmission disturbances such as myasthenia gravis and Lambert–Eaton myasthenic syndrome. Mier et al. (1992) found that five of 13 patients with generalized myasthenia gravis and dyspnea had a significant decrement of the diaphragmatic amplitude, 15%–43%, during 3 s phrenic nerve stimulation. The various technical variations of the technique have not been fully explored, nor have normal values been established. However, the technique may well be ultimately shown to be of value in clinical situations.

Intercostal Nerve Conduction

Intercostal nerve conduction (Pradhan and Taly 1989) may also be of value but we have found the marked variability of the compound muscle action potential (CAP) from the rectus abdominus muscle requires multiple recording sites. Thus, it is a time consuming technique we rarely use.

Needle Electromyography of the Diaphragm

We had originally believed that needle EMG of the diaphragm was too risky for fear of inadvertent puncturing of lung, liver, spleen or colon (Bolton 1987). However, the results of such a technique would clearly be of great value. The technique of Goodgold (1984) and Saadeh et al. (1987) in which the needle is inserted through the abdominal wall and angulated upward under the costal margin, was technically difficult in our hands. Therefore, we developed a technique, briefly described many years ago by Koepke (1958, 1960) which is safe, causes little discomfort, and gives excellent recordings of diaphragm activity (Bolton et al. 1992). It consists of the introduction of the recording needle through any interspaces between the anterior axillary and medial clavicular lines. The needle should be introduced just above the costal margin, where there is an approximately 1.5-cm distance between the pleural reflection and the lower costal cartilage upon which the diaphragm inserts. Thus, the needle does not traverse either the pleural space or the lung. Recordings can be made as the needle passes through external oblique or rectus abdominus muscles, external and internal intercostal muscles, and finally, diaphragm. With quiet respiration, the chest wall muscles do not fire, or only a few units fire, but will do so with coughing or twisting of the trunk. There is regular firing from the diaphragm with each inspiration and the firing pattern and other features of motor unit potentials can be observed. Motor unit potentials in the diaphragm are of shorter duration and smaller amplitude, but more numerous than chest wall muscles, suggesting a relatively low innervation ratio. Abnormal spontaneous activity can be detected in these various muscles, including the diaphragm.

In the ICU, in ventilated patients, we temporarily discontinue intermittent mandatory ventilation and reduce pressure support to a level which will just overcome ventilator–airway resistance (approximately 8–10 cm H_2O). While the patient is being closely monitored, recordings from the diaphragm are made during voluntary respirations. This brief respiratory challenge is often enough to increase diaphragmatic drive, thereby allowing an assessment of diaphragmatic activity. If there is total denervation, motor units will not fire in the diaphragm, and an important sign that one is in the diaphragm will be lost. The presence or absence of insertional activity and knowledge of the local anatomy must then be used to define location.

Pneumothorax is a rare complication of the Koepke technique of needle EMG of the diaphragm. A telephone survey of those currently using the technique indicates that among 1000 subjects, only two have had this complication. Both were patients with severe, chronic obstructive pulmonary disease and on ventilators who responded promptly to treatment. No instances have occurred in out-patients. Nonetheless, we recommend all persons be observed for a period of 1 h following this procedure, to observe pain, shortness of breath, increased heart rate and blood pressure, or decreased breath sounds on auscultation, as early signs of pneumothorax. If present, prompt hospital admission and emergency treatment is indicated.

This technique, therefore, is of great value in further establishing the presence of denervation of the diaphragm. It adds valuable information to the phrenic nerve conduction study since the compound muscle action potential from the diaphragm has such a wide range of normalcy. It may be difficult to interpret in an individual patient; that is, an amplitude within the low normal range may still occur in the presence of denervation. This may be detected by observing fibrillation potentials and positive sharp waves on needle EMG of the diaphragm. Observations of the size, complexity and the number of motor unit potentials firing may indicate the presence of chronic denervation and collateral reinnervation; i.e., large complex units in decreased numbers suggest this phenomenon.

Computer Analysis of Needle EMG of the Diaphragm

However, a major difficulty with needle EMG of the diaphragm is that motor unit potentials in the diaphragm are normally of low amplitude and complex with more high frequency components, as compared to chest wall or limb muscles. Distinguishing normal recordings from patients with a myopathy may be extremely difficult. To investigate further methods of assessing motor unit potentials in the diaphragm, we have turned to computer methods.

In a study of 43 diaphragms in 23 healthy volunteers, Chen et al. (1995b) established the mean ± standard deviation of the median frequency of the power spectrum of the diaphragm to be 233.3 ± 58.1 Hz. The median frequency tends to increase with age and decrease with forced vital capacity. The integrated EMG with each inspiration strongly correlated with the tidal volume and duration of inspiration. Studies in patients have shown that median frequency can be high, normal or low in patients with neuropathy and may be elevated in patients with myopathy. The technique may be useful in studying patients with diaphragmatic fatigue (Chen et al. 1995b).

Another approach to this problem is to utilize the automated electromyographic interference pattern analysis of Nandedkar and colleagues (1995). We modified the computer software to take into account the normally low amplitude and increased complexity of the diaphragm EMG and, hence, the technique may now be useful in distinguishing between patients with myopathy and normal diaphragmatic muscle (Collins et al. 1994).

Finally, utilizing the techniques of computer analysis by wavelet transforms and neural net, it may ultimately be possible to classify complicated EMG patterns into normals, neuropathic and myopathic. The neural net may then be successfully trained to distinguish between these three groups in individual patients being investigated (McKeown et al. 1995).

The Application of Electrophysiological Respiratory Techniques in Various Conditions

We have just begun to apply these techniques, but already they have proven to be valuable, particularly in the ICU setting where clinical assessment is difficult.

Utilizing the techniques of phrenic nerve conditions and needle EMG of the diaphragm, it has been possible to more precisely discover the neuromuscular causes of difficulty in weaning from the ventilator (Fig. 6; Maher et al. 1995). Patients with amyotrophic lateral sclerosis may present for the first time with acute respiratory insufficiency whose cause is not immediately apparent; these techniques accurately establish the diagnosis (Chen et al. 1996). In the acute stages of Guillain–Barre syndrome, the likelihood of ventilator assessment can be more accurately predicted (Zifko et al. 1996b). Serial electrophysiological studies will identify the causes of

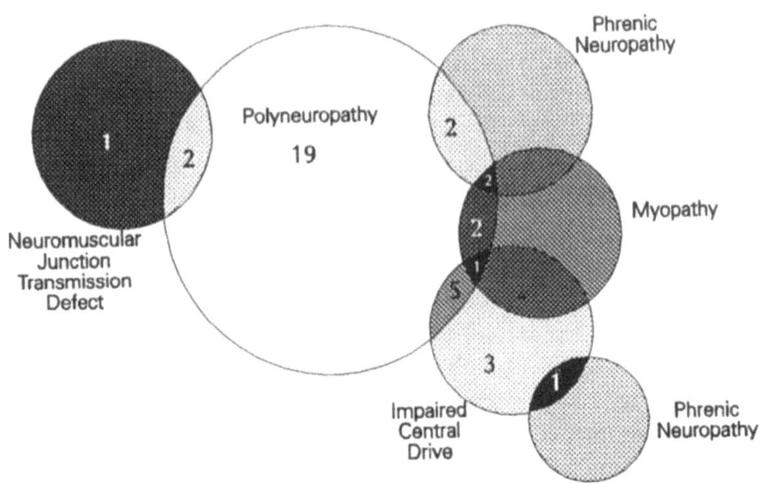

Phrenic
Neuropathy
Polyneuropathy
19
2
Myopathy
2
2
1
5
Neuromuscular
Junction
Transmission
Defect
1
2
3
1
Impaired
Central
Drive
Phrenic
Neuropathy

Bolton CF (1994) Muscle weakness and difficulty in weaning from the ventilator in the critical care unit. Chest 106:1–2 (editorial)

Bolton CF (1996) Sepsis and the systemic inflammatory response syndrome (SIRS): neuromuscular manifestations. Crit Care Med 74:1408–1416

Bolton CF, Laverty DA, Brown JD, Witt NJ, Hahn AF, Sibbald WJ (1986) Critically ill polyneuropathy: electrophysiological studies and differentiation from Guillain-Barre syndrome. J Neurol Neurosurg Psychiatry 49:563–573

Bolton CF, Grand'Maison F, Parkes A, Shkrum M (1992) Needle electromyography of the diaphragm. Muscle Nerve 15:678–681

Bolton CF, Young GB, Zochodne DW (1994) Neurological changes during severe sepsis. Curr Top Intensive Care 1:180–217

Chen R, Collins S, Remtulla H, Parkes A, Bolton CF (1995a) Phrenic nerve conduction study in normal subjects. Muscle Nerve 28:330–335

Chen R, Remtulla H, Power K, Collins S, Bolton CF (1995b) Needle EMG of the human diaphragm: power spectral analysis in normal subjects and in patients with respiratory failure. Can J Neurol Sci 22[Suppl 1]:22

Chen R, Grand'Maison F, Strong MJ, Ramsay DA, Bolton CF (1996) Motor neuron disease presenting as acute respiratory failure: a clinical and pathological study. J Neurol Neurosurg Psychiatry 60:455–458

Clowes GHA, George BC, Villee CA (1983) Muscle proteolysis induced by a circulating peptide in patients with sepsis or trauma. New Engl J Med 308:545–552

Collins SJ, Chen RE, Remtulla H, Parkes A, Bolton CF (1994) Novel parameters for automated electromyographic interference pattern analysis of the diaphragm: Results in normal subjects. Muscle Nerve 17(9)1098–1099

Danon MJ, Carpenter S (1991) Myopathy and thick filament (myosin) loss following prolonged paralysis witn vecuronium during steroid treatment. Muscle Nerve 14:1131–1139

Douglass JA, Tuxen DV, Horne M et al (1991) Myopathy in severe asthma. Am Rev Respir Dis 146:517–519

Faragher MW, Day BJ, Dennett X (1996) Critical care myopathy: an electrophysiological and histological study. Muscle Nerve 19:516–518

Fong Y (1989) Cachectin/TNF or II-1a induces cachexia with redistribution of body proteins. Am J Physiol 256:659–665

Gandevia SC, Rothwell JC (1987) Activation of the human diaphragm from the motor cortex. J Physiol 384:109–118

Giostra E, Magistris MRI, Pizzolato G, Cox J, Chevrolet J-C (1994) Neuromuscular disorders in intensive care unit patients treated with pancuronium bromide. Chest 106:210–220

Gooch JL, Suchyta MR, Balbierz JM (1991) Prolonged paralysis after treatment with neuromuscular junction blocking agents. Crit Care Med 9:1125–1131

Goodgold J (1984) Anatomical correlates of clinical electromyography, 2nd edn. Williams and Wilkins, Baltimore, p 41

Hirano M, Ott BR, Raps EC (1992) Acute quadriplegic myopathy: complication of treatment with steroids, nondepolarizing blocking agents, or both. Neurology 42:2082–2087

Karpati G, Carpenter S, Eisen AA (1972) Experimental core-like lesions and nemaline rods: a correlative morphological and physiological study. Arch Neurol 27:247–266

Koepke GH (1960) The electromyographic examination of the diaphragm. Bull Am Assoc Electromyogr Electrodiagn 7:8

Koepke GH, Smith EM, Murphy AJ, Dickinson DG (1958) Sequence of action of the diaphragm and intercostal muscles during respiration. I. Inspiration. Arch Phys Med Rehabil 39:426–430

Lacomis D, Smith TW, Chad DA (1993) Acute myopathy and neuropathy in status asthmaticus: Case report and literature review. Muscle Nerve 16:84–90

Lagueny A, Ellie E, Saintarailles J, Marthan R, Barat M, Julien J (1992) Unilateral diaphragmatic paralysis: an electrophysiological study. J Neurol Neurosurg Psychiatry 55:316–318

Leijten FSS, de Weerd AW (1994) Critical illness polyneuropathy: a review of the literature, definition and pathophysiology. Clin Neurol Neurosurg 96:10–19

Lissens MA (1994) Motor evoked potentials of the human diaphragm elicited through magnetic transcortical brain stimulation. J Neurol Sci 124:204–207

Lissens MA, De Muynck M, Decleir A, Vanderstraeten GG (1995) Motor evoked potentials of the abdominal muscles elicited through magnetic transcranial brain stimulation. Muscle Nerve 18(11)1353–1354

Low PA, Tuck RR, Takeuchi M (1987) Nerve microenvironment in diabetic neuropathy. In: Dyck PJ, Thomas PK, Asbury AK et al. (eds) Diabetic neuropathy. Saunders, Philadelphia, pp 268–277

Maher J, Rutledge F, Remtulla H, Parkes A, Bernardi L, Bolton C (1995) Neuromuscular disorders associated with failure to wean from the ventilator. Intensive Care Med 21:737–743

Markand ON, Kincaid JC, Pourmand RA, Moorthy SS, King RD, Mahomed Y, Brown JW (1984) Electrophysiologic evaluation of diaphragm by transcutaneous phrenic nerve stimulation. Neurology 34:604–614

Maskill D, Murphy K, Mier A, Owen M, Guz A (1991) Motor cortical representation of the diaphragm in man. J Physiol (Lond) 443:105–121

McKeown M, Bolton CF (1995) Classification of diaphragmatic EMG by wavelet transforms and a neural net. Muscle Nerve 18(9)1065

Mier A, Brophy C, Moxham J, Green M (1992) Repetitive stimulations of phrenic nerves in myasthenia gravis. Thorax 47:640–644

Munro I (1987) Predictors of successful weaning in ventilated patients. Lancet i(8544)604–614

Nandedkar SD, Barkhaus PE (1995) Is the motor unit action potential rise time too restrictive. Muscle Nerve 18:9

Newsom-Davis J (1967) Phrenic nerve conduction in man. J Neurol Neurosurg Psychiatry 30:420–426

Penn AS (1986) Myoglobinuria. In: Engel AG, Banker BQ (eds) Myology, 2nd edn. McGraw-Hill, New York, pp 7792–7793

Plum F, Posner JB (1980) The diagnosis of stupor and coma (3rd ed). FA Davis, Philadelphia, p 34

Pradhan S, Taly A (1989) Intercostal nerve conduction study in man. J Neurol Neurosurg Psychiatry 52:763–766

Pringle CE, Bolton CF, Ramsay DA et al (1992) Muscle biopsy in critical illness: electrophysiological and morphological correlations. Can J Neurol Sci 2:297

Ramsay DA, Zochodne DW, Robertson DM, Nag S, Ludwin SK (1993) A syndrome of acute severe muscle necrosis in intensive care unit patients. J Neuropathol Exp Neurol 52:4:387–398

Rich MM, Teener JW, Raps EC, Schotland DL, Bird SJ (1996) Muscle is electrically inexcitable in acute quadriplegic myopathy. Neurology 46:731–736

Roumen RM, Redl H, Schlag G, Zilow G et al (1995) Inflammatory mediators in relation to the development of multiple organ failure in patients after severe blunt trauma. Crit Care Med 23(3):474–480

Saadeh PB, Posner J, Wolf E (1987) Needle EMG of the diaphragm: a new technique. Arch Phys Med Rehabil 68:599

Segredo V, Caldwell JE, Matthay MA et al (1992) Persistent paralysis in critically ill patients after long-term administration of vecuronium. New Engl J Med 327:524–528

Sitwell LD, Weinshenker BG, Monpetit V, Reid D (1991) Complete ophthalmoplegia as a complication of acute corticosteroid- and pancuronium-associated myopathy. Neurology 41:921–922

Spitzer AR, Maher L, Awerbuch G, Bowles A (1989) Neuromuscular causes of prolonged ventilator dependence. Muscle Nerve 12(9)775

Swenson MR, Rubenstein RS (1992) Phrenic nerve conduction studies. Muscle Nerve 15:597–603

Tracey KJ, Lowry SF, Beutler B et al (1988) Cachectin/tumour necrosis factor mediates human muscle denervation: topical 31-P spectroscopy studies. Magn Reson Med 7:373–383

Wernig A, Pecot-Dechavassine M, Stover H (1980) Sprouting and regression of the nerve at the frog neuromuscular junction in normal conditions and after prolonged paralysis with curare. J Neurocytol 9:277–303

Witt NJ, Zochodne DW, Bolton CF, Grand'Maison F, Wells G, Young GB, Sibbald WJ (1991) Peripheral nerve function in sepsis and multiple organ failure. Chest 99:176–184

Zifko UA, Bolton CF (1996) Electrophysiological monitoring in neurological respiratory insufficiency. J Neurol Neurosurg Psychiatry (in press)
Zifko UA, Young BG, Remtulla H, Bolton CF (1995b) Somatosensory evoked potentials of the phrenic nerve. Muscle Nerve 18:1487–1489
Zifko UA, Chen R, Remtulla H, Hahn AF, Koopman W, Bolton CF (1996a) Respiratory electrophysiologic studies in Guillain-Barre syndrome. J Neurol Neurosurg Psychiatry 60:191–194
Zifko UA, Remtulla H, Power K, Harker L, Bolton CF (1996b) Transcortical and cervical magnetic stimulation with recording of the diaphragm. Muscle Nerve 19:614–620
Zochodne DW, Bolton CF, Wells GA, Gilbert JJ, Hahn AF, Brown JD, Sibbald WJ (1987) Polyneuropathy associated with critical illness: a complication of sepsis and multiple organ failure. Brain 110:819–842
Zochodne DW, Ramsay DA, Saly V, Shelley S, Moffatt S (1994) Acute necrotizing myopathy of intensive care: electrophysiological studies. Muscle Nerve 17:285–292

Discussion

Traber:

In the peripheral nerve myopathies that you saw in sepsis, have you identified any functional changes in the sensory portion of the phrenic nerve, and how does the feedback work?

Bolton:

These are good questions. We have not studied that, so I cannot answer any of your questions. We really do not have any idea how practical these somatosensory evoked potential (SEP) studies will be. At the moment, these results are only of theoretical interest.

Zornow:

Most of your studies suggest that defect occurs at the neuromuscular junction. Have you done nerve conduction velocity studies to look at actual neruopathies in these patients, or is it primarily a neuromuscular junction type of phenomenon?

Bolton:

We feel that difficulty in weaning from the ventilator is almost always due to a critical illness polyneuropathy. A small number of the patients have had defects in their muscular transmission, in one case due to the use of vecuronium. But in most of our cases it has been difficult to prove that these neuromuscular blocking agents have actually caused the problem. This observation has been recently confirmed in two prospective studies in Europe. These studies could not find any correlation between the use of steroids or neuromuscular blocking agents and critical illness polyneuropathy.

Shackford:

The observation that albumin is inversely related to nerve function and that glucose appears to be directly related, suggests that either the lack of nutrition or the catabolic response to critical illness may play a role. For example, you would see albumin catabolism and protein wasting if gluconeogenesis were occurring. To what extent do you think nutrition is causing this problem and have you done any studies or is there any literature on this in patients who actually have voluntarily starved themselves? I wonder if the cause of death following starvation is respiratory arrest.

Bolton:
A very good question. I am not sure if I can answer that, from my own experience anyway. I think the bottom line is that we have no proof yet that nutrition actually is a factor in any of the muscle problems, although it was widely studied. If you have disuse atrophy of the muscle or if you have a patient with anorexia nervosa, a good example, your electrical studies are entirely normal, nerve conduction, the amplitude of the compound muscle action potential, etc. The creatine phosphokinase is normal. If you biopsy the muscle it will either be normal or you may see a type II fiber atrophy, a nonspecific result. So you can identify the neuromuscular problem by doing these studies, and when you do it, it is hard to prove that nutrition or prolonged recumbancy are much of a factor. Now in disuse atrophy, as the muscle wastes away, down to 20% of its previous size, the muscle strength decreases, but other assessments of muscle are relatively normal.

Prough:
I was curious about your patient with reversible spinal cord ischemia. What was the pathogenesis of that?

Bolton:
I do not know precisely the pathogenesis, but the MRI showed increased uptake anterially in the cord indicating anterior cord infarction. Brian, it was your patient, what do you think was the pathogenesis?

Young:
We could not determine it; spinal cord dysfunction came on very abruptly in this man. He sat down in a lounge chair and never got up again. We thought it must be ischemic, but we could not prove it. He was in his late sixties or early seventies, as I remember, and probably there was some atherosclerosis. We looked at his heart in various ways for an embolism source, but could not find it. With the rapidity of the onset and the early signal changes on the MRI and the lack of preceding infection or injury, we thought it must be ischemic.

Morganti:
As a neurologist you may know that tumor necrosis factor (TNF)-α plays an important role in demyelinating diseases like multiple sclerosis. My question is whether you have measured any TNF-α in these patients and whether you have found any correlation to polyneuropathy.

Bolton:
No, we have not done any of those studies. There has been almost no basic work done on critical illness polyneuropathy.

Regel:
What do you do in those cases with critical illness polyneuropathy that have this prolonged weaning? Is there any therapeutic approach to this problem?

Bolton:
I think it is much like the septic encephalopathy. There isn't anything you can do except to treat the sepsis, the multiorgan failure and hope they recover. From the point of view of prognosis, the weaning will be much longer the more severe the critical illness polyneuropathy. Another practical implication is that respiratory muscle training, used in many ICUs, is useless in patients who have critical illness polyneuropathy.

Regel:
That is the same experience we made. Do you stimulate the diaphragm by means of taking a kind of pacemaker?

Bolton:
We stimulate the phrenic nerve, we do not stimulate the diaphragm. But it is helpful to know the response when you stimulate the phrenic nerve, because if there is a poor response from the diaphragm, you know there has been an axonal degeneration or some involvement of phrenic nerve and phrenic nerve pacing is not going to help.

Sprung:
You call this critical illness polyneuropathy. Do you think it is sepsis-related? Of the patients you have seen, what percentage of those patients did in fact receive neuromuscular blocking agents?

Bolton:
We think it is one of the complications of sepsis or the systemic inflammatory response syndrome. We have not found any relationship to the use of neuromuscular blocking agents and the incidence and severity of the polyneuropathy.

Sprung:
But what was the percentage? You said you get about ten to 15 patients a year, what percentage of those patients had received neuromuscular blocking agents?

Bolton:
I cannot remember the percentage. But basically in our unit, neuromuscular blocking agents are not used very much. They are used as a single injection for some procedure. Occasionally, they will be used for 1 or 2 days, rarely for longer than that. We look at the hospital chart to see if these agents have been given. If there is any chance they have been given, we routinely do repetitive nerve stimulation studies to detect the presence of neuromuscular transmission defects. We have had only single case where we could have said the polyneuropathy was due to the use of neuromuscular blocking agents.

Changes in Cerebral Blood Flow After Endotoxin in Humans and Sheep

V. Pollard, B. Conroy, D.S. Prough, D.J. Deyo, L. Traber, and D. Traber

Summary

Neurologic dysfunction is common in early sepsis. To better understand cerebral autoregulatory responses during sepsis, we studied cerebral hemodynamics, cerebral oxygen delivery (CDO_2), and the cerebral metabolic rate for oxygen ($CMRO_2$) in volunteers and in unanesthetized sheep during experimental endotoxemia. In ten healthy volunteers, we used a Kety-Schmidt technique to measure cerebral blood flow (CBF) at baseline and at hourly intervals for 5 h after a bolus of *Escherichia coli* endotoxin (4 ng/kg). We also measured $CMRO_2$, CDO_2, and cerebral vascular resistance (CVR) at these time points. Volunteers developed marked systemic and hemodynamic responses after endotoxin, including an elevated body temperature, cardiac index (CI), and heart rate (HR), and a decreased mean arterial pressure (MAP) and systemic vascular resistance index (SVRI). CBF, CDO_2, $CMRO_2$, and CVR were unchanged throughout the 5-h study period. In a separate study, we measured CBF (using radiolabeled or colored microspheres), and $CMRO_2$, CDO_2, CVR, and cerebral perfusion pressure (CPP) at baseline and at 1.5, 4, and 24 h in 18 sheep during continuous *E. coli* endotoxin infusion (10 ng/kg per hour). Eight sheep became hyperdynamic with an increased body temperature, CI, and HR, and a decreased SVRI. In the hyperdynamic sheep, CBF, CDO_2, $CMRO_2$, and CPP were elevated and CVR was decreased after 4 h of continuous endotoxin. Ten sheep did not become hyperdynamic although body temperature, white cell count, and pulmonary artery pressure had significantly increased. CBF, CDO_2, $CMRO_2$, CPP, and CVR were unchanged in these sheep.

We conclude that cerebral hemodynamics and oxygenation variables are unchanged after a bolus of endotoxin in volunteers although marked systemic responses are apparent. However, CBF, $CMRO_2$, CDO_2, and CPP are elevated and CVR is reduced in hyperdynamic sheep but unchanged in nonhyperdynamic sheep after 4 h of continuous endotoxin infusion. The responses to endotoxin may be species- or dose-dependent.

Introduction

Survival in sepsis is improved by early diagnosis before multiple system organ failure occurs [1]. Although neurologic involvement increases mortality [2,3] and is common in early sepsis [4,5], studies on brain dysfunction in sepsis are limited and are confounded by the presence of many underlying variables that make the interpretation of results difficult. CBF and $CMRO_2$ are reduced in patients with established sepsis [6,7]; however, cerebral hemodynamics during early hyperdynamic sepsis have not been thoroughly studied in humans or animals.

The hemodynamic and inflammatory changes that accompany early hyperdynamic sepsis in humans have been duplicated and studied in volunteers [8–12]. CI increases and systemic vascular resistance decreases after endotoxin [8,9], and inflammatory cytokine responses are similar to those seen during early clinical sepsis [10–12]. Endotoxin is known to induce altered nocturnal sleep patterns [13], but CBF has never been measured in volunteers after endotoxin administration. We used a Kety-Schmidt technique [14] to measure CBF and study cerebral oxygenation during early hyperdynamic experimental endotoxemia in healthy volunteers. We also measured hemodynamic and hematological variables to confirm a systemic response to the endotoxin bolus (*Escherichia coli* endotoxin, 4 ng/kg).

The ovine model of endotoxemia is an excellent model in which to study the hemodynamic responses during early hyperdynamic sepsis [15–17]. With continuous low-dose endotoxin administration, a hemodynamic state may be reproduced in sheep that closely mimics the hyperdynamic responses seen in clinical sepsis [15–17]. Moreover, sheep may be studied in the awake state, thus negating the influence of anesthetic drugs [18] or mechanical ventilation [19] on hemodynamic responses. Although the ovine model has been used by many investigators to study cardiovascular [16,17,20] and pulmonary [16,17,21] responses during sepsis, cerebral autoregulation has not been studied in awake sheep. We used this model to study cerebral hemodynamics and oxygenation variables during experimental sepsis. Over a 24-h period, we measured CBF in awake sheep using radiolabeled or colored microspheres, and calculated $CMRO_2$, CDO_2, CVR, and CPP during continuous low-dose endotoxin infusion (*E. coli* endotoxin, 10 ng/kg per hour). We also characterized the hemodynamic profile during endotoxin infusion, and used this response to differentiate hyperdynamic from nonhyperdynamic sheep.

Materials and Methods

Studies in Volunteers

Ten healthy volunteers (six males and four females), with a mean age of 30 years (age range 22–42 years) participated in a study approved by the institutional review board. All subjects were in good health based on clinical history, physical examination, hematological and biochemical profiles, urine analyses, and electrocardiographic (ECG) findings. After written informed consent was obtained, volunteers had a peripheral intravenous catheter inserted through which 0.9% saline, 2 ml/kg per hour, was infused throughout the study period. Additional fluid boluses of 500 ml/h of 0.9% saline were given as needed to maintain intravascular volume. All volunteers had radial arterial, right jugular bulb, and right internal jugular pulmonary artery catheters inserted for continuous invasive hemodynamic monitoring and intermittent blood sampling. Body temperature, MAP, central venous pressure (CVP), pulmonary artery pressure (PAP), CI, and systemic vascular resistance index (SVRI) were measured at 15-min intervals from the time of insertion of the catheters. CBF, $CMRO_2$, CDO_2, CVR, arterial and jugular bulb blood gases, and differential leukocyte and hemoglobin (Hb) counts were obtained at baseline, and at hourly intervals for 5 h after the endotoxin bolus. All volunteers received U.S. Reference *E. coli* endotoxin 4 ng/kg (Lot EC-5, Bureau of Biologics, Food and Drug Administration, Bethesda, MD, USA). After completion of the study, volunteers were monitored for a further 3 h until hemodynamics approached baseline values.

CBF was measured using a Kety-Schmidt inhalation technique. Volunteers breathed a mixture of 10% nitrous oxide (N_2O), oxygen, and air delivered from an anesthesia machine through a tight-fitting face mask and closed circuit-system over a 16-min period. Simultaneous arterial and jugular bulb blood samples were slowly drawn at over 20 sec 0, 1, 2, 4, 8, and 16 min and analyzed in a nondispersive trace N_2O gas infrared spectrophotometer (Dynatech Electro-optics, Saline, MI, USA), with a self-contained gas pump. The output from the spectrophotometer was integrated and analyzed, and global CBF (ml/100 g per minute) was calculated from the difference in area of N_2O concentration between the arterial and jugular venous curves.

Studies in Sheep

In an approved protocol, 18 range ewes of the Merino breed were surgically prepared under halothane anesthesia. Catheters were placed in the femoral vein and artery, and pulmonary artery and left atrium for monitoring pressures and obtaining blood samples for analysis. A midline craniotomy was performed and the sagittal sinus and lateral ventricle were cannulated. Sheep were allowed a 7-day recovery period during which they were allowed free access to food and water in metabolic cages. The animals were attached to transducers 1 day before the experiment began, and central venous, mean arterial, pulmonary artery, and left atrial pressures (LAP) were monitored continuously. A continuous infusion of 0.9% saline (2 ml/kg per hour) was begun at this time and continued for the duration of the study. After a 24-h stabilization period, baseline measurements, including body temperature, HR, MAP, CVP, LAP, PAP, CI, SVRI, CBF, $CMRO_2$, CDO_2, CVR, intracranial pressure (ICP), arterial and sagittal sinus blood gases and whole blood counts were taken. Sheep were then given *E. coli* endotoxin (10 ng/kg per hour) as a continuous infusion over 24 h and the intravenous fluid infusion was increased to 5 ml/kg per hour to prevent a decrease in CVP. All measurements were repeated 1.5, 4, and 24 h after the endotoxin infusion was begun. Cardiac index was calculated using a standard formula for sheep body surface area [$0.082 \times$ body weight $(kg)^{2/3}$]. CBF was measured using radiolabeled or colored microspheres. Microspheres were injected via the left atrial line and withdrawal samples were obtained from the femoral artery. At autopsy the brain was homogenized and whole brain blood flow was determined.

Data Analysis

Data are summarized in the text as mean ± the standard error (SE) of the mean. Data concerning each outcome variable were analyzed using repeated-measures analysis of variance for a single-factor experiment. The mean at each time point was compared with the baseline mean using Fisher's least significant difference procedure with a Bonferroni adjustment for the number of comparisons. Statistically significant differences were accepted at $p \le 0.05$.

Results

Volunteers

Volunteers developed marked "flu-like" responses after endotoxin, including rigors, headache, muscle pains, abdominal cramping, nausea, and vomiting, beginning 1 h after endotoxin administration and lasting approximately 1 h. Hemodynamic variables and body temperature are shown in Table 1. HR, CI, MAP, and body temperature were significantly elevated and SVRI, PAP, and CVP were significantly reduced after endotoxin. Hematological parameters are shown in Table 2. White cell and granulocyte counts were significantly elevated, and serum Hb, lymphocyte, and monocyte counts were significantly reduced after endotoxin. Cerebrovascular variables are shown in Fig. 1. CBF, CDO_2, CVR, and $CMRO_2$ were statistically unchanged after endotoxin. However, had we performed an analysis on the baseline and 3- and 5-h data only, $CMRO_2$ would have decreased significantly from 3.8 ± 0.4 ml/100 g per minute to 3.14 ± 0.3 ml/100 g per minute and 2.97 ± 0.3 ml/100 g per minute 3 and 5 h after endotoxin.

Sheep

Sheep were divided into two groups based on hemodynamic responses as follows: Group 1 ($n = 8$): Hyperdynamic sheep, defined as having an increase in CI > 15% from baseline after 24 h of endotoxin infusion. Group 2 ($n = 10$): Nonhyperdynamic sheep, defined as having a CI close to baseline after 24 h of endotoxin infusion.

Hemodynamic and hematological variables are shown in Table 3. All sheep developed rigors, and somnolence accompanied by an elevation in body temperature and PAP beginning approximately 1 h after the endotoxin infusion was begun. White blood cell count was significantly decreased in both groups after 4 h and significantly increased after 24 h of endotoxin infusion. HR was significantly elevated in hyperdynamic sheep after 1.5 h of endotoxin. CI was significantly elevated in hyperdynamic sheep after 8 h of endotoxin, but was significantly reduced in nonhyperdynamic sheep after 4 h of endotoxin; however, the decrease in CI was not sustained. SVRI was significantly elevated in both groups after 4 h, and significantly reduced in the hyperdynamic group after 8 h of endotoxin.

Table 1. Hemodynamic variables in volunteers after endotoxin

Variable	Baseline	Time (h after endotoxin)				
		1	2	3	4	5
Temp (°C)	36.6 ± 0.1	36.7 ± 0.1	37.6 ± 0.1*	37.9 ± 0.1*	37.8 ± 0.1*	37.6 ± 1
HR (beats/min)	69.5 ± 2.6	76.9 ± 3.4	89.1 ± 2.9*	95.8 ± 2.6*	95.8 ± 3*	93 ± 2.9*
MAP (mm Hg)	99.3 ± 2.2	102.6 ± 4.3	92.7 ± 3.8*	84.4 ± 2.8*	84 ± 3.1*	84 ± 3.4*
CVP (mm Hg)	5.6 ± 1.1	4.1 ± 0.9	2.1 ± 0.5*	1.4 ± 0.4*	2.1 ± 0.6*	1.8 ± 0.4*
PAP (mm Hg)	15.9 ± 1.2	13.9 ± 0.8	11.6 ± 0.8*	12.9 ± 1*	15 ± 1.2	14.7 ± 1.1
CI ($l \cdot min^{-1} \cdot m^{-2}$)	3.7 ± 0.2	4.1 ± 0.3	5.8 ± 0.4*	6.2 ± 0.2*	6 ± 0.3*	5.7 ± 0.2*
SVRI ($dynes \cdot sec^{-1} \cdot cm^{-5} \cdot m^{-2}$)	1498 ± 53	1422 ± 83	938 ± 53*	788 ± 37*	813 ± 56*	849 ± 36*

Temp, body temperature; HR, heart rate; MAP, mean arterial pressure; CVP, central venous pressure; PAP, pulmonary artery pressure; CI, cardiac index; SVRI, systemic vascular resistance index.
*$p < 0.05$ compared with baseline values; mean ± SEM.

Table 2. Hematological variables in volunteers after endotoxin

Variable	Baseline	Time (h after endotoxin)				
		1	2	3	4	5
Hb (g/dl)	13.6 ± 0.2	13.3 ± 0.3	13.3 ± 0.4	$12.9 \pm 0.4^*$	$12.8 \pm 0.3^*$	$12.5 \pm 0.4^*$
WBC (cells/mm^3)	6.5 ± 0.4	4.8 ± 0.6	8.2 ± 0.9	$9.3 \pm 1^*$	$10.9 \pm 0.9^*$	$11.6 \pm 0.8^*$
Gran (cells/mm^3)	62.6 ± 3.6	63.1 ± 4.3	$85.1 \pm 2.9^*$	$91.8 \pm 0.9^*$	$93.3 \pm 0.6^*$	$91.7 \pm 0.7^*$
Lymph (cells/mm^3)	26.7 ± 3	30.1 ± 3.4	$12.3 \pm 2.5^*$	$5.7 \pm 0.9^*$	$3.5 \pm 0.5^*$	$4.7 \pm 0.6^*$
Mono (cells/mm^3)	7.4 ± 0.9	$2.7 \pm 0.5^*$	$0.6 \pm 0.2^*$	$0.5 \pm 0.2^*$	$1.2 \pm 0.4^*$	$2.4 \pm 0.4^*$

$^*p < 0.05$ compared with baseline values; mean $\pm$ SEM.
Hb, serum hemoglobin; WBC, white blood cell count; Gran, granulocyte count; Lymph, lymphocyte count; Mono, monocyte count.

Global brain blood flow is shown in Fig. 2. CBF was elevated in hyperdynamic sheep, but unchanged in nonhyperdynamic sheep after 4 h of endotoxin. Cerebrovascular and cerebral oxygenation variables are shown in Fig. 3. The $CMRO_2$, CDO_2, and CPP were significantly elevated and CVR was significantly reduced in hyperdynamic sheep but unchanged in nonhyperdynamic sheep after 4 h of endotoxin. ICP was unchanged in both groups throughout the study period.

Discussion

Sepsis remains a major cause of morbidity and mortality, with an incidence of more than 500 000 cases in the United States every year [2]. Although it is estimated that approximately 100 000 deaths will result from septic shock and multisystem organ failure this year [2,22], little progress has been made in understanding the complex pathophysiological changes that contribute to increased mortality. Of major relevance is the need for an appropriate experimental model in which to study the relevant changes in sepsis, as many animal models do not reproduce the clinical conditions seen in human sepsis [23]. Both models used in our study generate a hyperdynamic profile similar to that which accompanies early human hyperdynamic sepsis, with an elevated CI and decreased SVRI [8,9,15–17]; thus, both may provide relevant information when used to determine cerebral autoregulatory responses in sepsis.

Neurologic dysfunction in sepsis has not been well defined. Indeed, cerebrovascular responses in experimental endotoxemia may differ considerably between models depending on the species studied [24–26], dose of endotoxin administered [27,28], and whether or not the animals are studied in an anesthetized state [29,30]. In our studies in volunteers, CBF, CDO_2, CVR, and $CMRO_2$ were unchanged after endotoxin, despite a significant increase in CI and white cell count, and a decrease in SVRI. Our results may reflect a dose-related response to endotoxin, as CBF and $CMRO_2$ are

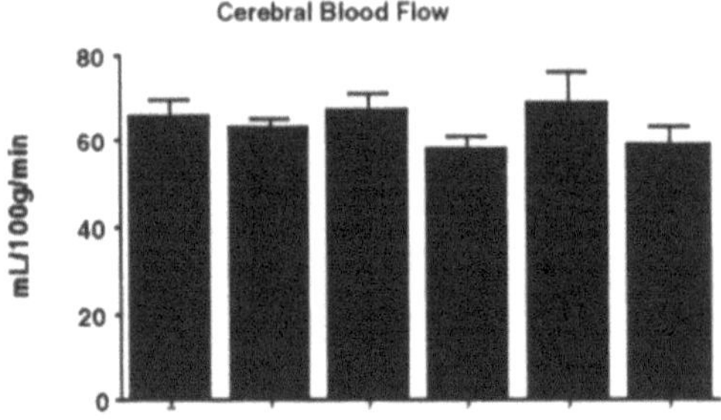

Cerebral Blood Flow
80
60
40
20
0
mL/100g/min

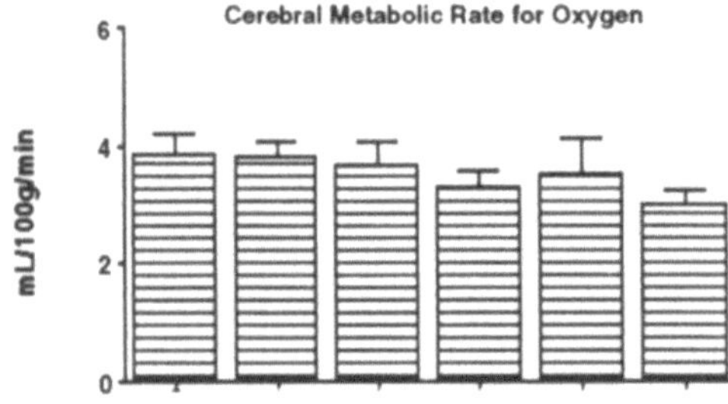

Cerebral Metabolic Rate for Oxygen
6
4
2
0
mL/100g/min

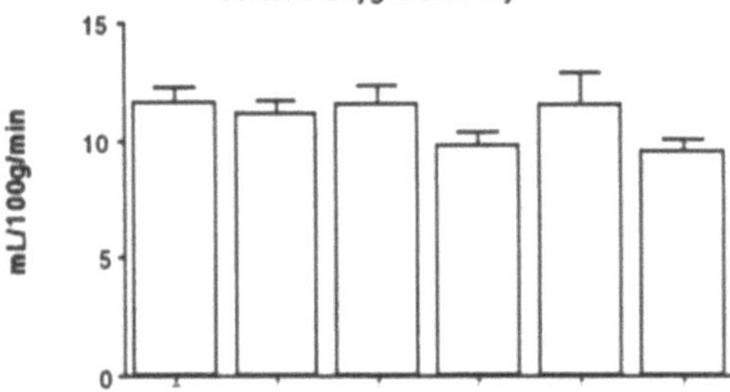

Cerebral Oxygen Delivery
15
10
5
0
mL/100g/min

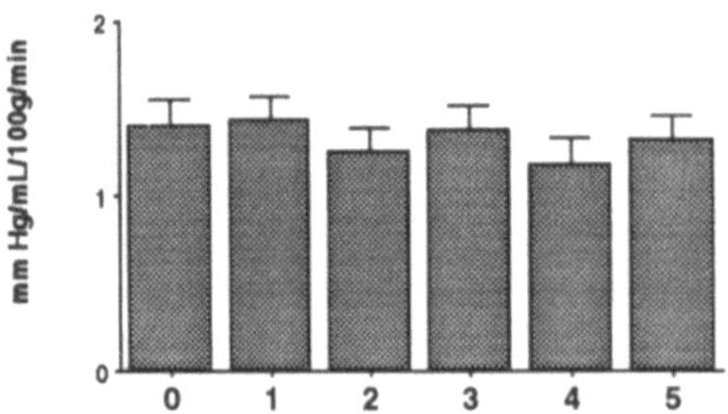

Cerebral Vascular Resistance
2
1
0
mm Hg/mL/100g/min
0 1 2 3 4 5
Time (hours after endotoxin)

Table 3. Hemodynamic and hematological variables in sheep receiving endotoxin

Variable	Group	Baseline	Time (h after endotoxin)			
			1.5	4	8	24
Temp (°C)	Hyperdynamic	39.3 ± 0.1	40.1 ± 0.2*	40.7 ± 0.2*	40.5 ± 0.2*	40.3 ± 0.2*
	Nonhyperdynamic	39.3 ± 0.1	40.5 ± 0.2*	41.4 ± 0.2*	40.9 ± 0.2*	40.4 ± 0.2*
HR (beats/min)	Hyperdynamic	94.3 ± 6	117 ± 7*	115 ± 7*	130 ± 0.8*	128 ± 10*
	Nonhyperdynamic	97.6 ± 4	117 ± 6	103 ± 5	145 ± 0.4*	112 ± 6
MAP (mm Hg)	Hyperdynamic	98.9 ± 4	98.4 ± 3	112 ± 5*	98.1 ± 6	99 ± 6
	Nonhyperdynamic	92.0 ± 4	93.0 ± 4	101 ± 5	86.8 ± 3*	89 ± 4
CVP (mm Hg)	Hyperdynamic	5.9 ± 1.2	5.4 ± 1	6.6 ± 1.6	6.3 ± 1.1	4.5 ± 1.3
	Nonhyperdynamic	6.0 ± 1.2	5.0 ± 2.5	7.4 ± 1.5	6.7 ± 1.2	6.4 ± 1.3
PAP (mm Hg)	Hyperdynamic	17.7 ± 1.6	27.8 ± 1.6*	25.4 ± 2.3*	27.5 ± 1.5*	22.6 ± 2*
	Nonhyperdynamic	17.4 ± 1.6	31.2 ± 2.6*	25.0 ± 1.8*	25.0 ± 1.7*	22.0 ± 1.8*
CI ($1 \cdot min^{-1} \cdot m^{-2}$)	Hyperdynamic	6.3 ± 0.5	6.5 ± 0.6	6.2 ± 0.6	8.3 ± 0.9*	8.1 ± 0.7*
	Nonhyperdynamic	7.7 ± 0.4	7.6 ± 0.8	6.1 ± 0.4*	8.5 ± 0.8	7.4 ± 0.3
SVRI ($dynes \cdot sec^{-1} \cdot cm^5 \cdot m^{-2}$)	Hyperdynamic	1237 ± 121	1215 ± 129	1456 ± 160*	958 ± 138*	1004 ± 113*
	Nonhyperdynamic	1031 ± 624	1033 ± 67	1438 ± 135*	813 ± 92	1018 ± 65
WBC (cells/mm^3)	Hyperdynamic	6.0 ± 0.6	2.8 ± 0.6*	3.3 ± 1.1*	–	10.4 ± 1.2*
	Nonhyperdynamic	6.6 ± 0.8	7.5 ± 4.3	3.2 ± 0.7*	–	10.4 ± 1.9*

*$p < 0.05$ compared with baseline values; mean ± SEM.
Temp, body temperature; HR, heart rate; MAP, mean arterial pressure; CVP, central venous pressure; PAP, pulmonary artery pressure; CI, cardiac index; SVRI, systemic vascular resistance index; WBC, white blood cell count.

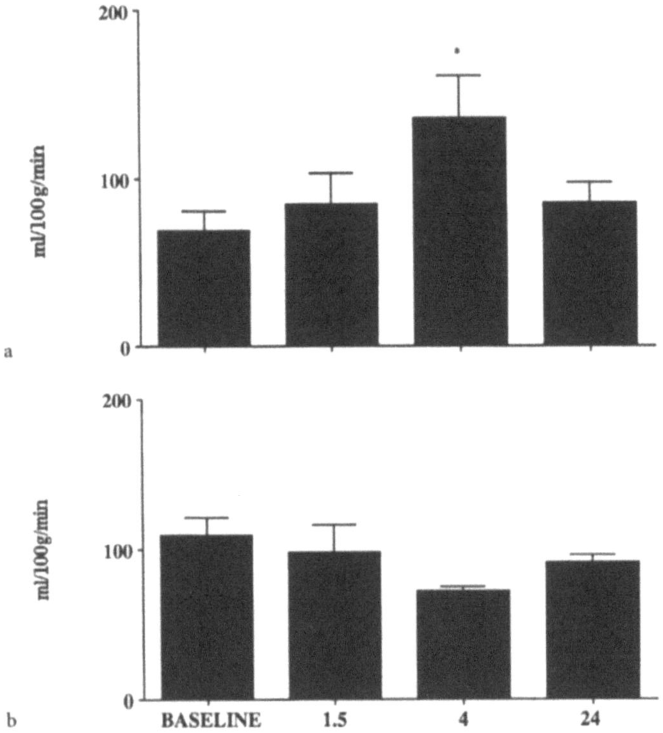

Fig. 2a,b. Whole brain blood flow was increased in sheep with hyperdynamic sepsis (**a**; $n = 8$), but unchanged in sheep with nonhyperdynamic sepsis (**b**; $n = 10$) after 4 h of continuous endotoxin (*E. coli*, 10 ng/kg per minute). Values are expressed as mean ± SEM. *$p < 0.05$ from baseline

decreased after high-dose endotoxin [26], and unchanged or elevated during low-dose endotoxin infusion in sheep [27]. Alternatively, cerebral autoregulation may be unchanged in human experimental endotoxemia.

We used a Kety-Schmidt technique to measure CBF. Because this technique provides a global measurement of CBF, it is also feasible that regional changes in CBF, known to occur in animal models of endotoxemia [26,30], may not have been detected by this method. $CMRO_2$ was also unchanged in the study. Post-hoc interval testing comparing the 3- and 5-h data with the baseline data revealed a significant reduction in $CMRO_2$; consequently, a decrease that was not detected by our analysis may have been present. Volunteers were apprehensive at the beginning of the study and were more relaxed and sleepy after the systemic symptoms had subsided; thus, baseline $CMRO_2$ may have been artificially elevated, although after instrumentation all volunteers were given a rest period of 1 h before the study began. However, as endotoxin is known to cause changes in human sleep patterns with a relative reduction in wakefulness that is related to body temperature and inflammatory cytokine release [13], it is also possible that $CMRO_2$ was reduced.

In contrast to the human studies, sheep demonstrated different hemodynamic and cerebrovascular profiles, as two distinct responses developed with administration

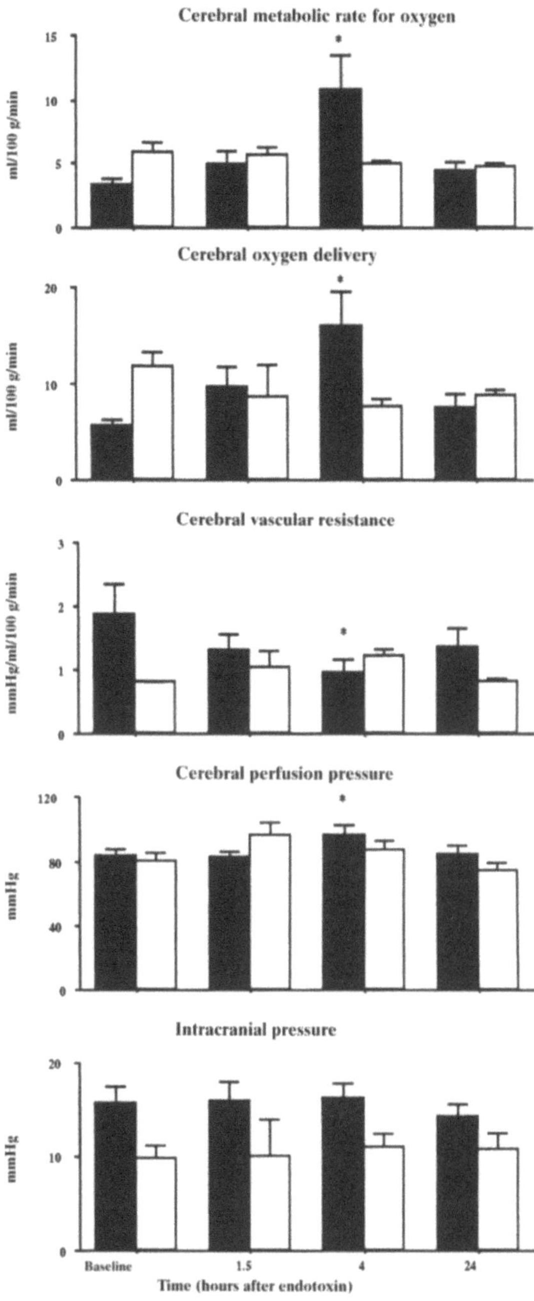

Fig. 3. Cerebrovascular parameters during hyperdynamic (*solid bars*; $n = 8$) and non-hyperdynamic (*open bars*; $n = 10$) sepsis in sheep. The cerebral metabolic rate for oxygen, cerebral oxygen delivery, cerebral vascular resistance and cerebral perfusion pressure were increased in hyperdynamic sheep and unchanged in nonhyperdynamic sheep 4h after the endotoxin infusion (*E. coli*, 10 ng/kg per minute) was begun. Intracranial pressure was unchanged in both hyperdynamic and nonhyperdynamic sheep. Values are expressed as mean ± SEM. *$p < 0.05$ from baseline

of endotoxin. Both hyperdynamic and nonhyperdynamic sheep developed early systemic signs of shivering, and obtundation, and body temperature and PAP were significantly elevated in both groups. The early depression in white blood cell count may indicate a more pronounced response to endotoxin in the hyperdynamic group, as CI was significantly increased and SVRI was significantly decreased after 8 h in this group. HR was also significantly elevated in hyperdynamic sheep, but was unchanged in nonhyperdynamic sheep. Variations in response to endotoxin may reflect a difference in individual susceptibility to endotoxin, as all sheep were managed and resuscitated equivalently, and received similar doses of endotoxin. However, because inflammatory cytokine responses were not assessed, it is not known whether the hyperdynamic sheep developed a more profound response. CBF was elevated in hyperdynamic sheep 4 h after endotoxin was begun. $CMRO_2$, CDO_2, and CPP were also elevated and CVR was significantly reduced. At this time sheep were recovering from the systemic manifestations of endotoxin and were more alert, and cerebral autoregulation may have been preserved through the release of cerebral vasodilator metabolites such as the endothelial-derived relaxant factor, which produces cerebral vasodilation, a decrease in CVR, and an increase in CBF. Indeed, in rabbits, topical lipopolysaccharide (LPS) causes cerebral arteriolar vasodilation, which is inhibited by N^G-monomethyl-L-arginine (L-NMMA), a nitric oxide synthase (NOS) inhibitor, dexamethasone, and indomethacin, suggesting an important role for both nitric oxide and cyclooxygenase products in LPS-induced cerebral arteriolar dilatation [31]. Pretreatment with a NOS inhibitor prevents the increase in CBF seen after intracisternal injection of live *pneumococci* in rats [32], while N^G-nitro-L-arginine methylester (L-NAME) restores CBF to baseline after 24 h of continuous endotoxin infusion in sheep [33].

In summary, CBF was unchanged during experimental hyperdynamic endotoxemia in volunteers, but was elevated after 4 h of continuous endotoxin infusion in hyperdynamic sheep. Cerebral hemodynamics, including CVR and CPP, and cerebral oxygenation parameters, including $CMRO_2$ and CDO_2, were unchanged in volunteers, but CVR was decreased, and CPP, $CMRO_2$, and CDO_2 were increased in hyperdynamic sheep. Although body temperature and PAP were elevated in nonhyperdynamic sheep, CI and SVRI were unchanged. Similarly, cerebral hemodynamics and cerebral oxygenation variables were unchanged in these sheep. Clearly, the mechanisms governing cerebral autoregulation during sepsis are complex. LPS-induced responses may be dose-dependent, and species differences and genetic susceptibility may influence both systemic and cerebral responses. Further studies are essential to determine the specific vasodilator metabolites and inflammatory mediators released in the cerebral and systemic circulation during endotoxemia, as changes in these mediators may allow modulation therapies to be investigated and developed that may ultimately improve survival in multiple system organ failure.

References

1. Sprung CL, Peduzzi PN, Shatney SN, Schein RMH, Wilson MF, Sheagren JN, Hinshaw LB, The Veterans Administration Systemic Sepsis Cooperative Study Group (1990) Impact of encephalopathy on mortality in the sepsis syndrome. Crit Care Med 18:801–806

2. Barriere SL, Lowry SF (1995) An overview of mortality risk prediction in sepsis. Crit Care Med 23:376–393

3. Pine RW, Wertz MJ, Lennard EP, Dellinger CJ, Carrico CJ, Minshew BH (1983) Determinants of organ malfunction or death in patients with intraabdominal sepsis: a discriminate analysis. Arch Surg 118:242–249

4. Young GB, Bolton CF, Austin TW, Archibald YM, Gonder J, Wells GA (1990) The encephalopathy associated with septic illness. Clin Invest Med 13:297–304

5. Jackson AC, Gilbert JJ, Young GB, Bolton CF (1985) The encephalopathy of sepsis. Can J Neurol Sci 12:303–307

6. Bowton DL, Bertels NH, Prough DS, Stump DA (1989) Cerebral blood flow is reduced in patients with sepsis syndrome. Crit Care Med 17:399–403

7. Maekawa T, Yukimasa F, Daikai S, Yokata K, Soejima Y, Ishikawa T, Miyauchi Y, Takeshita H (1991) Cerebral circulation and metabolism in patients with septic encephalopathy. Am J Emerg Med 9:139–143

8. Martich GD, Parker MM, Cunnion RE, Sufferedini AF (1992) Effects of ibuprofen and pentoxifylline on the cardiovascular response of normal humans to endotoxin. J Appl Physiol 73:925–931

9. Sufferedini AF, Fromm RE, Parker MM, Brenner M, Kovacs JA, Wesley RA, Parillo JE (1989) The cardiovascular response of normal humans to the administration of endotoxin. N Engl J Med 321:280–287

10. Revhaug A, Michie HR, Manson JM, Watters JM, Dinarello CA, Wollf SM, Wilmore DW (1988) Inhibition of cyclo-oxygenase attenuates the metabolic response to endotoxin in humans. Arch Surg 123:162–170

11. Cannon JC, Tompkins RG, Gelfand JA, Michie HR, Stanford GG, van der Meer JWM, Endres S, Lonnemann G, Corsetti J, Chernow B, Wilmore DW, Wolff SM, Burke JF, Dinarello CA (1990) Circulation interleukin-1 and tumor necrosis factor in septic shock and experimental endotoxin fever. J Infect Dis 161:79–84

12. Spinas GA, Bloesch D, Kaufmann MT, Keller U, Dayer JM (1990) Induction of plasma inhibitors of interleukin 1 and TNF-α activity by endotoxin administration to normal volunteers. Am J Physiol (Regulatory Integrative Comp Physiol 28) 259:R993–R997

13. Pollmacher T, Schreiber W, Gudewill S, Vedder H, Fassbender K, Wiedemann K, Trachsel L, Galanos C, Holsboer F (1993) Influence of endotoxin on nocturnal sleep in humans. Am J Physiol (Regulatory Integrative Comp Physiol 28) 264:R1077–R1083

14. Kety SS, Schmidt CF (1945) The determination of cerebral blood flow in man by the use of nitrous oxide in low concentrations. Am J Physiol 143:53–66

15. Traber DL, Traber LD (1989) Sheep as a cardiopulmonary model. Prog Clin Biol Res 299:253–263

16. Sugi K, Newald J, Traber DL, Maguire JP, Herndon DN, Schlag G, Traber DL (1991) Cardiac dysfunction after acute endotoxin administration in conscious sheep. Am J Physiol 260:H1474–H1481

17. Traber DL, Flynn JT, Herndon DN, Redl H, Schlag G, Traber LD (1989) Comparison of the cardiopulmonary responses to single bolus and continuous infusion of endotoxin in an ovine model. Circ Shock 27:123–138

18. Booke M, Armstrong C, Hinder F, Traber LD, Traber DL (1994) Anesthesia in ovine sepsis: fentanyl propofol in contrast to propofol alone worsens hemodynamics and myocardial performance. Anesthesiology 81:A458 (abstr)

19. Beach T, Millen E, Grenvik A (1973) Hemodynamic response to discontinuance of mechanical ventilation. Crit Care Med 1:85–90

20. Talke P, Dunn A, Lawlis L, Sziebert L, White A, Herndon D, Flynn JT, Traber DL (1985) A model of ovine endotoxemia characterized by an increased cardiac output. Circ Shock 17:103–108

21. Demling RH, Lalonde CC, Jin L-JJ, Albs J, Fiori N (1986) The pulmonary and systemic response to recurrent endotoxemia in the adult sheep. Surgery 100:876–883

22. Centers for Disease Control (1990) Increase in national hospital discharge survey rates for septicemia – United States 1979–87. MMWR Morb Mortal Wkly Rep 39:31–34

23. Traber DL, Traber LD, Redl H, Schlag G (1993) Models of endotoxemia in sheep. In: Schlag G, Redl H (eds) Pathophysiology of shock, sepsis and organ failure. Springer Berlin Heidelberg New York, pp 1031–1047

24. Kreimeier U, Ruiz-Morales M, Messmer K (1993) Comparison of the effects of volume resuscitation with dextran 60 vs. Ringers lactate on central hemodynamics, regional blood flow, pulmonary function and blood composition during hyperdynamic endotoxemia. Circ Shock 39:89–99
25. Hariri RJ, Ghajar JBG, Bahramian K, Sharif S, Barie PS (1993) Alterations in intracranial pressure and cerebral blood volume in endotoxemia. Surg Gynecol Obstet 176:155–166
26. Miller CF, Breslow MJ, Shapiro RM, Traystman RJ (1987) Role of hypotension in decreasing cerebral blood flow in porcine endotoxemia. Am J Physiol 253:H956–H964
27. Pollard V, DeMelo E, Prough DS, Traber LD, Traber DL (1993) Cerebral metabolic rate and cerebral blood flow are uncoupled during endotoxemia in sheep. Anesthesiology 79:A784 (abstr)
28. Parker JL, Emerson TE (1977) Cerebral hemodynamics, vascular reactivity, and metabolism during canine endotoxin shock. Circ Shock 4:41–53
29. Weiner DE (1970) Effects of endotoxin on cerebral blood flow in the monkey. Am J Physiol 218:160–164
30. Wyler F, Forsyth RP, Nies AS, Neutze JM, Melmon KL (1969) Endotoxin-induced regional circulatory changes in the unanesthetized monkey. Circ Res 24:777–786
31. Brian JE, Heistad DD, Faraci FM (1995) Dilatation of cerebral arterioles in response to lipopolysaccharide in vivo. Stroke 26:277–281
32. Haberl RL, Anneses F, Ködel U, Pfister HW (1994) Is nitric oxide involved as a mediator of cerebrovascular changes in the early phase of experimental pneumococcal meningitis? Neurol Res 16:108–112
33. Booke M, Meyer J, Lingnau W, Hinder F, Traber LD, Traber DL (1995) Use of nitric oxide synthase inhibitors in animal models of sepsis. New Horiz 3:123–138

Discussion

Sprung:
Those were elegant studies. I have two questions: the first relates to the methodology. There are those who have suggested that the infusion of endotoxin and various bacteria may not mimic the clinical picture as much as perhaps the cecal ligation model or an infective clot. The question is, do you have any data in that model looking at these types of issues, and could that perhaps explain the differences between the increased cerebral blood flow that you saw as opposed to the decreased cerebral blood flows that were seen in the clinical model? Number two: I am frankly surprised that the IRB allowed you to place pulmonary catheters in human volunteers. That has come up in several IRBs I have been involved in, and was flatly refused. I am just interested in your comments.

Traber:
We have not done cecal ligation and puncture, but of course Dr. Sibbald in London, Ontario, has, and in his situation he did not measure cerebral blood flow. He did measure blood flow to other organs using radioactive microspheres, and his data are quite similar to those we have for other organs. So I suspect that those two models are similar. We did not elect to do cecal ligation and puncture, because we thought we could have a much more quantitative model if we gave a continuous infusion of bacteria or their toxins. And then we had some reluctance to create peritonitis in our animals in the unanesthetized state, feeling that there was some possibility for pain.

We have not investigated the clot model. We do have a hyperdynamic situation, as Dr. Parrillo's group did. Dr. Parrillo has examined our data and he has not questioned the validity of our model in comparison to his. But it is certainly something that would be worthwhile for us to test. It is just very difficult, as you know, once you have got something that works, to change that. As they say, if it ain't broken, don't fix it. But you are suggesting that it might be broken, so therefore we might have to have another comparative study.

The IRB approval for placement of the Swan-Ganz catheter: we did not bribe them or anything. However, these were all medical personnel, most of them were from the operating room, certainly all of them knew what a Swan-Ganz catheter was and the risks that were involved. And we did advise them of those risks as we did of course advise them about the jugular bulb catheter placement. I think most anaesthesiologists would rather get the endotoxin than the Swan-Ganz catheter, as you have already indicated, because you did not seem to be very concerned about getting endotoxin. The amount of endotoxin that is given here actually is not such a tremendous amount. Those of you who grew up in a tropical climate, as I did, probably received that much endotoxin every year when you went in to get your shots for prevention of typhoid fever, since that is what typhoid fever shots were, giving the *Salmonella typhimurium* endotoxin.

Shackford:

Dan, a normal response when patients get septic is that they hyperventilate. When you drop the blood pressure in experimental animals, occasionally they would hyperventilate. Hyperventilation can reduce the PCO_2 and could lower cerebral blood flow. These animals were awake, is that correct, and did you monitor the PCO_2?

Traber:

That is right. And we did the same with the volunteers.

Shackford:

And the arterial pH?

Traber:

At a 24-h time period there was no change in pH. Earlier, around 3 h in the sheep, there was a trend to show some metabolic acidosis, but at the 24-h time period they are pretty much similar to the baseline values. PO_2, on the other hand, is reduced.

Shackford:

And the PO_2? When you were looking at the difference between the animals receiving the L-NAME and the L-NMMA, were there any differences in PO_2 or hemoglobin concentration?

Traber:

It is not stable; hemoglobin concentration drops. Because they are receiving about 5 ml/kg per hour of fluid resuscitation, and the same in the volunteers. We have to give them fluid to maintain filling pressures — of course we did not have left atrial pressures — in the volunteers we used the pulmonary capillary wedge pressure for resuscitation.

Baethmann:

My questions are concerned with two points. One is the significance of NO as a mediator of the systemic cardiovascular response acutely after endotoxin administration, as you have described, versus its role in a chronic state of sepsis, whether NO is still responsible. And the second point is that you have observed in your experiments that some animals were in a hyperdynamic state without increase of the cerebral blood flow and oxygen uptake, while other animals were not and had no cerebral hyperemia. What factors were influencing whether an animal became hyperdynamic or not after infusion of *Pseudomonas*?

Traber:

We go back to the first question, that is, the significance of nitric oxide in chronic sepsis. The data to support that from the clinical situation, there are one or two studies to demonstrate an elevation in nitrates and nitrites in chronic sepsis, one from Pittsburgh and one from the pediatric literature showing the same. Dr. Robert Kilbourn has done some stable isotope studies in which he used isotopically labeled arginine, and was able to show that in patients receiving interleukin (IL)-2, who develop a similar type of situation where they become hyperdynamic, as you see here, the level for arginine falls and the label for nitrate goes up, suggesting an in vivo elevation in nitrate, and then isolation of cells and tissues from animals, especially rats, who are chronically septic, and show elevation of nitrates and nitrites and a conversion of arginine to citrulline and that elevation is not affected by giving calcium-chelating compounds, suggesting that a nitric oxide synthesis is involved. Lastly, there have been numerous animal studies that have shown nitrate levels to be elevated by both the grease technique and chemiluminescence technique. In our animals, we do not show an elevation in total nitrates at a 24-h time period. However, we do show a fall in nitrates when we give a nitric oxide synthase inhibitor. Now, as you know, the nitrates have sources other than the metabolism of arginine, and so consequently it could be related to the diet or adsorption of the animals. These animals are ruminants; they have the capability of fixing nitrogen. You can feed them urea and they can make amino acids out of it, so it is a complex kind of situation. We presently have data that are being analyzed using stable isotopically labeled arginine and we have only data from two animals that show that as we give L-NMMA 24 h after sepsis, labeled arginine levels rise, suggesting that we are seeing an effect upon that. Those are the data that support that nitric oxide, and they are strong enough data that Glaxo-Wellcome is going forward with a clinical trial with L-NMMA; another company, Apex Pharmaceuticals, is going along with another trial using hemoglobin as a scavenger for nitric oxide.

Now, as to why some animals get hyperdynamic and others do not, this was not a phenomenon that we saw in our other studies except of course in some of the *Pseudomonas* animals. They were resistant to *Pseudomonas* because when you are using bacteria in a laboratory even though you may take care it is possible that an animal would be exposed to *Pseudomonas* and therefore be resistant to it, but in the other animals that we studied, we did not have such an instance of resistance. This could be related to the preparation of the brain, as you have noted, there appeared to be higher cerebral pressures in the animals that were hyperdynamic and lower in the others, perhaps there is some relationship between cerebral and spinal fluid pressure and this is something that we are presently at a loss to explain. We base it upon perhaps the animal sensitivity to the materials, either the cytokines or the endotoxin that is administered.

Schlag:
I think the difference between humans and sheep is just a question of dosage. Because you use 4 ng in humans and you use much more in the sheep, so that the increase in cerebral blood flow in the sheep is really related to the dosage of endotoxin.

Traber:
That is what we feel at the present time. Of course, we also have a time factor. If we were able to give 4 ng/kg per minute to the volunteers we probably would see a similar phenomenon as we saw with continuous endotoxin in sheep. But, on the other hand, when we give 4 ng or 10 ng/kg per minute we have about a 20% mortality rate in the sheep, and I do not think that those would be acceptable to most IRBs.

Schlag:
Another question on the dosage of the endotoxin in sheep: Morell used, I think, 50 ng/kg.

Traber:
In his first studies, those where he was showing the expression of endothelin, he used 10 ng/kg per minute. It is a rather interesting phenomenon, because he based his dosage on a paper we had written in which we showed a hyperdynamic situation with a continuous infusion of 10 ng/kg. But we were giving 10 ng/kg per hour and it was a transient phenomenon and not sustained. And he misinterpreted our paper and gave 10 ng/kg per minute and the hyperdynamic state was sustained, and so in later studies he gave it at higher doses. Those were papers that he published with Dr. Pellet.

Schlag:
What is the mortality with your dosage of 24 ng/kg per minute?

Traber:
There was no mortality from that dosage of endotoxin.

Schlag:
You know our problems with this dosage: our sheep died. Maybe that is a difference between the sheep in the USA and in Europe.

Traber:
I do not remember the breed of sheep that we worked with here in Vienna. But there are two major differences. Number one, we were working with a different breed of sheep; in the USA we use the Merino type of sheep, which is a Spanish breed that is pretty universal in Australia, England, and New Zealand. In Europe we used another strain, I do not recall what it was. And there is a difference in age. The animals that we used in these studies were 3–6 years old, whereas the animals that we used here in Vienna were somewhat younger and there may be age differences in responsiveness to the endotoxin.

Bolton:

These are interesting investigations. Just a few thoughts. First of all, I was wondering how closely your measurements of cerebral blood flow reflect changes in the micro-circulation in the brain, which is the likely site of dysfunction. Then, I wonder, in the animal and the human experiments, if you are measuring changes early in the course of sepsis. Later on at the microvascular level, adhesion molecules, cellular elements begin to take part. I believe some investigators have shown in microcirculation of other organs there may actually be occlusive phenomena toward the venous end of the capillaries, which would produce even more profound changes. The other thought is that it would be nice if you could get some measurement of the cerebral function during the course of the experiments. Dr. Young has shown that changes in EEG are very sensitive in sepsis. I believe Dr. Young has been approached about recording the EEG in sheep, and I do not believe that he was very enthusiastic, but he may want to comment on that.

Traber:

Before we get into EEG, let me discuss the circulation question. The blood flows in these experiments were measured using either radioactively labeled microspheres or fluorescent microspheres. As you know we are going away from radioactive microspheres in the sheep and are going to colored microspheres, because of the cost of getting rid of the carcass of radioactive animals and environmental problems that are involved with it. So, therefore, we are looking at blood flow to vessels that are in the order of 15 µg, so we are down at the arteriolar level; we are not in the capillary level, but we certainly are very close to it with our measurements. As far as chronic versus acute, we have data that go up to 48 h, so I would suggest that is pretty chronic. As far as the microcirculation is concerned, the data here are somewhat difficult, I think, to interpret, because it is based upon rats that are getting huge dosages of endotoxin; they are not sure in a hyperdynamic state. There is surely adhesion of polymorphonuclear cells in the microcirculation, and that is in a very acute situation. However, with the chronic situation, we have been unable to show that a large amount of polymorphonuclear cells adhered at the microcirculation after that particular point in time, and I think that would be what you would suggest would be occurring. There are, however, a large number of patients who become septic who have no polymorphonuclear cells. And it would be also suggested that in chronic sepsis polymorphonuclear cells would be in the microcirculation or would have already diapedesed down or are in the process of diapedesing, so our data looking at the microcirculation suggest that macrophages might be something that might be in-creasing microvascular resistance. And of course these cells, for the most part, do leave on the venule side of the circulation, so your suggestion that there could be emboli is one that could be taken into advisement, but on the other hand, perhaps that in one area the circulation has the least resistance because it has the largest cross sectional area. So now the EEG. We did not try to measure EEGs, but I understand that Dr. Young did.

Young:

We have not, for logistical reasons, studied EEG in the sheep. There were just several problems in getting around this. One was that our technologists had to receive rabies inoculation, because the sheep were wild sheep that were studied in Dr. Sibbald's laboratory, and they were not keen on receiving rabies prophylaxis. The other problem in recording scalp EEG in the sheep was the very large frontal sinus over the brains of the sheep that markedly attenuates the scalp EEG. I think if you were to put drills through the skull of the sheep and implant electrodes, you could probably do it. It would be useful to monitor frequency changes in the EEG to give you an idea of what was happening, at the tissue level anyway, to the brain function. I suppose regional cerebral blood flow would also be of interest, although you did look at flow in cortical and other areas. I was interested that the cortical blood flow did not really change all that much, while areas in the cerebellum and brain stem did, in one of your slides. Would you comment?

Traber:
That was in one of the slides I did not show, a really large elevation in cortical blood flow, that seemed to be a freakish phenomenon, because all of the other data did, and the data from the endotoxin groups that we showed you, the first group that was from Dr. Jörg Mayer, and then the later ones for *Pseudomonas* which were data from Dr. Booke, both of those showed an increase in cortical blood flow, just diversely to the same extent. So I am at a loss to explain why in that one study they did not. I must admit that our analysis for microspheres were done, that is, the colored microspheres (the one study that did not show a very good effect). I said that was an early study. Those data were examined at the same time as the earthquake in San Francisco. So it could be that those data are a little different from the others because of the earthquake; I do not know.

Histological Aspects of Sepsis-Induced Brain Changes in a Baboon Model*

K. Zarkovic, N. Zarkovic, G. Schlag, H. Redl, and G. Waeg

Introduction

Encephalopathy is one of the organ dysfunctions seen in critically ill patients with multiple organ dysfunction syndrome (MODS) secondary to sepsis (defined as the systemic response to infection).

Neurological or central nervous system (CNS) status is usually included in multiple organ dysfunction scores [14], based in part on the Glasgow Coma Score (see Oppenheim, this volume). It is often difficult to evaluate the CNS status in patients due to sedation, intubation, etc., and some other studies use the EEG pattern as an evaluation criteria (see Young, this volume). There are few studies available, however, in which changes were observed at the cellular level of septic CNS disorders. This is partly because of the limited possibilities for monitoring and the limited access to sample material, e.g., from the brain. On the other hand, the problem in clinical studies is the undefined time course of sepsis. Therefore, experimental studies with a defined time course are a valuable supplement to clinical studies. We have previously set up a nonhuman primate model of sepsis [32], which involves infusion of *Escherichia coli* in baboons. The baboon, a nonhuman primate which is phylogenetically very similar to humans, offers many advantages as an experimental animal [30]. In addition to our previous studies in which we have primarily investigated heart, lung, liver, and gut dysfunction [31], and mediator systems (e.g., phospholipase A) [29] we have now broadened our approach to include the brain.

Possible reasons for brain dysfunction are numerous and probably interrelated including multiple brain microabscesses (see Young, this volume) or the action of bacterial toxins on the brain macrophage system, which induces the inflammatory reactions. This network of reactions includes cytokines, neutrophils, and the release of cytotoxic reactive oxygen species (ROS) and proteinases. The other source of ROS can be ischemia-reperfusion as a result of sepsis-induced microcirculatory mismatch.

Due to their toxicity, ROS produced by the inflammatory cells and the endothelial cells play a crucial role in the body's defense against germs [28,41]. Yet ROS also induce peroxidation of the lipids (cellular membrane lipids or circulating lipoprotein molecules), generating highly reactive aldehydes, which are considered "secondary toxic messengers" of free radicals [11,41]. Aldehydes produced in this way are very toxic and damage tissue [10], meaning that various organs are damaged simultaneously by infective agents as well as by the toxic products of sepsis. The permeability

---

* This paper is dedicated to Prof. Hermann Esterbauer. We lost a fantastic colleague and wonderful friend.

of the blood vessels both for bacteria and for the toxic mediators of the oxidative stress is thus of crucial importance for determining the outcome of sepsis [1,33]. Highly reactive aldehyde 4-hydroxynonenal (HNE) is one of the most important products of lipid (i.e., polyunsaturated fatty acids, PUFAs) peroxidation [11,12]. Very recently [38], specific monoclonal antibodies have been developed against HNE-protein (or peptide) conjugate(s) that allow morphological analysis of the tissue distribution of aldehyde. Data now indicate that HNE and related aldehydes are involved in ROS induced damage to various organs, particularly the brain, after different pathological events [3,4,16,40]. It was impossible to analyze the cascade of events leading to oxidative damage to brain tissue during sepsis from neither a dynamic or a morphologic point of view since the data indicating the involvement of ROS and their secondary toxic messengers in different diseases of the brain (as well as the other organs) were obtained by biochemical analysis of the activity of enzymes involved in ROS production or their detoxification or by determination of the presence of HNE or related aldehydes in serum, cerebrospinal fluid (CSF), or the tissue homogenates [13,19,40]. This of course precluded morphologic evaluation of the tissue and cellular distribution of the mediators of oxidative stress that might show differences between the different types of cells or parts of organs involved in pathological events.

In addition to inflammatory processes, systemic metabolic abnormalities such as abnormal amino-acid patterns may also account for brain alterations (e.g., neutrotransmitter) [20].

Studies on the pathophysiology of sepsis that focus on brain damage are complex due to the specific permeability of the brain–blood barrier, unique inflammatory responses (engagement of the glial cells), and the specific anatomy and histology of different brain regions. To gain an insight into the role of oxidative stress in the pathophysiology of brain damage caused by sepsis involving one of two strains of *E. coli*, we have performed an immunohistochemical analysis of the distribution of HNE in the brain of the septic baboons and investigated whether the morphologically defined brain damage was also reflected in plasma markers of brain damage, e.g., neuron specific enolase (NSE). NSE is the neuronal form of the glycolytic enzyme 2-phospho-D-glycerate hydrolase, which is used in the CSF as an index of neuronal damage [6], in serum as a marker of cerebral injury after head trauma [9], Creutzfeld-Jacob disease [39], and hypoxic brain damage [3], and a marker of tumors with neuroendocrine properties [36].

Materials and Methods

Experimental Procedure

Male animals of the species *Papio ursinus* (baboon) with a weight of about 20 kg were investigated. Fasting animals were sedated with 6–8 mg/kg ketamine hydrochloride (Ketalar, Parke Davis Co., Ann Arbor, MI), placed in the supine position. Following intubation, the tube was connected to an oxygen blender via a T-piece. The FiO$_2$ was kept within 23% ± 2%. Anesthesia was maintained with pentobarbital at a dosage of 2–4 mg/kg per hour.

Following exposure of the right femoral vein, an introducer for a heparinized Swan-Ganz catheter (7 F) was positioned in the pulmonary artery. A catheter was introduced into the right brachial artery for blood withdrawal and for pressure monitoring. At the end of the acute study catheters were filled with 500 U heparin and placed in a subcutaneous pouch; the wound was closed with stitches. A triple lumen catheter was inserted into the right brachial vein for infusion (anesthesia, medication, venous blood withdrawal), which was withdrawn at the end of the acute study (4 h after the start of *E. coli* infusion).

Baboons were infused with either serum-sensitive (SS) 2×10^9 cfu live *E. coli*/kg [Hinshaw's strain B7 (086a:61) ATCC 33985] or non-serum-sensitive (SNS) $2 \times$ 109 cfu live *E. coli*/kg (0.18:K1:H7 strain Bort) [8] intravenously over a 2-h period according to our sepsis protocol [32]. To maintain the fluid balance and compensate for losses, the animals received 5 ml Ringer's solution/kg per hour, which was further adapted to the wedge pressure (baseline) during the course of the experiment. In addition, during the 72-h recovery period animals were administered additional intravenous fluid, depending on the measured pulmonary wedge pressure assessed at 10, 24, and 48 h following recovery.

For each measurement and for infusion therapy after the acute phase of the study, the animals were sedated with ketamine hydrochloride (Ketalar) 6–8 mg/kg, placed in supine position, and intubated. The subcutaneous pouch was opened under sterile conditions and the catheters connected to the measurement lines or to the infusion pump. The wound was reclosed after the procedure and the animals were further kept without anesthesia. Blood samples were drawn in ethylenediaminetetraacetate (EDTA) and serum vacuum tubes (Greiner, Kremsmünster, Austria) centrifuged at 3500 g for 10 min and stored at –30°C.

Total blood counts, hemoglobin, and hematocrit were determined by a coulter T890 (Coulter Electronics Inc., Hialeah, FL, USA). NSE was measured using a commercial radioimmunoassay (RIA) kit (Pharmacia, Uppsala, Sweden). Briefly, this RIA is a double antibody assay. NSE in the sample competes with a fixed amount of ^{125}I-labeled NSE for the binding sites of the specific antibodies. Bound and free NSE are separated by the addition of a second antibody immunoadsorbent followed by centrifugation and decanting. The radioactivity in the pellet is then measured. The radioactivity is inversely proportional to the quantity of NSE in the sample.

Escherichia coli Preparation

E. coli was grown in a fermenter using Tryptone soy broth for 150 min at 37°C with agitation, aeration, and pH control to maximize living cell counts and to minimize free lipopolysaccharide (LPS) levels as previously described [32].

Brain Fixation and Morphological Analysis

The material for the study consisted of 14 baboon brains which were examined by the method of subserial consecutive paraffin section as modified by Grcevic [15]. The brain was removed by autopsy within 1 h after death and fixed in 10% formalin. Upon fixation, the brains were grossly inspected and cut by consecutive coronal section into slabs of about 5 mm thickness. After detailed examination, the material was photographed. The samples of brain tissue fixed in 10% buffered formalin were dehydrated in graded ethanol, and embedded in paraffin.

Paraffin blocks of different sizes, corresponding to the sizes of the brain slabs, were cut subserially by a large Tetraner-Jung microtome into sections of 5 μm and used for histological and immunohistochemical analysis.

Monoclonal Antibodies Against HNE

Monoclonal antibodies that detect HNE-modified proteins were obtained from the culture medium of the clone "HNE 1g4" which was derived from a fusion of Sp2-Ag8 myeloma cells with B-cells of a BALBc mouse immunized with HNE modified keyhole limpet hemocyanine [39]. The antibody is specific for the HNE-histidine epitope in HNE-protein (peptide) conjugates. HNE-lysine and HNE-cysteine give 5% and 4% cross-reactivity with HNE 1g4.

Immunohistochemical Analysis

For the immunohistochemical detection of HNE adducts, the immunoperoxidase technique was used, with secondary rabbit-anti-mouse antibodies (Dako, Denmark). Nonspecific binding was prevented by the use of normal, nonimmunized rabbit serum while endogenous peroxidase reactions were prevented by H_2O_2 treatment of the sections using a 1% BSA solution as scavenger for washing the slides (three times). The affinity of the HNE 1g4 antibody was determined by testing the serial dilutions of the antibody on HeLa cells fixed in 4% buffered paraformaldehyde that had been treated by HNE in vitro for 1 h with concentrations of the aldehyde ranging between 0.1 and 100 μM. The specificity of HNE 1g4 monoclonal antibody was previously verified by adsorption with its primary antigen (HNE-histidine epitope) in the form of an HNE–BSA conjugate (100 μM HNE/25 mg BSA/ml saline solution). The HNE–BSA conjugate was washed of the excess of free aldehyde by filtering it on the Amicon membrane ultrafiltration system using an 0.5 kDa membrane (Amicon, Ireland) under pressure of nitrogen, with the sample being constantly stirred an immunohistochemically positive reaction to HNE was stained by 3,3′-diaminobenzidine tetrahydrochloride (DAB, Dako, Denmark) and nickel chloride $(NiCl_2$, Kemika, Croatia). Contrast staining was done using 1% acridine orange solution (Sigma, USA) and 1% Safranin-O-stock solution (Sigma, USA). Positive immunostaining thus produced a dark gray-to-black color, with contrast of a light yellow-to-orange staining.

Results and Discussion

Experimental sepsis caused the death of the experimental animals within 2 days, irrespective of the strain of *E. coli* used to induce sepsis. The *E. coli* strain did influence the inflammatory response to the bacteria within the blood vessels, as

Table 1. Distribution of the inflammatory cells in the brain of baboons with experimental sepsis

Animal no.	Survival (h)	Experimental treatment	Inflammatory cells in the			
			Blood vessels	V-R space	Subarachnoidal space	Brain tissue
55	48	SNS *E. coli*	Pl, Ly, Mc, Ne	Pl, Ly, Mc	–[a]	–
56	148	SNS *E. coli*	Pl, Ly, Mc, Ne	Pl, Ly, Mc, Ne	Pl, Ly, Mc, Ne	–
57	40	SNS *E. coli*	Pl, Ly, Mc	Pl, Ly, Mc	Pl, Ly, Mc	–
59	17	SNS *E. coli*	Pl, Ly, Mc, Ne	Pl, Ly, Mc, Ne	Pl, Ly, Mc, Ne	Mg, NF
65	16	SNS *E. coli*	Pl, Ly, Mc	–	–	–
66	43	SS *E. coli*	Mo	Mo	–	–
67	53	SS *E. coli*	Mo	–	–	–
69	21	SS *E. coli*	Mo	Mo	–	–
73	28	SS *E. coli*	Mo, Ne	–	–	–

SNS, serum non-sensitive; SS, serum sensitive; Ne, neutrophils; Pl, plasma cells; Mc, macrophages; Mo, monocytes; Ly, lymphocytes; Mg, microglial cells; NF, neuronophagia.
[a] No inflammatory cells present.

presented in Table 1. Hence, brain blood vessels of the control septic baboons injected with SNS *E. coli* contained mainly lymphocytes (including plasma cells), neutrophils, and macrophages. The blood vessels of the brains of animals injected with SS *E. coli* contained mainly neutrophils and monocytes, while lymphocytes were only found occasionally. The V-R and subarachnoidal spaces were infiltrated by the leukocytes in the SNS *E. coli* injected control animals. It can therefore be assumed that the strain of bacteria plays a role in the induction of the systemic inflammatory response and its consequences on the brain. However, as could be expected, there were no prominent inflammatory cells found in the brain tissue itself, except in the brain of one baboon, in which the phenomenon of neuronophagia was manifested. As can be seen from Table 2, very strong immunohistochemical staining on HNE was observed for almost all the animals in the subarachnoidal space and the brain white matter (Fig. 1). In contrast, the presence of the aldehyde was less obvious in the gray matter of the brain and could not be even detected for some animals. Interestingly, the animals in which there was no positive testing for HNE in gray matter were those who lived for a relatively short time (16–30 h).

The difference in HNE content observed for the white and gray matter of septic baboons was even more obvious if the positive HNE testing stemmed from astrocytes in the gray and white matter respectively (Table 3, Fig. 2). Numerous astroglial cells in the white matter were HNE positive although the presence of HNE could hardly be detected for the same glial cells in the white matter. While the strain of *E. coli* used to induced sepsis did not seem to be of importance concerning astroglial "oxidative burst" in white matter, it seemed to be of relevance for the HNE positivity of astrocytes in gray matter. Thus, weak HNE positivity was seen for the astrocytes in the gray matter of 3 of 5 baboons infected with SNS *E. coli* but only in 1 of 5 baboons infected with SS *E. coli*.

Table 2. The effects of experimental sepsis on the presence of the lipid peroxidation product 4-hydroxynonenal (HNE) in the brain blood vessels

Animal no.	Survival (h)	Experimental treatment	Position of the blood vessels		
			Subarachnoidal space	White matter	Gray matter
55	48	SNS *E. coli*	+++	+++	++
56	148	SNS *E. coli*	+++	++	+
57	40	SNS *E. coli*	++	++	+
59	17	SNS *E. coli*	++	+	−
65	16	SNS *E. coli*	++	+	−
66	43	SS *E. coli*	++	++	+
67	53	SS *E. coli*	++	+	+
69	21	SS *E. coli*	++	++	+
73	28	SS *E. coli*	++	++	−

SNS, serum non-sensitive; SS, serum sensitive; Immunohistochemical positivity to HNE: +++ very strong; ++ moderate; + weak; − negative.

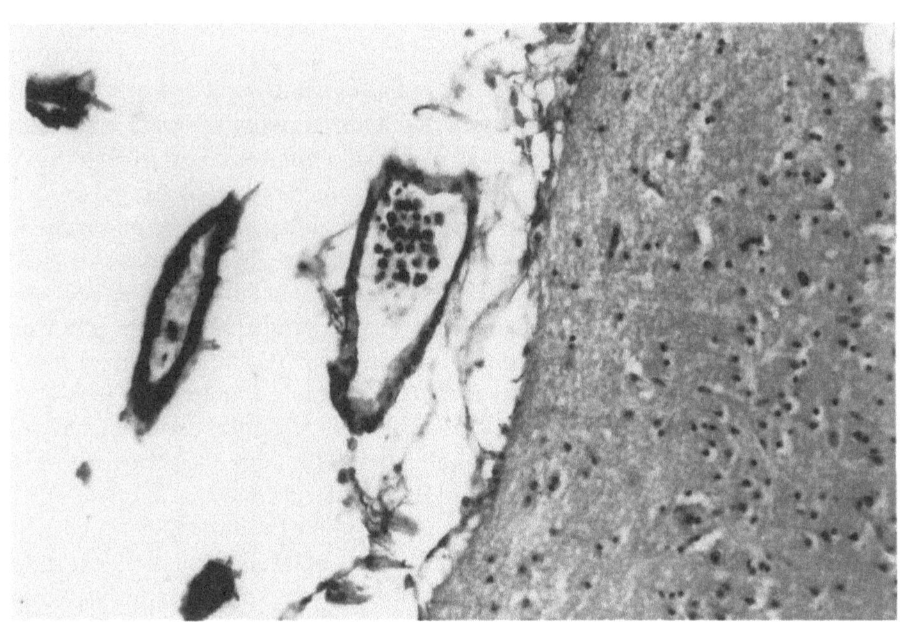

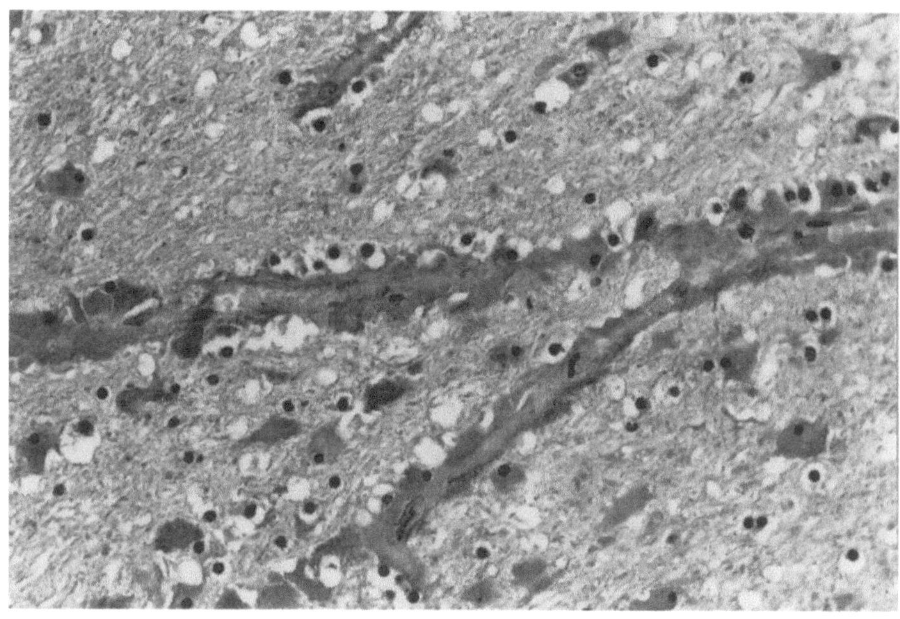

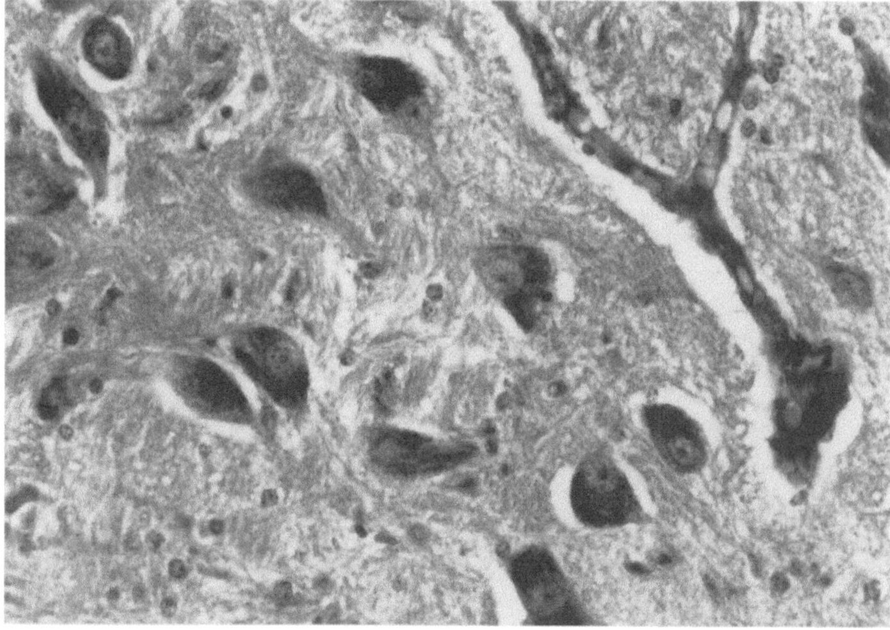

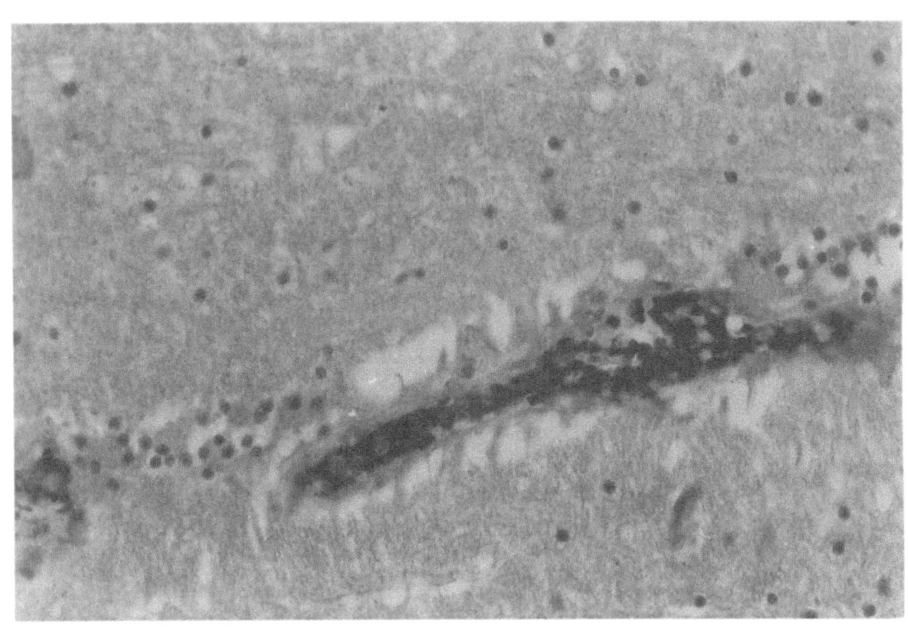

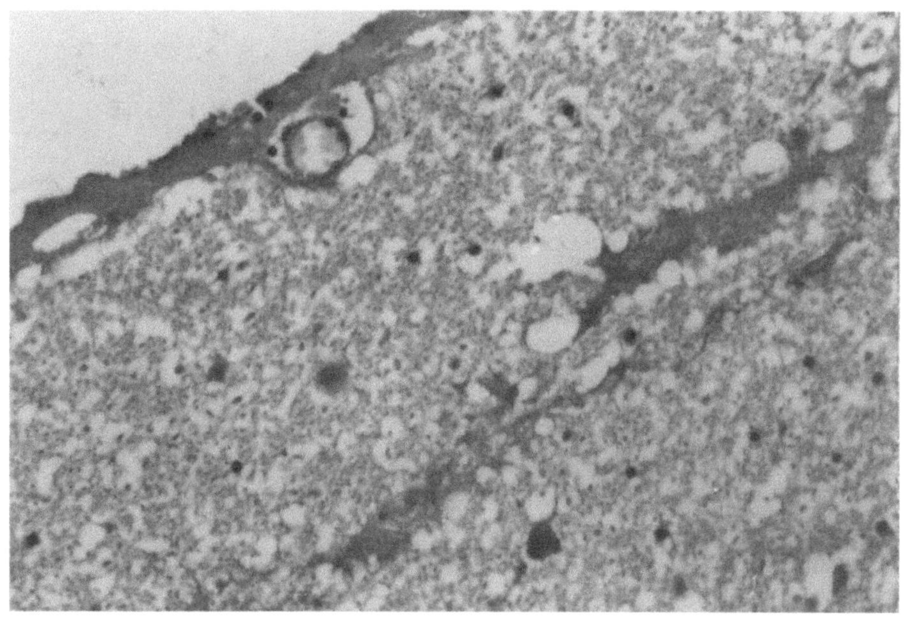

Table 4. Particular observations on the presence of the lipid peroxidation product 4-hydroxynonenal (HNE) in the brain tissue of septic baboons

Animal no.	Survival (h)	Experimental treatment	Meninges[b]	Pio-glial border[a]	Ependim chorioid plexus[a]	Subependimal white matter[a]	Hemolytic content of the blood vessels[b]	Edema fluid[b]
55	48	SNS *E. coli*	+++	−	+++	+++	+	+
56	148	SNS *E. coli*	+++	−	++	−	+	−
57	40	SNS *E. coli*	++	−	−	−	+	−
59	17	SNS *E. coli*	++	++	++	++	+	+
65	16	SNS *E. coli*	++	−	−	−	−	−
66	43	SS *E. coli*	++	−	−	−	+	+
67	53	SS *E. coli*	++	++	+	+++	+	−
69	21	SS *E. coli*	++	−	−	−	−	−
73	28	SS *E. coli*	++	++	+	++	−	−

[a] HNE positivity: +++, more than ten HNE-positive cells per high magnification (×400) field (HMF); ++, five to ten HNE-positive cells per HMF; +, less than five HNE-positive cells per HMF; −, no HNE-positive cells.
[b] +, moderate to strong intensity of the HNE immunopositive staining, −, no HNE positivity.

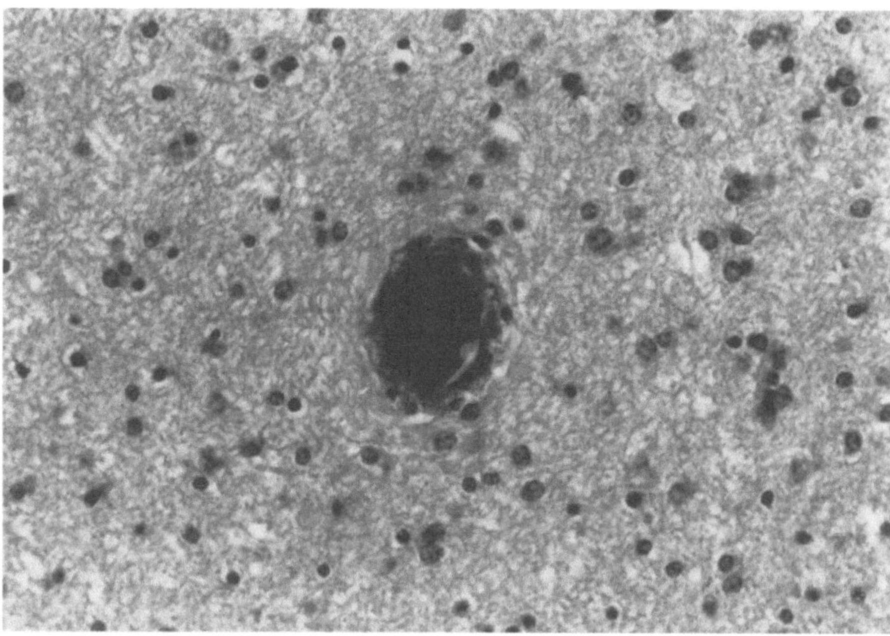

Fig. 6. The minute brain blood vessel and its hemolytic content are very stronly positive to HNE (*black*) (×400)

E. coli Cross (four of five animals) than by SS *E. coli* (in two of four animals). This is the opposite of the incidence of HNE-positive glial cells at the pio-glial border, while it does not show any relationship to the HNE positivity of the perivascular edema fluid. It therefore seems that both the nature of the HNE adducts (their biochemical origin, structure, molecular mass or size) produced during sepsis within the blood vessels as well as the "functional integrity" of the brain–blood could be of great importance for the determination of spread of the mediators of oxidative stress (such as HNE) from blood into brain tissue. Further analysis of the biochemical and biological features of HNE adducts in plasma of septic baboons is needed.

Finally, the strain of germs used to induce sepsis did not influence the HNE positivity of the chorioid plexus (Table 4; Fig. 7). The individual differences in the HNE content of the chorioid plexus that were seen were also found in the subependimal white matter. Hence, it can be assumed that the possible presence of HNE adducts or of other mediators of oxidative stress in the CSF of the septic baboons (which could not be studied so far) depend on the individual abilities for cleavage of the ROS diffusing out of the blood, brain tissue, and membranes into the CSF and back into the blood. Evaluation of this possibility requires further studies on the nature of HNE adducts in CSF and their comparison with the HNE adducts in blood.

The analysis of NSE (Fig. 8), the marker of CNS damage, revealed an interesting time course, where elevated levels were not seen in the first 11 h after the assault and trendwise higher levels were seen in animals that died early after sepsis induction.

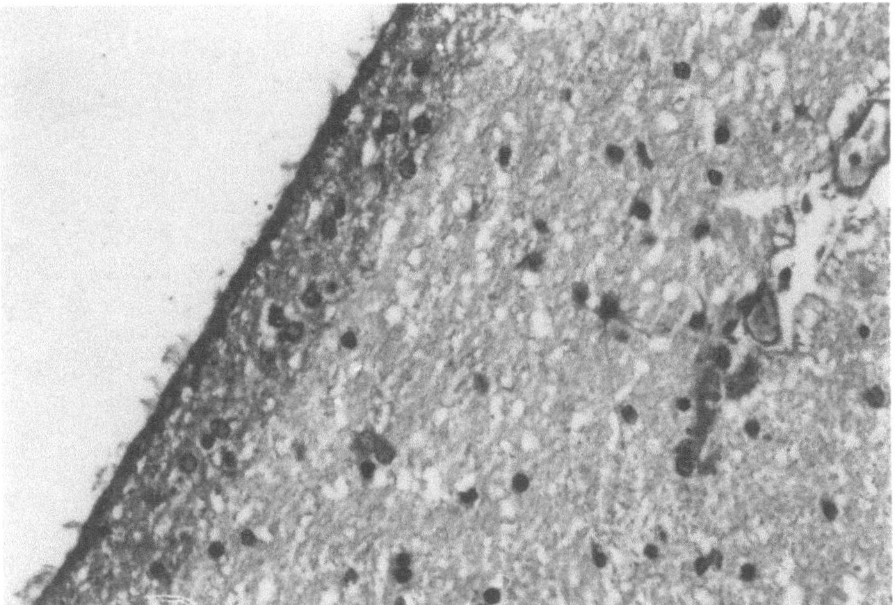

Fig. 7. Positive immunohistochemical reaction to HNE (*dark staining*) of the ependimal cells and subependimal white matter (×400)

Although this marker has previously been used in traumatic brain injury [9], reports of its use in the context of sepsis are scarce; it nonetheless appears to be a promising tool for further sepsis studies.

It cannot be ruled out that the observed NSE levels are from sources other than damaged neurons, since NSE has been described as endogenous to erythrocytes and platelets [18,22] it may thus be misleading as a marker of brain damage. Brown et al. [6] however, suggest that a 1% degree of hemolysis would still account for a normal serum level of NSE. The observed kinetics of the NSE release is at least not obviously related to a loss of platelets or a change in erythrocytes. A comparison of enolase plasma levels with platelet or red blood cell count does not indicate that blood cells are a source of increased enolase plasma levels unrelated to brain damage due to the completely different kinetic behavior.

Conclusions

The results of this study can be summarized as follows:

1. The perivascular edema fluid of the brain and the hemolytic content of the blood vessels were rich in HNE-protein adducts.
2. Strong HNE positivity was noticed in the brain membranes and blood vessels, particularly in the subarchnoidal space.

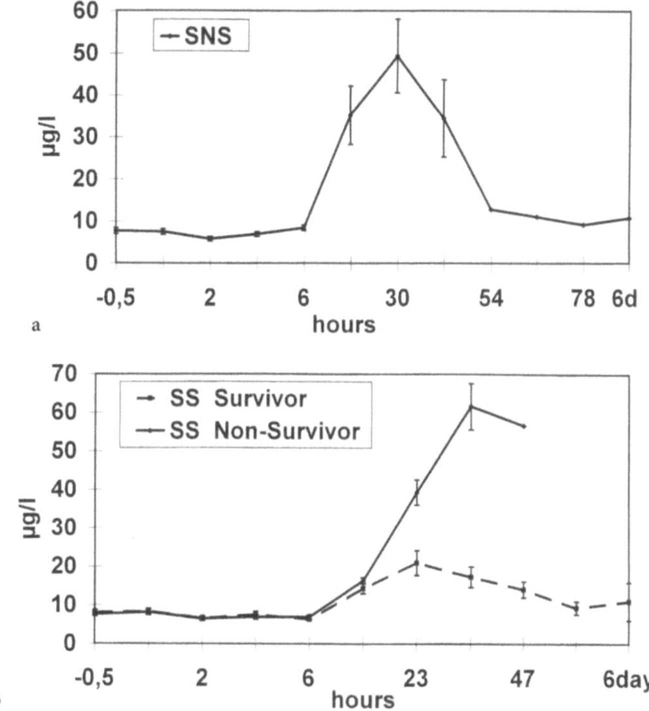

Fig. 8a,b. Plasma levels of neuron specific enolase (NSE) in baboons subjected to *Escherichia coli* sepsis. Five surviving animals (of which no histology is available) have less enolase release. *SS*, serum sensitive *E. coli*; *SNS*, serum non-sensitive *E. coli*. $^{*}p < 0.05$ versus baseline

3. Swelling of astrocytes was associated with the presence of HNE and was much more pronounced in the midbrain than in the other brain regions.
4. Similarly, more HNE-positive neurons were found in the midbrain than in the other parts of the brain.
5. Sepsis-induced oxidative stress of the brain did not depend on the cellular inflammatory response but on the blood supply.
6. These findings lead us to suppose that the brain damage induced by sepsis could be based on the oxidative damage to the blood–brain barrier and on the release of the secondary toxic messengers of free radicals (such as HNE) from the blood vessels into the brain.
7. Sepsis-induced brain damage can be seen in the plasma enolase values, which could be employed as a useful marker for longitudial studies.

Acknowledgments. We thank James Davies for his support performing the animal experiments and Eva Paul for enolase measurements.

References

1. Beerthuizen GIJM (1993) Response of the microcirculation: Tissue oxygenation. In: Schlag G, Redl H (eds) Pathophysiology of shock, sepsis, and organ failure. Springer Berlin Heidelberg New York, pp 230–256
2. Booke M, Traber LD, Traber DL (1994) Vasodilatators in sepsis. In: Schlag G, Redl H, Traber DL (eds) Shock, sepsis and organ failure-nitric oxide. Fourth Wiggers Bernard Conference. Springer Berlin Heidelberg New York, pp 243–258
3. Bradley HE, Fitch W (1994) Biochemical markers of cerebral ischaemia. In: Sebel PS, Fitch W (eds) Monitoring the cerebral nervous system. Blackwell, London, pp 26–50
4. Braughler JM, Hall ED (1989) Central nervous system trauma and stroke I. Biochemical considerations of oxygen radical formation and lipid peroxidation. Free Radic Biol Med 6:289–301
5. Breslow MJ, Traystman RJ (1993) Neurologic abnormalities in sepsis. In: Schlag G, Redl H (eds) Pathophysiology of shock, sepsis, and organ failure. Springer Berlin Heidelberg New York, pp 996–1003
6. Brown KW, Kynoch PAM, Thompson RJ (1980) Immunoreactive nervous system specific enolase (14-3-2 protein) in human serum and cerebrospinal fluid. Clin Chim Acta 101:257–264
7. Campbell IL, Chiang CS (1995) Cytokine involvement in central nervous system disease. Ann N Y Acad Sci 771:301–312
8. Cross A, Asher L, Seguin M, Yuan L, Kelly N, Hammack C, Sadoff J, Gemski P (1995) The importance of a lipopolysaccharide initiated cytokine mediated host defense mechanism in mice against extraintestinally invasive Escherichia coli. J Clin Invest 96:676–686
9. Dauberschmidt R, Marangos PJ, Zinsmeyer J, Bender V, Klages G, Gross J (1983) Severe head trauma and the changes of concentration of neuron specific enolase in plasma and in cerebrospinal fluid. Clin Chim Acta 131:165–170
10. Esterbauer H (1993) Cytotoxicity and genototxicity of lipid-peroxidation products. Am J Clin Nutr 57[Suppl]:779S–786S
11. Esterbauer H, Weger W (1967) Über die Wirkungen von Aldehyden auf gesunde und maligne Zellen; Synthese von homologen 4-Hydroxy-2-alkenalen. Chem Monthly 98:1884–1891
12. Esterbauer H, Schaur RJ, Zollner H (1991) Chemistry and biochemistry of 4-hydroxynonenal, malonaldehyde and related aldehydes. Free Radic Biol Med 11:81–128
13. Freeman BA, Topolosky MK, Crapo JD (1982) Hyperoxia increases oxygen radical production in rat lung homogenates. Arch Biochem Biophys 216:477–484
14. Goris RJA, Nuytinck HKS, Redl H (1986) Scoring system and predictors of ARDS and MOF. Prog Clin Biol Res 236B:3–15
15. Grcevic N (1982) Topography and pathogenic mechanisms of lesions in "inner cerebral trauma". Rad JAZU 402:265–331
16. Hall ED, Braughler JM (1989) Central nervous system trauma and stroke II. Physiological and pharmacological evidence for involvement of oxygen radicals and lipid peroxidation. Free Radic Biol Med 6:289–301
17. Hasselgren PO, Fischer JE, Meyer TA, Tiao G (1994) Inhibition of nitric oxide synthase during sepsis and endoxemia may be detrimental. In: Schlag G, Redl H, Traber DL (eds) Shock, sepsis and organ failure-nitric oxide. Fourth Wiggers Bernard Conference, Springer Berlin Heidelberg New York, pp 198–213
18. Hullin DA, Brown KB, Knoxh PAM, Smith C, Thompson RJ (1980) Human 14-3-2 protein: purification, radioimmunoassay and distribution in human tissue. Biochim Biophys Acta 628:98–108
19. Jamieson D, Chance B, Cadenas E, Boveris A (1986) The relation of free radical production to hyperoxia. Annu Rev Physiol 48:703–719
20. Jellinger K (1978) Brain mono-amines in human hepatic encephalopathy. Acta Neuropathol (Berl) 43:63–68
21. Katusic ZS, Schugel J, Consentino F, Vanhoutte PM (1993) Endothelium-dependent contractions to oxygen-derived free radicals in the canine basilar artery. Am J Physiol 257:H859–H864

22. Marangos PJ, Schmechel D, Parma AM, Clark RL, Goodwin FK (1979) Measurement of neuron specific enolase (NSE) and non neuronal specific enolase (NNE) isoenzymes in enolase of rat, monkey and human nervous tisse. J Neurochem 33:319–329
23. Martinez MC, Bosch-Morell F, Raya A, Roma J, Aldasoro M, Vila J, Lluch S, Romero FJ (1994) 4-Hydroxynonenal, a lipid peroxidation product, induces relaxation of human cerebral arteries. J Cereb Blood Flow Metab 14:693–696
24. McCann SM, Lyson K, Karanth S, Gimeno M, Belova N, Kamat A, Rettori V (1995) Mechanisms of action of cytokines to induce the pattern of pituitary hormone secretion in infection. Ann N Y Acad Sci 771:386–395
25. Meyer J, Stothert JC Jr, Pollard V (1993) Nitric oxide synthesis inhibition in ovine endotoxemia: effects on brain blood flow. Anesth Analg 76:S264
26. Parrat JR (1994) Nitric oxide and cardiovascular dysfunction in sepsis and endotoxaemia. In: Schlag G, Redl H, Traber DL (eds) Shock, sepsis and organ failure-nitric oxide. Fourth Wiggers Bernard Conference, Springer Berlin Heidelberg New York, pp 1–29
27. Parrat JR, Stoclet JC, Fleming I (1993) The role of L-arginine nitric oxide pathway in sepsis and endotoxaemia with special reference to vascular impairment. In: Schlag G, Redl H (eds) Pathophysiology of shock, sepsis, and organ failure. Springer Berlin Heidelberg New York, pp 575–592
28. Redl H, Gasser H, Hallström S, Schlag G (1993) Radical related cell injury. In: Schlag G, Redl H (eds) Pathophysiology of shock, sepsis, and organ failure. Springer Berlin Heidelberg New York, pp 92–110
29. Redl H, Dinges HP, Buurman WA, van der Linden C, Pober JS, Cotran RS, Schlag G (1991) Expression of endothelial leukocyte adhesion molecule-1 in septic but not traumatic/hypovolemic shock in the baboon. Am J Pathol 139:461–466
30. Schlag G (1994) Shock models – relevance for human studies. Shock 2[Suppl]:41
31. Schlag G, Redl H, van Vuuren CJJ, Davies J (1992) Hyperdynamic sepsis in baboons: II. Relation of organ damage to severity of sepsis evaluated by a newly developed morphological scoring system. Circ Shock 38:253–263
32. Schlag G, Redl H, Davies J, van Vuuren CJJ, Smuts P (1993) Live Escherichia coli sepsis models in baboons. In: Schlag G, Redl H (eds) Pathophysiology of shock, sepsis, and organ failure. Springer Berlin Heidelberg New York, pp 1076–1107
33. Seyr M, Mutz NJ (1993) Permeability changes. In: Schlag G, Redl H (eds) Pathophysiology of shock, sepsis, and organ failure. Springer Berlin Heidelberg New York, pp 176–193
34. Stratakis CA, Chrousos GP (1995) Neuroendocrinology and pathophysiology of the stress system. Ann N Y Acad Sci 771:1–18
35. Strieter RM, Colletti LM, Metinko AP, Rolfe MW, DeMeester SR, Standiford TJ, Kunkel SL (1993) The role of cytokine networks mediating inflammation and ischemia-reperfusion injury. In: Schlag G, Redl H, Traber DL (eds) Shock, sepsis and organ failure. Third Wiggers Bernard Conference. Springer Berlin Heidelberg New York, pp 205–227
36. Tapia FJ, Polak JM, Barbosa AJA, Bloom SR, Marangos PJ, Dermody C, Pearse AGE (1981) Neuron-specific enolase is produced by neuroendocrine tumours. Lancet I:808–811
37. Vincent JL, Bakker J, Silance PG (1993) Relationship between oxygen demand and oxygen supply in severe sepsis. In: Schlag G, Redl H (eds) Pathophysiology of shock, sepsis, and organ failure. Springer Berlin Heidelberg New York, pp 908–914
38. Waeg G, Dimsity G, Esterbauer H (1996) Monoclonal antibodies for detection of 4-hydroxynonenal modified proteins. Free Radic Biol Med 25:149–159
39. Wakayama Y, Shibuya S, Kawase J, Sagawa F, Hashizume Y (1987) High neuron specific enolase level in cerebrospinal fluid in the early stage of Creutzfeld-Jakob disease. Klin Wochenschr 65:798–801
40. Waterfall AH, Singh G, Fry JR, Marsden CA (1995) Detection of the lipid peroxidation product malondyaldehyde in the rat brain in vivo. Neurosci Lett 200:69–72
41. Zarkovic N, Ilic Z, Jurin M, Schaur RJ, Puhl H, Esterbauer H (1993) Stimulation of HeLa cell growth by physiological concentrations of 4-hydroxynonenal. Cell Biochem Funct 11:279–286
42. Zarkovic N, Schaur RJ, Puhl H, Jurin M, Esterbauer H (1994) Mutual dependence of growth modifying effects of 4-hydroxynonenal and fetal calf serum in vitro. Free Radic Biol Med 16:877–884

43. Zollner H, Schaur RJ, Esterbauer H (1991) Biological activities of 4-hydroxyalkenals. In: Sies H (ed) Oxidative stress. Academic London, pp 337–369

Discussion

Traber:
You mention that in the first set of slides, which I think were describing swelling, that there appeared to be less injury in the animals that received N^G-monomethyl-L-arginine (L-NMMA) and I noticed the same as you progressed along. Did you have any conclusions from your histological material that you would like to make in regard to nitric oxide synthase or nitric oxide and possible interactions with damage that you observed?

K. Zarkovic:
That may be possible, but we have observed only inflammatory cellular reaction. We have made only inflammatory cellular reaction analysis and in these cases with L-NMMA we have seen only lower intensity of this reaction in brain tissue and around the vessels.

Traber:
What would you conclude from that? That there was less cellular interaction with inhibition of nitric oxide synthase?

K. Zarkovic:
Yes.

Redl:
Our conclusion is that it is too early to draw conclusions, because it is an ongoing study, and we have only first preliminary results.

Traber:
It is very interesting, because the data are similar to those that Thiemermann presented last year at this time at the Forum, related to the liver.

Baethmann:
What is your current interpretation of the data? Are the pathological changes in the brain due to intoxication from endotoxin, or other bacterial products, or due to blood flow alterations, i.e., progressing ischemia?

Redl:
I think you are absolutely right that it might be mainly due to blood flow changes by itself and then some kind of local ischemic reperfusion, in addition to the inflammatory reaction. What we see in terms of endotoxin or cytokine action is, for instance, up-regulation of adherence molecules like VCAM-1. So, definitely, like Dr. Zarkovic pointed out, there is a lot going on on the vessel wall and it might be that really the changes in the blood–brain barrier are decisive.

Bolton:
Very interesting results. The thing that I was struck by was the amount of cerebral edema. Clinically, or in the pathological studies that we have observed in humans, we do not see cerebral edema in septic encephalopathy. We have, however, had at least one patient, where cerebral edema occurred, and advanced rapidly and caused the death of the patient. I believe Allan Roper and his group have collected four more cases from around the world. It is almost like a Reye syndrome, but affecting adults. Cultures have been negative, too; I know they were in ours. The patient had all the systemic signs of sepsis. But in general, I do not think cerebral edema in humans has been observed in septic encephalopathy.

Schlag:
But you have to consider that we have a big bacterial challenge, so we infuse 10^9 and we have a level of about 10^5 in the blood stream. It is not comparable with humans, where there are about 10^3 bacteria. So we have much more toxicity.

Kochanek:
It is interesting, because what you are describing reminds me of a combination that we can see in children, and that is of meningitis plus overwhelming septic shock. This is a group of patients that is particularly vulnerable to mortality. In that setting, even moderate hypotension can lead to cerebral ischemia because of loss of autoregulation. It seems somewhat reminiscent. Do you see any meningeal involvement in this model; is the bacterial challenge great enough that you actually see meningitis develop in these animals?

K. Zarkovic:
Maybe this is an effect of endotoxin, and maybe of "second toxic messengers" for free radicals such as HNE, which damage the blood–brain barrier.

Schlag:
But our baboons, if they die, they die of adrenal bleedings, so they are really comparable with the Waterhus-Fridreichs syndrome in children with meningococci; that is very interesting. But the reason is the great challenge. We use the bacterial challenge, it is to a certain degree comparable to children with meningococci sepsis.

Kochanek:
I think it would be very interesting also to see what nitrite and nitrates were in your model.

Schlag:
We measured it. We see an increase.

Kochanek:
Again, thinking about this with regard to Dr. Traber's presentation, there have been several reports particularly of an association between elevations of nitrite and nitrates in pediatric septic shock and the development of multiple organ failure. Many of these children have overwhelming infections and we obviously go to the wall for them "try anything you can", massive doses of pressors, etc. Have you modeled the situation, where you produce what would be an overwhelming insult with a need for

critical care intervention, in sheep, i.e., producing a situation where the sheep are so sick they need to be intubated and require inotropic support. I wonder if you have ever taken your model to that extent, almost turn it in an overwhelming septic shock analogue?

Traber:
Yes, but we do not have nitrites and nitrates of those animals. We have had them to the point of having to put them on oxygen, these animals are not included in the groups we presented. We have had to give inotropic support, we have taken them to those situations in which they had volume resistance and pressure resistance.

Schlag:
In certain animals we also see disseminated intravascular coagulation with a severe development of purpura fulminans, which also corresponds to what we see in these children.

Recommendation

C.F. Bolton, D.S. Prough, C.L. Sprung, and G.B. Young

At present, the Glasgow Coma Score (GCS) can be used to assess brain dysfunction in septic patients. The rationale for its continued use in septic patients is:

1. The demonstrated correlation of scores with outcome
2. Its standardization
3. Its ease of use
4. Its universal application around the world.

Problems with the GCS are found with:

1. Assessment in sedated patients
2. Intubated patients
3. Patients whose eyes are swollen shut
4. GCS design: Fragmentation into subcategories rather than comprising a single ordinal scale.

Other scoring systems, e.g., the Reaction Level Scale-85, that do not have these problems should be compared with GCS in large comparative studies. Electro-psychological monitoring, e.g., continuous or serial EEG, is a valuable supplement to clinical assessment, especially in the evaluation of cerebral cortical function in comatose patients.

Brain Damage Secondary to Traumatic Brain Injury

Mechanisms of Secondary Brain Damage in Severe Head Injury: A Clinical Perspective

A. Baethmann, N. Plesnila, J. Eriskat, and M. Stoffel

Introduction

Severe head injury with and without peripheral trauma is the most frequent cause of death and morbidity within the age bracket of up to 45 years [1,2]. The medical and psychosocial consequences for the patient and family, together with the burden on society, are extraordinary. Victims of accidents with head injury are often young persons, requiring in many cases life-long care. Expenses are incurred not only for the medical treatment and subsequent rehabilitation, but also through financial losses, e.g., from the futile investments in education and professional training and those concerning the expected income. The significance of the problem in Germany can be deduced from data obtained by the Federal Bureau of Statistics, Wiesbaden for the Year 1993 [3] reporting all cases with head injury admitted to a hospital. The sampling efficiency was no less than 96.3%. Altogether, more than 270 000 patients were referred to hospitals with (a) intracranial injuries ($n = 220\,393$), or (b) skull fractures ($n = 52\,781$). Although the diagnosis of head injury was not utilized, it can be concluded that a poor outcome in patients with either intracranial injuries or skull fracture is attributable to severe head injury. In total 10 584 patients died in 1993 from severe head injury. Estimates concerning the frequency of cases with severe head injury according to the internationally accepted definition of a Glasgow Coma Score of 8 points (or less) for at least 6 h (or longer) approach 20 000–30 000 cases per year, of which probably 2400–4800 survive with severe disabilities, requiring life-long care as dependants in nursing homes. In other words to the preexisting number of severely disabled patients no less than 2400, probably even more, new cases are annually added with all the misery for the patient and families and expense for the society.

Clinical and experimental findings have made it clear that outcome in severe head injury is determined not only by the primary traumatic insult – the resulting brain injury at the moment of an accident – but also by the subsequently evolving complications leading to and summarized as secondary brain damage [4,5]. The clear distinction between primary and secondary brain damage in head injury is of major clinical significance, since the latter might be influenced by therapeutical interventions, in the preclinical emergency phase and after admission to the hospital. Hence, an improvement in the alarming statistics on outcome in severe head injury can alone be expected by an increased efficacy of preventing or attenuating secondary brain damage from extra- and intracranial origin.

The importance of secondary brain damage in head injury is perfectly illuminated by "patients who talk and die" [6]. The capability to talk after head injury not only requires at least some consciousness but also the integrity of many brain areas indicating that large parts of the brain remain undamaged from the primary impact, in principle being compatible with survival of the patient. If such a patient nevertheless dies, the development of avoidable or non-avoidable complications must be held liable, not the severity of the primary impact. Consequently, the identification of avoidable and non-avoidable complications underlying secondary brain damage and contributing to a poor outcome takes on highest priority. These considerations lead to the question of how the incidence and severity of secondary complications can be reduced by adjustments in management and treatment. This includes implementation of prompt and appropriate diagnostic measures, as well as administration of therapy modalities which, more selectively than modalities so far available, inhibit the mechanisms of secondary brain damage in severe head injury. A reduction of "talk and die" patients in severe head injury would be exemplary for progress in both the prevention of avoidable complications and in general management and treatment. The most important examples of primary and secondary brain damage will be discussed here.

Primary Brain Lesions from Severe Head Injury

Brain damage from severe head injury, in simple terms, is caused by either acceleration or deceleration of the skull (inertial loading) in a linear or angular mode, or also occurring in combination [7]. Other mechanisms are associated with impression of the skull with and without fracture. The linear (translational) or angular acceleration (or deceleration) of the skull results in movements of the brain relative to the cranial vault, leading to contusions at the site of the *coup*, also sometimes in the opposite brain, the so-called *contre coup*. Noticable in this context are also so-called gliding contusions, attributable to the movement of the basal brain surface over the rough protuberances of the skull base, as for example the petrosal processes. Evidence is available that angular, rotatory movements of the skull are more damaging than mere translational acceleration or deceleration [7]. Rotatory movements are considered to be more effective to rupture blood vessels, for example the fragile bridging veins passing through the subdural space to the cerebral sinus system. The presence of subdural hemorrhage indicates that a traumatic impact was particularly severe leading also to the damage of brain parenchyma – not only of blood vessels. Accordingly, head injury patients with subdural hemorrhage belong to the group with the worst outcome [8].

Another manifestation of primary brain damage is diffuse axonal injury (see also Gennarelli, this volume [8–11]). This type of lesion has been overlooked for quite a while for various reasons. One is that its recognition requires histological assessment of the brain which is not done on a routine basis during autopsy. Another reason is that the histological changes characteristic of diffuse axonal injury only evolve with time until becoming visible after trauma, notwithstanding that the lesion is induced upon impact by shearing and tearing of the long nerve fibers in the white matter, which could encompass the cerebral hemispheres down to the upper cervical spinal cord. Based on electron microscopical investigations evidence has been provided that the axonal fine structure is subjected to characteristic cell biological alterations evolving during the posttraumatic course [12,13]. This may be suggestive of an involvement of secondary processes deserving investigation to discover whether therapeutical measures could be influential. Altogether, contusions, rupture of blood vessels leading to hematoma, and diffuse axonal injury comprise the most significant manifestations of primary brain damage in severe head injury [8,9].

Manifestations and Mechanisms of Secondary Brain Damage

Cerebral ischemia and hypoxia must be considered as the most pertinent cause of secondary brain damage in severe head injury. This has been born out by neuropathological and other investigations, demonstrating that the hallmarks of ischemia (and hypoxia) are present in the postmortem brain in approximately 90% of patients falling victim to a severe head injury [14,15]. Graham et al. [14,15] have conducted two serial investigations, one in the early 1970s, another approximately 10 years later, on the frequency of secondary ischemic changes in the brain of patients dying from severe head injury. A total of 151 patients were investigated in the first study and 112 patients in the latter. Accordingly, the incidence of secondary ischemic brain lesions was almost identical, namely 90% (Table 1).

As seen in Table 1, diffuse ischemic damage of cerebral cortex was found in 28%, boundary zone infarction in 25%, with territorial infarctions in 17%. Of these patients 38% were talking prior to death. In the latter study conducted in the early 1980s only 22% of patients were talking after trauma. The difference in this category between

Table 1. Frequency of ischemic brain damage in fatal head injury: an up-date [15]

	1968–1972 ($n = 151$)	1981–1982 ($n = 112$)
Patients with secondary ischemia	$n = 137$ (92%)	$n = 97$ (87%)
Diffuse cortical damage	28%	42%[a]
Arterial boundary zones	25%	13%[a]
Arterial territories	17%	19%
Talked and died	38%	22%[a]
Supratentorial hematoma	70%	82%[a]
ICP ↑	87%	87%

[a] Values significantly different from those in 1968–1972.
Comparison of the frequency of ischemic brain damage in cases with fatal head injury studied between 1968 to 1972, and 1981 to 1982 by the Department of Neuropathology, University of Glasgow. As seen, histological findings indicating ischemia (hypoxia) were present in approximately 90% of patients who died from severe head injury. Nevertheless, the incidence of "talk and die" patients as well as of ischemic boundary zone damage was significantly reduced 10 years later, suggestive of improvements in management with reduction of avoidable complications. The increase of supratentorial hematomas can be attributed to an adjustment of the referral practice in this region to the neurotrauma center at the University of Glasgow. As seen, the predominant influence of intracranial hypertension was unabating. (From [14,15])

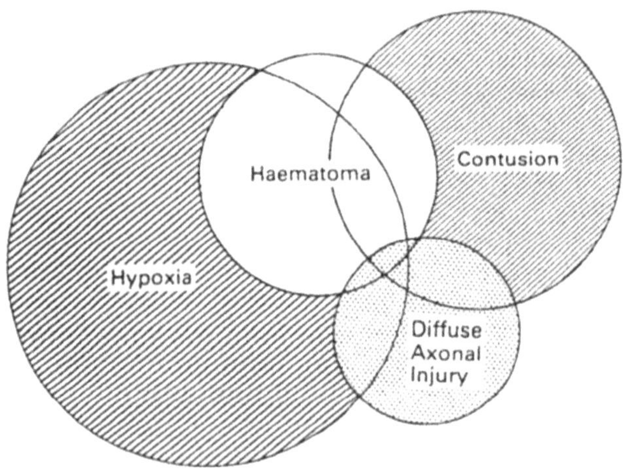

Hypoxia
Haematoma
Contusion
Diffuse
Axonal
Injury

Table 2. Clinical outcome of patients entered into the US Traumatic Coma Data Bank Study ($n = 746$) [22]

Mortality	36%
Vegetative survival	5%
Severe disability	16%
Moderate disability	16%
Good outcome or minimal neurological deficit	27%

preclinical emergency phase, but also plays a role after patient admission to the hospital. This conclusion can be drawn from evidence provided by retro- and prospective studies on the frequency of avoidable factors in children dying from severe head injury, or the incidence of adverse events associated with patient transfer in the hospital [19,20].

A useful source of prospectively collected data on risk factors in severe head injury is the US Traumatic Coma Data Bank Study carried out by four major neurotrauma centers in the United States [21,22] . Patient recruitment was carried out from 1984 to 1987. A total of 60% of the patients were admitted to the hospital within 1 h, 75% within 3 h. One third of the patients was admitted to another clinic prior to referral to the study hospital, while 63% were admitted directly to the neurotrauma center from the accident scene. The final outcome was assessed using the Glasgow Outcome Scale (Table 2).

Information emerging from this study emphasizes the prognostic influence of a treatment-refractory intracranial pressure rise as well as the significance of arterial hypotension – most frequently from cardiovascular failure in polytraumatized patients with hemorrhagic shock – both important mechanisms of secondary brain damage. Patients with systolic blood pressure of <90 mm Hg on admission to the hospital have a doubly high mortality rate [23,24] (Marmarou, personal communication). A promising result is that the mortality of patients with subdural bleeding, thus with the highest risk, was decreased [22]. The most important extracranial risk factors were pulmonary infections with an incidence of 41%, cardiovascular failure or shock at 29%, disturbances of coagulation at 19%, and the development of sepsis at 10% [24].

Mutual Interactions of Severe Head Injury and Cardiovascular Failure

Only few experimental studies have systematically analyzed the potentially fatal interactions between cardiovascular failure, hemorrhagic shock, and severe head injury. DeWitt et al. [25] carried out experiments in mongrel cats subjected to fluid percussion of the skull for assessment of the regional cerebral blood flow (rCBF) with radioactive microspheres. rCBF was measured prior to and after fluid percussion (2.2 atmosphere impact pressure) combined with a gradual lowering of the systemic blood pressure by incremental exsanguination. Initially, the blood pressure was decreased to 80 mm Hg, then to 60 mm Hg, and finally to 40 mm Hg for approximately 30 min at each level. The resulting intracranial pressure (ICP) rise and rCBF were more adversely affected in animals with hemorrhagic hypovolemia plus fluid percussion compared to the control animals with hypovolemia alone. ICP rose to almost 20 mm Hg in the combined brain trauma plus hemorrhagic shock group during arterial hypotension (60 or 40 mm Hg), whereas the ICP remained within the control range in animals with hemorrhagic shock only. Similar observations were made on the maintenance of rCBF. In the combined (trauma + shock) group cerebral blood flow was significantly decreased upon lowering blood pressure, i.e., to <20 ml/100 g per minute from approximately 90 ml/100 g per minute during control. In animals with hemorrhagic shock only, rCBF remained above >35 ml/100 g per minute at the same level of arterial hypotension [25]. The findings indicate that head injury markedly impairs the cardiovascular competence in hemorrhagic shock. Conversely, impairments of the cardiovascular compensatory capacity in shock can be expected to enhance traumatic brain injury. Corresponding observations were made by Yuan and Wade [26] who examined the outcome in rats with traumatic brain injury (fluid percussion). Animals with hemorrhagic shock (blood pressure 70–24 mm Hg) had a poorer survival with brain injury compared to those with hemorrhagic shock alone [26].

Obviously, brain trauma worsens the course of hemorrhagic shock, while hemorrhagic shock enhances traumatic brain injury by cerebral ischemia. Consequently, the maintenance or reestablishment of a competent cardiovascular function in head injury is the highest priority in emergency care at the scene of an accident and during transport to prevent secondary ischemic brain damage.

Significance of Hemorrhagic Hypotension and Intracranial Hypertension in Head Injury Patients

Any assessment of the prognostic significance of hemorrhagic hypotension in severe head injury also requires attention to interactions of the blood pressure with the ICP. In a specific analysis of the US Traumatic Coma Data Bank findings, Marmarou et al. [27] investigated in 428 cases the impact of both low blood pressure and intracranial hypertension with regard to patient outcome (Glasgow Outcome Scale at 6 months). A sophisticated methodology was utilized for that purpose, i.e., a stepwise ordinal logistic regression for identification of descriptors of a poor outcome. Major prognostic determinants were the pupil response on admission to the hospital, the proportion of the temporary increases of the ICP above 20 mm Hg at hourly readings, as well as the frequency and duration of periods with decreases in the systemic blood pressure (<80 mm Hg). The individual contribution of these partly interacting factors determining cerebral perfusion pressure was selectively analyzed, elucidating the specific influence of a high ICP vs a low blood pressure. Accordingly, a low blood pressure alone (i.e., without elevation of ICP) increasingly contributed to poor outcome once it decreased below 80 mm Hg. Such a threshold could also be recognized for the ICP rise. The frequency of a poor outcome started to increase (without low blood pressure) once an ICP threshold of 20 mm Hg was reached and eventually passed [27].

The enormous significance of intracranial hypertension for the outcome in severe head injury was already recognized by the clinical observations of the late Douglas Miller et al. [28]. The authors observed that in approximately 50% of patients dying from severe head injury intracranial hypertension could not be therapeutically controlled. Thus, intracranial hypertension as well as arterial hypotension constitute the most important determinants of secondary cerebral ischemia in severe head injury.

Cardiovascular Stabilization in Severe Head Injury

It is obvious from the above that establishing cardiovascular function by volume replacement and surgical hemostasis is of greatest significance in head injury. As to the fluid resuscitation in patients with hemorrhagic shock and "unstable circulatory conditions" evidence has been provided, however, that a vigorous volume therapy on the scene may adversely affect outcome [29]. This is attributed to an additional secondary blood loss from injured organs (e.g., liver, spleen) once the blood pressure rises again by the infusion regimen. Such a situation is exemplary for the preclinical management dilemma of either "scoop and run" or "stay and play".

This being as it is, normalization of the blood pressure >80 mm Hg [cf. 27] in severe head injury is certainly one of the most important objectives of the prehospital emergency care, together with of course maintenance or reestablishment of respiration. When using electrolyte solutions such as Ringer's lactate, a major problem in efficient fluid resuscitation in severe hemorrhagic shock is, however, that enormous amounts must be infused in the shortest possible time – practically an impossible requirement. An interesting alternative is provided by the "small volume resuscitation" fluids [30–33], i.e., mixtures of hypertonic saline (e.g., 7.2% NaCl) and hyperoncotic colloids, such as 10% Dextran 60. No other infusion regimen normalizes cardiac output in severe hemorrhagic shock as efficiently and promptly. A major advantage is that, independent of the lost blood volume, only a small bolus of fluid is required, i.e., 4 ml/kg bw, which can be rapidly administered. Actually, infusion of only 10% of the volume of the shed blood suffices to nearly normalize cardiac output and markedly increase systemic blood pressure. Such an amount can be infused within minutes. The efficacy of this treatment modality is explained by the hypertonic–oncotic components immediately attracting water from the extravascular compartments into blood vessels, remaining there for a while as it is bound to the colloid component. It is, however, recommended that administration of the "small volume resuscitation" bolus is always followed by infusion of isotonic fluids (electrolytes, colloids). This is not only to enhance the therapeutic effect on the blood volume but also for dilution of the hypernatremic blood plasma.

The impressive effectiveness of the "small volume resuscitation" treatment in hemorrhagic shock notwithstandig, apprehensions have been raised as to potential side effects, if the blood–brain barrier is damaged. Under these circumstances hypertonic fluid might enter the brain parenchyma enhancing traumatic brain edema. This question has been intensively examined in various experimental programs of this laboratory. Schürer et al. [32] have assessed the rCBF and O_2 supply of the brain in rabbits with and without hemorrhagic shock and infusion of hypertonic-hyperoncotic saline–dextran (7.2 NaCl/10% dextran 60). Hemorrhagic shock by withdrawal of approximately one third of the circulating blood volume resulted in a blood pressure of 40 mm Hg for 30 min. Infusion of hypertonic–oncotic NaCl/dextran (4 ml/kg bw) afforded rapid normalization of cardiac output and a marked recovery of the systemic blood pressure. Cardiac output was studied by an electromagnetic flow probe around the pulmonary artery, while rCBF by H_2 clearance at the brain surface, and the cerebral O_2 supply by a multiwire PO_2 electrode according to Kessler et al. [34].

Infusion of small volume resuscitation fluid significantly increased cerebral perfusion in animals with shock ($p < 0.01$), although hemorrhagic hypotension (blood pressure 40 mm Hg) before treatment did not affect rCBF. On the other hand, rCBF remained unchanged in the normovolemic control animals also receiving hypertonic–oncotic saline–dextran. The maintenance of cerebral blood flow during shock may explain why the cerebral O_2 supply measured by registration of the regional PO_2 at the brain surface was not significantly changed, although the frequency of "hypoxic" PO_2 (<5 mm Hg) values in hemorrhagic shock increased from 5% (normovolemic control) to 10.6%. Hypertonic saline–dextran also led to recovery of this parameter at 60 and 120 min after treatment. Since, however, rCBF was increased by the fluid regimen above the control level prior to exsanguination from 50 ml/100 g per minute (control) to ca. 60 ml/100 g per minute (after treatment), enhancement of vasogenic edema cannot be ruled out once the blood–brain barrier is broken. This aspect was scrutinized by additional experiments utilizing a corresponding protocol in animals with an additional focal brain trauma (cold injury).

Hypertonic Fluid Resuscitation in the Presence of an Open Blood–Brain Barrier

Former observations have already indicated that infusion of "small volume resuscitation" fluid does not enhance posttraumatic brain edema at 24 h after trauma [35]. Experiments were carried out in this laboratory to elucidate whether hypertonic-oncotic saline–dextran enhances brain edema within 4 h in animals with a focal brain lesion and hemorrhagic shock in addition [36]. Briefly, albino rabbits (2.6–3.5 kg bw) were anesthesized and paralyzed for artificial ventilation. The skull was trephined for the measurement of rCBF by H_2 clearance. A cryogenic lesion according to Klatzo [37] was then made at the left parietal brain surface by a stainless steel cylinder filled with a dry ice–acetone mixture at a temperature of −68°C. The brain lesion was followed by withdrawal of approximately one third of the circulating blood volume to lower blood pressure to 40 mm Hg for 30 min. The shock period was terminated by infusion of hypertonic–oncotic saline–dextran (4 ml/kg bw) within 2 min. Additional infusions (e.g., isotonic fluid) were not administered. Administration of the hypertonic–oncotic fluid bolus was thus made at 60 min after induction of the focal brain lesion, corresponding to the preclinical situation of fluid resuscitation. Formation of brain edema was assessed by measurements of the specific gravity of cortical and white matter tissue samples. The specific gravity (SG) was determined by a Percoll-density gradient after slicing the brain hemispheres into 2 × 4 × 4-mm blocks, which were placed onto the surface of the gradient column. Based on the SG data of cerebral cortex and white matter a topographical SG distribution map of the brain was established, indicating spread of vasogenic brain edema from the site of the lesion. Animals with trauma (without additional shock or fluid infusion) had the highest water content in grey matter in the lesion and in perifocal white matter. Infusion of hypertonic saline–dextran alone (without trauma or shock) did not significantly affect the brain water content in these areas, but appeared to inhibit spread of edema from the lesion into the surrounding grey and white matter.

Altogether, the experimental data rule out that hypertonic–oncotic saline–dextran administered in the critical early posttraumatic period in severe head injury in patients with hemorrhagic shock enhances traumatic brain edema [36]. It is, therefore, concluded that this treatment, which is unmatched to normalize cardiac output and blood pressure in severe hemorrhagic shock, does not adversely affect the formation of traumatic brain edema nor the cerebral blood and O_2 supply in patients with head injury. On the contrary, it can be expected that the risk of secondary cerebral ischemia from arterial hypotension is substantially reduced by the rapid recovery of cardiac output and systemic blood pressure. Beneficial effects of this treatment concept have been confirmed in additional studies demonstrating that hypertonic–oncotic saline–dextran is nearly as effective as hypertonic mannitol to lower the ICP in the presence of an intracranial space-occupying process [38].

Avoidable Factors Involved in Secondary Brain Damage from Severe Head Injury

A delicate issue is the contribution of avoidable complications to an adverse outcome in severe head injury. A clear identification is nevertheless required in order to attenuate or even eliminate their impact by adjustments of the organization and logistics of patient management. This, however, necessitates a careful analysis of the causes and mechanisms involved. The problem of avoidable factors in severe head injury has been recognized for quite a while [17], yet only few investigations have been made, probably for obvious reasons. A significant study has been conducted in the United Kingdom based on retrospective assessment of patient records [20]. In children with head injury with a fatal outcome coroners' reports were analyzed in a large northern region of England covering the period 1979–1989 during which altogether 25 134 children died. The authors attempted to identify the frequency of avoidable complications in a subgroup of 255 children with fatal outcome from severe head injury. Of the young patients 19% were a priori admitted to a neurosurgical department, whereas the remaining 81% intermittently to a general trauma hospital followed by secondary transport to a neurosurgical department. Avoidable complications probably determining outcome were found in 81 patients, i.e., in approximately one third of all fatal cases during this period. The most important were:

- Failure of appropriate diagnosis
- Delayed recognition of an intracranial bleeding
- Delayed recognition of peripheral injuries

- Inadequate airway managment and/or aspiration, and finally
- Poor management of patient transfer between hospitals.

In view of the above considerations on preclinical patient management one result is of major significance, namely that avoidable factors occurred in 22% of cases during the prehospital rescue phase, whereas in no less than 42% after hospital admission. This demonstrates that in an apparently better controlled environment, as for example in a trauma center with an emergency room (shock room), an intensive care unit and other facilities, avoidable complications are by no means a smaller problem than under preclinical conditions.

Respective conclusions can be drawn from an intrahospital study on the incidence of adverse events in the care of head injury patients [19]. A group of 50 patients was prospectively observed with regard to the development of secondary insults during intrahospital transport, for example from the intensive care unit to the computed tomography (CT) scan. The patients were in a severity range of <8 points to >12 points on the Glasgow Coma Score. The study cases were intensively monitored during intrahospital transfer, including ICP, arterial pCO_2, systemic blood pressure, and jugular venous O_2 saturation. A number of abnormal changes occurred as given in their order of frequency:

- Arterial hypertension
- Arterial hypotension
- Intracranial hypertension, and
- Cerebral hypoxia.

Most importantly, almost 90% of all patients had at some point during intrahospital transfer one or more of the above events [19].

Results emerging from these retrospective and prospective assessments of complications being avoidable or not in severe head injury and their significance for outcome highlight the fact that the whole system of patient management and organization, including the prehospital rescue phase, should repeatedly be subjected to an efficiency control to discover and, if necessary, correct shortcomings. In essence, the medical treatment of secondary brain damage by specific antagonization of, e.g., mediator mechanisms including brain protection, might benefit the patient only if all components of patient management are executed on an optimal level.

Analysis of Organization and Logistics of Patient Management

The challenge of improving outcome in head injury is enormous as well as complex as it requires not only more effective, specific forms of medical treatment, but also perfect organization and management of the patient in the prehospital emergency phase as well as on admission to hospital. It encompasses, among others, an up-to-date communication and transportation network, professional dispatch and rescue services, cooperation and interaction of the medical and non-medical staff at the scene, comprehensive patient monitoring during the prehospital phase and, most importantly, prompt referral to a competent neurotrauma center with experienced neurosurgeons and the necessary diagnostic equipment. The attention given to a head injury patient during prehospital care must not decrease on admission to hospital. The early phase of clinical management in severe head injury is as critical as the preclinical resuscitation, as delays in recognition and correction of life-threatening complications, such as hypovolemic shock, pulmonary hypoventilation, cerebral herniation, or other confounding factors, impairing the blood and oxygen supply to the brain further increase damage to the injured brain. Pre- and early clinical management personnel must be aware that a head injury patient is in an unstable dynamic situation, liable to change at any moment into a hopeless catastrophic condition and, thus, need to be continuously alert and ready. Obviously, the advanced management of severe head injury patients is comprehensive and complex as medical care is not restricted to diagnosis and surgical or medical treatment. The care system comprises much more. In view of these considerations, careful assessment ("system analysis") of all major components involved in the management of head injury patients beginning at the scene of an accident seems to be mandatory.

For that purpose a study group has been established at the University of Munich as part of a research consortium "Neurotraumatologie und Neuropsychologische Rehabilitation" in Munich, which is supported by the German Federal Department of Education, Technology, and Research [39]. The objective of this project is a comprehensive analysis of "state of the art" logistics and organization of head injury patient management in the prehospital and early clinical phase. Pertinent yard sticks include outcome-relevant time intervals of providing life-saving care, monitoring the patient at the scene, during transport, and after admission to the hospital. Recording all this relevant information for evaluation of the management efficiency is carried out by specially trained documentation assistants who escort the rescue team upon dispatch of the emergency vehicle to the site of an accident utilizing a specifically designed protocol. Their assignment does not involve providing medical care in order not to interfere with the quality of the prospective documentation. The colleague on duty also escorts the patient in the ambulance helicopter to the hospital, assuming responsibility for a smooth transition of the documentation procedure during early clinical care.

It is hoped that, by establishing this elaborate manpower-dependent protocol mechanism, it will be possible to gather valid information on important details of patient management and its organization and logistics which are not obtained by evaluation of routine protocols completed by the rescue team or routine personnel in the hospital, sometimes according to memory. Emerging data from this stady may be useful for a variety of purposes, such as identification of avoidable complications, faulty management design, and/or shortage of care capacity. In addition, the study logistics established for the above assessment might also be useful for prospective controlled trials on specific treatment measures.

Acknowledgments. The secretarial assistance of Helga Kleylein and Edith Martin in the preparation of this manuscript is gratefully acknowledged.

This work was supported by the Bundesministerium für Bildung und Forschung, Verbund "Neurotrauma" München, Grant No. 01 K0 9402.

References

1. Runyan CW, Gerken EA (1989) Epidemiology and prevention of adolescent injury. A review and research agenda. JAMA 262:2273–2279
2. Jennett B (1996) Epidemiology of head injury. J Neurol Neurosurg Psychiatr 60:362–369
3. Statistisches Bundesamt (1993) VII-D M, Fachserie 12 Gesundheitswesen, Reihe 4. Statistisches Bundesamt, Wiesbaden
4. Baethmann A, Go KG, Unterberg A (eds) (1986) Mechanisms of secondary brain damage. Plenum, New York (NATO ASI series A: Life sciences, vol 115)
5. Baethmann A, Kempski O, Plesnila N, Staub F (eds) (1996) Mechanisms of secondary brain damage in cerebral ischemia and trauma. Acta Neurochir Suppl (Wien) 66
6. Reilly PL, Adams JH, Graham DI, Jennett B (1975) Patients with head injury who talk and die. Lancet 2:375–377
7. Ommaya AK, Gennarelli TA (1974) Cerebral concussion and traumatic unconsciousness – correlation of experimental and clinical observations on blunt head injuries. Brain 97:633–654
8. Strich SJ (1976) Cerebral trauma. In: Blackwood W, Corsellis JAN (eds) Greenfield's neuropathology. Arnold, London, pp 327–360
9. Adams JH, Graham DI, Scott G, Parker LS, Doyle D (1980) Brain damage in fatal non-missile head injury. J Clin Pathol 33:1132–1145
10. Adams JH, Graham DI, Gennarelli TA (1986) Primary brain damage in non-missile head injury. In: Baethmann A, Go KG, Unterberg A (eds) Mechanisms of secondary brain damage. Plenum, New York, pp 1–13 (NATO ASI series A: Life sciences, vol 115)
11. Gennarelli TA, Adams JH, Graham DI (1986) Diffuse axonal injury – a new conceptional approach to an old problem. In: Baethmann A, Go KG, Unterberg A (eds) Mechanisms of secondary brain damage. Plenum, New York, pp 15–28 (NATO ASI series A: Life sciences, vol 115)
12. Povlishock JT, Jenkins LW (1995) Are the pathobiological changes evoked by traumatic brain injury immediate and irreversible? Brain Pathol 5:415–426
13. Povlishock JT, Pettus EH (1996) Traumatically induced axonal damage: evidence for enduring changes in axolemmal permeability with associated cytoskeletal change. Acta Neurochir Suppl (Wien) 66:81–86
14. Graham DI, Adams JH, Doyle D (1978) Ischaemic brain damage in fatal non-missile head injuries. J Neurol Sci 39:213–234
15. Graham DI, Ford J, Adams JH, Doyle D, Teasdale GM, Lawrence AE, Mc Lellan DR (1989) Ischaemic brain damage is still common in fatal non-missile head injury. J Neurol Neurosurg Psychiatr 52:346–350
16. Bullock R (1992) Introducing NMDA antagonists into clinical practice: why head injury trials? Br J Clin Pharmacol 34:396–401
17. Jennett B, Teasdale G (1981) Management of head injuries. Davis, Philadelphia (Contemporary neurology series, vol 20)
18. Jennett B (1992) Minimising brain damage from head injury by appropriate early management. In: von Steinbüchel N, von Cramon DY, Pöppel E (eds) Neuropsychological rehabilitation. Springer, Berlin Heidelberg New York, pp 139–145
19. Andrews PJD, Piper IR, Dearden NM, Miller JD (1990) Secondary insults during intrahospital transport of head-injured patients. Lancet 335:327–330
20. Sharples PM, Storey A, Aynsley-Green A, Eyre JA (1990) Avoidable factors contributing to death of children with head injury. Brit Med J 300:87–91
21. Foulkes MA, Eisenberg HM, Jane JA, Marmarou A, Marshall LF and the Traumatic Coma Data Bank Research Group (1991) The Traumatic Coma Data Bank: design, methods, and baseline characteristics. J Neurosurg 75:S8–S13
22. Marshall LF, Gautille T, Klauber MR, Eisenberg HM, Jane JA, Luerssen TG, Marmarou A, Foulkes MA (1991) The outcome of severe closed head injury. J Neurosurg 75:S28–S36
23. Michaud LJ, Rivara FP, Grady MS, Reay DT (1992) Predictors of survival and severity of disability after severe brain injury in children. Neurosurgery 31:254–264

24. Piek J, Chesnut RM, Marshall LF, van Berkum-Clark M, Klauber MR, Blunt B, Eisenberg HM, Jane JA, Marmarou A, Foulkes MA (1992) Extracranial complications of severe head injury. J Neurosurg 77:901–907
25. DeWitt DS, Prough DS, Taylor CL, Whitley JM, Deal DD, Vines SM (1992) Regional cerebrovascular responses to progressive hypotension after traumatic brain injury in cats. Am J Physiol 363:H1276–H1284
26. Yuan XQ, Wade CE (1991) Influence of traumatic brain injury on the outcomes of delayed and repeated hemorrhages. Circ Shock 35:231–236
27. Marmarou A, Anderson RL, Ward JD, Choi SC, Young HF, Eisenberg HM, Foulkes MA, Marshall LF, Jane JA (1991) Impact of ICP instability and hypotension on outcome in patients with severe head head trauma. J Neurosurg 75:S59–S66
28. Miller JD, Becker DP, Ward JD, Sullivan HG, Adams WE, Rosner MJ (1977) Significance of intracranial hypertension in severe head injury. J Neurosurg 47:503–516
29. Bickell WH, Wall MJ, Pepe PE, Martin RR, Ginger VF, Allen MK, Mattox KL (1994) Immediate versus delayed fluid resuscitation for hypotensive patients with penetrating torso injuries. N Engl J Med 331:1105–1109
30. Kramer GC, Perron PR, Lindsey DC, Ho HS, Gunther RA, Boyle WA, Holcroft JW (1986) Small-volume resuscitation with hypertonic saline dextran. Surgery 100:239–247
31. Kreimeier U, Meßmer K (1987) New perspectives in resuscitation and prevention of multiple organ system failure. In: Baethmann A, Meßmer K (eds) Surgical research: recent concepts and results. Springer, Berlin Heidelberg New York, pp 39–50
32. Schürer L, Dautermann C, Härtl R, Murr R, Berger S, Röhrich F, Meßmer K, Baethmann A (1992) Treatment of hemorrhagic hypotension with hypertonic/hyperoncotic solutions: effects on regional cerebral blood flow and brain surface oxygen tension. Eur Surg Res 24:1–12
33. Holcroft JW, Vassar MJ, Turner JE, Derlet RW, Kramer GC (1987) 3% NaCl and 7.5% NaCl/dextran-70 in the resuscitation of severely injured patients. Ann Surg 206:279–288
34. Kessler M, Höper J, Krumme BA (1976) Monitoring of tissue perfusion and cellular function. Anesthesiology 45:184–197
35. Walsh JC, Zhuang J, Shackford SR (1991) A comparison of hypertonic to isotonic fluid in the resuscitation of brain injury and hemorrhagic shock. J Surg Res 50:284–292
36. Härtl R, Schürer L, Götz C, Berger S, Röhrich F, Baethmann A (1995) The effect of hypertonic fluid resuscitation on brain edema in rabbits subjected to brain injury and hemorrhagic shock. Shock 3:274–279
37. Klatzo I (1967) Neuropathological aspects of brain edema (Presidential address). J Neuropathol Exp Neurol 26:1–14
38. Berger S, Schürer L, Härtl R, Meßmer K, Baethmann A (1995) Reduction of post-traumatic intracranial hypertension by hypertonic/hyperoncotic saline/dextran and hypertonic mannitol. Neurosurgery 37:98–108
39. Lehr D, Baethmann A, Reulen H-J, Steiger H-J, Huf R, Stummer W, Wirth A et al (1996) Management of patients with severe head injury in the preclinical phase – a prospective analysis. J Trauma (in press)

Discussion

Regel:
My question to you is: You mentioned that it is very important that you have an early diagnosis of hypoxia and of hypotension, so what is the monitoring system that you use; what do you prefer?

Baethmann:
The specific purpose is to uncover the development of cerebral ischemia or hypoxia as early as possible, which are separately mentioned here. An increasingly used

method is assessment of the jugular vein O_2 saturation, which still has some problems, and a recent development, near-infrared spectroscopy through the intact skull of the brain. I fear infrared spectroscopy is not yet a routine method, whereas the measurement of O_2 saturation in the jugular bulb in a variety of centers seems to have become routine. Of course, there are also indirect measures indicating whether the brain is at risk of ischemia. Particularly, the monitoring of ICP should be mentioned. More or less all advanced centers do ICP monitoring nowadays, and you can extrapolate that, if the ICP is increased and if this occurs for some duration, this sooner or later causes cerebral ischemia, particularly in traumatic brain injury with impaired cerebrovascular autoregulation.

Schlag:
I think the problem in polytrauma is that the hypoxia in the brain is not diffuse, it is distributed in certain areas, because otherwise it would be easy to measure the hypoxia just by the PO_2 in the brain. If there is a certain level of decreased blood pressure (40 mm Hg), then there is the possibility of ischemia and ischemic insult and the question is now, is it really so localized or is it more diffuse?

Regel:
Do you measure the tissue oxygen in your baboon experiments in the brain, and where do you measure it? Do you measure it directly in the environment of the primary insult?

Schlag:
I just want to point out that these baboons do not have a traumatic insult, they just have hemorrhagic shock. And even with the hemorrhagic shock we get distinct areas in the brain, that is also my question to Dr. Baethmann: Do you know some reports in the literature of severe hemorrhagic shock or traumatic hemorrhagic shock without brain injury, without ischemia in the brain or encephalomalacia in patients? Do you recall a report?

Baethmann:
I do not really recall whether in patients without brain damage respective measurements were made in hemorrhagic shock. If the brain is not damaged, it has a very powerful mechanism available to ensure its perfusion and O_2 supply by the cerebrovascular autoregulation, as long as the perfusion pressure, say the mean arterial blood pressure, is not below 60 or 55 mm Hg. However, once the brain is even minimally damaged, this capacity is impaired. Then even a moderate decrease of the systemic blood pressure may adversely affect brain perfusion.

Regel:
I just want to mention a study by Becker, I think, which showed even in multiple trauma patients without brain injury an effect on the Glasgow Outcome Scale.

Kossmann:
I want to congratulate Prof. Baethmann for his excellent contribution. He actually puts a lot of pressure on the clinicians.

Two things, first of all your last sentence, that you want the outcome to be actually dependent on the primary damage and to avoid secondary damage, and secondly, you showed very nicely how the first hours, the first minutes, are actually fundamental for the outcome. I think for myself as a trauma surgeon, it is very important to have a protocol on how to resuscitate these patients.

In my experience it is also very important to monitor patients with severe head trauma very early on, and we have to urge the clinicians to start monitoring these patients from the beginning and not on the second or third or fourth day when the patient is not waking up any more. So I think this is one of the things we should really work on, to give the people outside the research institutes something in their hands they can work with.

Baethmann:

I cannot agree more. Nowadays in Germany, as in other Western states, organization of the emergency systems is well developed. We have legally required time periods for the rescue team after alert, to be at the site of an accident within 10 or 12 min, which is usually met. The problem we have is that once a patient is stabilized at the scene to find the best possible center for referral. Not many centers are available with all necessary interdisciplinary departments, and often there is a shortage in intensive beds due to shortage in nursing staff. Recently, general trauma centers have increasingly available neurosurgical units with respective diagnostic facilities. We are currently conducting in the area of Munich, including smaller cities such as Augsburg and Murnau, a prospective and a retrospective analysis of the organization and management of prehospital and early hospital care in collaboration with many hospitals in these areas. The approach is mostly to document the various measures which are taken by employing a carefully worked out protocol. The time course, or time interval, when a patient is seen at the accident site after trauma, when he is intubated, stabilized for transport, etc., are highly interesting in this context. Based on this analysis we hope to obtain information on whether and where organization, logistics, management and other factors should be improved.

Kossmann:

We actually need very clear algorithms in the treatment of patients with severe traumatic brain injury. I have, for example, one experience myself. We had a traumatized patient coming in with a Glasgow Coma Scale <8, he was intubated then and in the first CT scan he did not have much. He also had a fractured femur. The first thing we did was to install an ICP device, then we stabilized his femur fracture. During this procedure his ICP rose, and then we rushed him back to the CT. He had developed an acute subdural hematoma and we could evacuate it without big problems. Ten days later this patient was sitting in bed reading the "Spiegel". This shows how important it is to control ICP immediately in order to avoid preventable death in the hospital, advocating that clinicians do an early ICP monitoring in patients with severe traumatic injury.

Sprung:

Just a comment about technology assessment. I think, around the room, we have physiologists, scientists and clinicians who desire more information which could help us understand the physiology of this disorder and do a better job to care for the patients. The question is: Have we to date and should we not in the future call not only for more physiological monitoring, be it ICP monitoring, jugular bulb saturation and the like, but call for studies to determine who are the patients who can really benefit, and who are the patients who cannot benefit from monitoring. We clearly monitor many patients in many different ways. I am not sure we have clearly identified the patients who benefit from the various types of monitoring or therapies. Until we in the clinical arena have done our job to determine which patients we can really help or not, just to call for the use of a lot more monitoring is not appropriate. In the future, as money becomes less available, unless we determine which patients will benefit from our monitoring, we may not be able to afford to monitor the patients who will really benefit.

Shackford:
I would like to raise two issues, one in response to Dr. Sprung. I think there are some patients that we can identify who would benefit from early ICP monitoring. I come from an area which is very rural and we frequently get patients who are transported for an hour or an hour and a half from the referral hospital. It would be immensely important for us to know the ICP so that patients with increased ICP can be treated. If an ICP monitor is placed and the ICP is normal, no treatment for increased ICP is needed. On the other hand, if the ICP is elevated, then hyperventilation or osmotherapy can be used to lower the ICP during transport.

The second issue I would raise is the one about hypovolemic shock in the absence of brain injury. Most of the patients that we take care of clinically who are in shock, even profound hypovolemic shock, do not develop cerebral blood flow which is below the ischemic threshold of 20 cc/100 min. There are occasional patients who are in such profound shock that cerebral blood flow is below the ischemic threshold. They are models of occlusive cerebral ischemia. One of the first patients that I ever took care of got me interested in this. I cared for a patient that was hit by a train who had partial traumatic amputations of both lower extremities. On admission, the patient had no blood pressure. We resuscitated the patient and amputated both legs in the resuscitation area. After resuscitation the patient was communicating with us. He had no brain injury on CT scan. We put in an ICP monitor, his ICP was 12, and in 36 h the patient's ICP precipitously rose, and the patient herniated with a severe reperfusion injury. So I think that, very rarely, profound hypovolemic shock will set up a model of occlusive cerebral ischemia, because cerebral blood flow goes below the ischemic threshold. Most of the shock patients that we take care of, in the absence of brain injury, do not develop cerebral blood flow which goes below the ischemic threshold.

Baethmann:
May I come back to the point of Dr. Sprung on which patient benefits from monitoring? As far as jugular vein O_2 saturation and other more novel technologies are concerned, an answer is difficult, whereas I am convinced that monitoring of ICP has improved the management of head injury patients. Almost all treatment currently administered in head injury patients is concerned with the management of ICP. For that purpose, ICP monitoring is indispensable, irrespective of whether such a patient eventually has a good or bad outcome.

The Processes Involved in Traumatic Axonal Injury

T.A. GENNARELLI, D.I. GRAHAM, and L.E. THIBAULT

Introduction

Brain injury can be viewed as several clinical syndromes that result from various combinations of neural or vascular events occurring after mechanical distortion of the head. The primary traumatic events appear to be mediated by four basic mechanisms, the consequences of which are not instantaneous. Thus, brain injury involves processes that are set in motion at the time of head injury, but may require hours or days for completion. These four mechanisms of cellular dysfunction are receptor dysfunction, free radical effects, inflammatory events, and calcium-mediated damage and they have the potential for causing delayed cell dysfunction or delayed cellular death. These events, depending on whether they are primarily to the neural or vascular tissues, may produce additional events or epiphenomena, such as brain swelling, cerebral edema, and increased intracranial pressure (see Fig. 1). These types of events are similar in focal and diffuse brain injuries, but their effects may appear to be different because of a different mixture of neural versus vascular tissue involvement, and because of a different combination of the four principal mechanisms of cell damage. This paper addresses the manner in which axons are damaged after injury by these mechanisms.

Origins of the Concept of Diffuse Axonal Injury as a Traumatic Entity

When the term diffuse axonal injury (DAI) was first utilized in the early 1980s, it provided an appealing explanation for the pathophysiology that occurred in the types of diffuse brain trauma in which little or no macroscopically-visible pathologic changes were present [1,2]. Subsequent to the initial definition, axonal damage was found to be present in human minor head injury, in human concussion, as well as in experimental minor head injury using acceleration or percussion concussion systems [3]. Additionally, in severe head injury, axonal damage was reported to have a 44% incidence in a large series, and axonal damage was associated with a 33% mortality. It should be pointed out that at that time, patients with severe diffuse brain injury (coma lasting longer than 6h, with no mass lesions to explain it) was considered, by definition, to be DAI [4]. Pathological series of nonsurvivors demonstrated axonal damage in 34% of all head injury deaths, and in 53% of deaths that occurred after 12h of survival. Additionally, it was found that diffuse axonal injury was the greatest

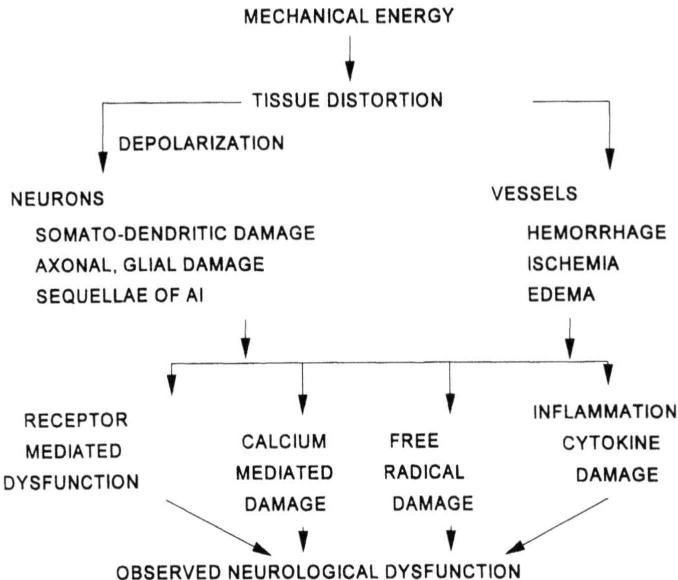

Fig. 1. Major events in the pathophysiology of traumatic brain injury

contributor to patients who survived and later died in a vegetative or severely impaired existence [5] and, more recently, axonal damage was found to be almost universally present after fatal head injury [6].

As originally described, diffuse axonal injury was used as a pathophysiological descriptor of a condition that was, in the early 1980s, known by numerous synonyms. These include diffuse damage to white matter, shearing injury, diffuse white matter shearing injury, central brain damage, diffuse brain injury, etc. However, as the concept of axonal damage and diffuse brain injury matured, the overriding hypothesis was that a spectrum of injuries occurred, all due to the same axonal pathology, but differing in amount, location and severity of axonal damage. Thus, it was postulated that, as physiological disturbances of function became more severely altered, there was a progressively larger amount of axonal damage. It therefore became possible to conceive of the spectrum of events that began with concussive syndromes and ended in the severe form of brain impairment which included promptly appearing coma associated with decerebrate posturing, long-lasting coma, and incomplete recovery. Thus, it was conceived that diffuse brain injury was a spectrum from a smaller to a larger amount of axonal damage associated with smaller and greater functional disturbance, similar to what had been previously described as concussive injuries [7].

This concept was also supported by pathological analysis from human nonsurvivors, as well as from experimental DAI in animals [1,2]. A pathological distribution of the severity of DAI was then proposed. Three grades were recognized; the first, DAI grade I was the least severe and was characterized by widespread abnormality of axonal morphology in the white matter of the cerebral hemispheres; in grade II DAI, there were, in addition to white matter axonal damage, similar axonal abnormalities in the corpus callosum, often associated with small hemorrhages which were called tissue tear hemorrhages (TTH). Grade III DAI, the most severe, had, in addition to the findings of grade II DAI, axonal abnormalities, and commonly, TTH, in the brainstem, particularly in the dorsolateral quadrant of the dorsal midbrain.

These concepts were rather widely embraced by several scientific communities, particularly those in neuropathology and experimental neurotrauma. It soon became evident, however, particularly because of the difficulty of making a clinical diagnosis objectively, that the finding of axonal damage was, at times, not associated with the clinical conditions originally proposed. Thus, it was observed that TTH seen on computed tomography (CT) scan could be found in conditions other than those associated with prompt, prolonged coma. It was further recognized that immediate coma was not always required to find the pathological spectrum, of at least grade I, DAI [8]. Other investigators began to use the term DAI for any finding of a morphologically abnormal axon, particularly if retraction bulbs were identified. It appears, however, that, although bulbs represent the worst condition of axotomy after injury, there are less severe types of traumatic axonal damage. This paper reviews the major types of traumatic axonal injury.

Types of Axonal Damage in the Brain

It must be recognized that all traumatic axonal damage may not be part of the DAI complex. Since the name diffuse axonal injury was coined, many have used this term to represent any condition in which axonal retraction bulbs are found. Confusion now exists regarding the clinical pathological syndrome of DAI which we defined as immediate, deep and prolonged coma not due to mass lesions and associated with widespread axonal damage. This definition was proposed at a time when no other alternative explanations were available to explain the clinical status of deep prolonged coma and when we recognized pathological gradations that appeared to be well correlated to the depth and duration of coma and to the quality of recovery in survivors. Soon, we and others began to recognize conditions with lesser amounts of axonal damage and it became clear that widespread axonal damage, albeit of lesser degree, could be present without instantaneous, deep or prolonged coma. Furthermore, new hypotheses, principally involving receptor mediated brain dysfuntion, appeared that possibly could provide alternate explanations for some phenomena of "diffuse brain injury" and the clinical syndromes that occurred [9]. Because the axonal damage is microscopic, the inability of diagnositic methods to objectively detect axonal damage was a limiting factor in the clinical categorization of diffuse brain injury, especially in survivors.

There are many types of axonal damage in the brain, all of which manifest as microscopic changes in axonal morphology. There appears to be a sequence of descriptive alterations that is common to many, if not all, types of axonal damage, similar to that first described by Cajal. The precise time-oriented presence of these changes may differ with the causal condition or the species, but, in general, first, irregular dilitations and increases in axonal diameters occur. These axonal swellings can be followed by retraction balls (bulbs) or axonal spheroids, the hallmark of axotomy in the brain. Once formed, the appearance of retraction balls does not appear to be different in various circumstances (although this has not yet been thoroughly documented by immunohistochemical methods), thus suggesting that this appearance represents a final common response to axonal damage caused by a variety of chemical, genetic, vascular, neoplastic or traumatic stimuli.

Clearly, traumatic axonal damage is not the only cause of axonal swellings or retraction balls (see Table 1). In fact, for many years, what is now recognized as DAI was argued to be a response to cerebral ischemia and not due to trauma. The reason is that neuropathologists have for quite some time recognized that retraction balls can arise in non-traumatic circumstances.

It should be noted, however, that not all axonal damage is to be equated with the term DAI. Many conditions not associated with trauma can produce axonal abnormalities of a morphology identical to that seen in traumatic conditions. These could be divided into two types: secondary and primary nontraumatic axonal damage. Secondary nontraumatic axonal damage is regularly seen associated with, or at the periphery of, cerebral infarctions of any cause, cerebral ischemia, brain abscesses, and many varieties of brain tumor. Primary axonal damage is seen in association with the normal aging process, with various intoxications, and with a class of primary axonal dysfunctions known as the neuroaxonal dystrophies (NAD). The latter was divided by Seitelberger into six categories that include: infantile NAD (Seitelberger's disease), late infantile NAD, juvenile generalized NAD, Hallervorden–Spatz disease, neuroaxonal leukoencephalopathy, and pre-senile NAD. Other primary non-traumatic types of axonal damage are seen in perinatal, periventricular leukomalacia, and in nutritional deficiencies, particularly those associated with deficiency of vitamin E. Severe forms of thiamin deficiency and Wernicke's encephalopathy can also be associated with primary axonal damage.

Table 1. Types of axonal damage in the brain

Primary axonal damage
  Non-traumatic
    Aging
    Primary axonal dystrophies
    Intoxications
  Traumatic
    Regional
    Diffuse (DAI)
Secondary axonal damage
  Non-traumatic
    Infarction
    Ischemia
    Abcess
    Tumor
  Traumatic
    Contusion
    Intracerabral hemorrhage
    Infarction

Numerous CNS intoxications also cause primary axonal damage. These include triorthocrecyl phosphate (TOCP), a plasticizer; iminodi-proprionitrile (IDPN), an agent which slows axonal transport; and the amoebicide clioquinol. Finally, some types of paraneoplastic cerebellar degeneration are associated with axonal damage as well.

Traumatic axonal damage, similarly, is not all associated with DAI. Secondary axonal damage may be produced secondary to other conditions seen with traumatic injury. These, similar to secondary nontraumatic axonal damage, may occur around contusions, intracerebral hemorrhages, infarctions or regions of ischemia. These conditions must be distinguished from primary traumatic axonal damage, which is seen not in association with any of the other conditions. Not all primary traumatic axonal damage is DAI, either. In some cases, only a few abnormal axons are seen in one, or perhaps two, distant regions. These may be best described as regional traumatic axonal damage, in distinction to the true condition of diffuse axonal injury, in which primary traumatic axonal damage is rather widespread throughout the brain. Of course, it is not homogeneously distributed, and in fact is usually more intense in some areas than in others. It is not present in absolutely every region of the brain, but the preponderance of damage is scattered sufficiently through the brain to warrant the term diffuse.

The general causes of axonal damage, whether primary or secondary, or traumatic or nontraumatic, are numerous and include: impairment of axoplasmic transport, such as occurs in IDPN intoxication; cytoskeletal damage, such as is present in many of the neuroaxonal dystrophies; and damage to the cell body, such as is probably the case in vitamin E deficiency. The causes of primary axonal damage, whether traumatic or nontraumatic, involve a disturbance within the axon itself, and can be thus viewed as equivalent to internal axonal disturbances. Secondary axonal damage, whether traumatic or nontraumatic can be viewed not as an internal, but rather as an external, influence on the axon.

Pathophysiology of Axonal Damage: Gradations of Severity of Damage to Axons

Traumatic axonal damage can be viewed as having four principal stages, each of increasing severity of damage. These are: (1) nodal membrane injury; (2) reversible cytoskeletal damage; (3) secondary axotomy; and (4) primary axotomy.

Stage I Axonal Injury: Nodal Ionic Fluxes

Because of the morphologic construction of most axons, it was originally felt that the node of Ranvier is the structurally weakest portion of the myelinated axon and that, therefore, mechanical perturbation involving stretching of the axon would most easily injure the node of Ranvier. Work in the unmyelinated giant axon of the squid and subsequently in the myelinated single sciatic nerve axon of the rat, as well as electron micrographic studies in stretch-injured optic nerve in the guinea pig, have corroborated the node of Ranvier as the principal, but not the sole, site of mechanical distortion of the axon [10]. In addition to the node of Ranvier, the paranodal region can be primarily damaged. These studies have demonstrated that there is a relationship between the amount of axonal stretch and the amount of axonal dysfunction. If an axon is stretched less than 15%–20% of its resting length (15%–20% strain), the axon usually will not tear, but will undergo various types of alteration of its function. At the lowest level of strain (5% or less), ionic influx of various species occurs and causes failure of the generation and propagation of action potentials. The ionic influxes of particularly sodium, calcium and chloride, and the efflux of potassium, at this level of injury, are fully restored in a matter of minutes, and the damaged axon recovers is function completely.

A new concept, that of *mechanoporation,* has recently been proposed to explain this initial event [11]. The development of transient defects in the cell membrane that are due to its mechanical deformation has been shown experimentally and analytically to explain the magnitude and kinetics of the brief ionic fluxes than are promptly restored. The defects or mechanically induced pores are usually transient, but occasionally may reach metastable conditions associated with long-lasting membrane leakage (see Stage II below). Because of its large gradient (10 000 : 1), calcium ion flux has been of particular interest and, based on direct intracellular measurements using either selective microelectrodes or fluorescent dyes, the magnitude and duration of rise of intracellular Ca^{+2} correlates well with pore theory and with axonal dysfunction.

Stage II Axonal Injury: Reversible Cytoskeletal Damage

If the level of axonal stretch is in the 5%–10% range, then additional ionic perturbations are associated with fluid fluxes to maintain osmotic balance. This causes local swelling and enlargement of the injured axon, and, perhaps, mild impairment of axoplasmic transport [12]. In an optic nerve stretch injury model, approximately 17% of the axons were found to be enlarged by 3 days after injury. Very few of these seemed to undergo secondary axotomy, and most recovered electrophysiologically [13]. Local architectural changes may also occur, such as membrane blebbing described at the node of Ranvier. It is apparant, however, that the overall disturbance of axonal cytoarchitecture is small and, thus, restitution of structure and function is expected.

Stage III Axonal Injury: Conditions Leading to Secondary Axotomy

At this level of injury, associated with a 15%–20% strain, sufficient ionic imbalance occurs so that the axoplasm cannot fully restore ionic and osmotic homeostatisis and as a consequence, numerous physiological and morphological changes begin. There may be an inability to buffer, extrude or bind intracellular calcium and the excess calcium load initiates autodestructive processes during which calcium-activated neutral proteases (CANPs, or calpains) are activated. Calpains have as their substrates the cytoskeletal proteins within the axon, and thus proteolysis of neurotubules, microtubule-associated proteins, fodrin (a subaxolemma structural protein) and neurofilaments begins. The dissolution of these structural components begins to impair axoplasmic transport locally and, as a consequence, accumulation of transported materials occurs at sites of maximal cytoskeletal damage. Associated with the cytoskeletal damage is membrane damage that occurs from lipolysis, due to calcium-activated phospholipases that attack membrane fatty acids. Arachidonic acid metabolism may then progress to the generation of numerous injurious compounds including free radical species and various inflammatory mediators including cytokines, prostaglandins, and leukotrienes. Thus, the axolemma becomes structurally less stable and the combination of swelling due to accumulated transported organelles and membrane weakness eventuates over 24–72 h in axonal separation and discontinuity or secondary axotomy [14].

This process, since it is not self-reparative, as are stages I and II of axonal damage, is potentially the most important to understand. If the process leading to secondary or delayed axotomy can be interrupted, then perhaps reparative mechanisms can rescue the axon from permanent disruptive damage.

Stage IV Axonal Injury: Primary Axotomy

Primary axotomy is the immediate structural disruption of the axon at the time of trauma. The mere fact that this occurs has been debated for some time, but it has now been established that primary axotomy, though rather unusual, occurs in certain instances [15]. This is probably associated with axonal strains exceeding 20%, and is, of course, associated with irreversible failure of action potentials and, in most cases, in cessation of all other neuronal function. Primary axonal tearing occurs in relatively few axons, compared to stages I, II, and III of axonal damage. The process appears to be most frequent at the nodal region but also occasionally is present in internodes. The process appears to be self-sealing and the torn axons, probably by an active process involving phospholipases, reseal themselves within 30–60 min [16,17].

Prevalence of Axonal Damage After Head Injury

As the spectrum of clinical injury progresses from less to more severe, greater amounts of damage to axons occurs and greater numbers of axons are involved. In reversible injuries (e.g., concussions), little stage III and IV damage is present, most changes being stages I and II. As the *clinical syndrome* of diffuse axonal injury (e.g., prolonged coma unassociated with mass lesions or ischemia) occurs, larger numbers of axons are injured and the distribution of injured axons is shifted to the more severe stages of damage. Here a distribution of the numbers of damaged axons in each severity stage is shifted to the right with a higher degree of clinical injury severity. More likely is a situation where different frequency distributions of axonal damage are associated with different clinical gradations of injury. In addition to the differing number and severity of axonal damage, there also is the variation in the sites (location) of axonal damage within the brain in each patient. These three factors, namely, severity of axonal damage (e.g., what proportion are damaged at each stage), total number of damaged axons and anatomic location (and networks disrupted), will determine the clinical syndromes and neurological deficits in any one patient. Thus, the number and location of permanently damaged axons (e.g., stage III and IV axonal damage) will determine whether permanent sequelae of head injury exist and will determine the nature and magnitude of those persisting neurological deficits. A better understanding of the details of the neurobiology of the progression of axonal damage from stages I through IV will allow the potential for intervention by neuroprotective agents that may halt or slow the mechanisms that produce delayed axonal and neuronal degeneration after head injury. These agents thereby offer the possibility of substantially reducing the sequelae and the magntidue of permanent congitive, behavioral, and neurological impairments from traumatic brain damage.

Axonal injury is almost always present after head injury and because of its frequency and its importance, a more detailed understanding of the pathobiology of axonal damage is required before further improvements in the care of head-injured patients can occur.

References

1. Adams JH, Graham DI, Murray LS, Scott G (1982) Diffuse axonal injury due to non-missile head injury in humans. Ann Neurol 12:557–563
2. Gennarelli TA, Thibault LE, Adams JH et al (1982) Diffuse axonal injury and traumatic coma in the primate. Ann Neurol 12:564–574
3. Gennarelli TA (1994) Animate models of head Injury. J Neurotrauma 11:357–368
4. Gennarelli TA (1983) Head injury in man and experimental animals: clinical aspects. Acta Neurochir Suppl (Wien) 2:1–13
5. McLellan DR, Adams JH, Graham DI et al (1986) Structural basis of the vegetative state and prolonged coma after non-missile head injury. In: Papo I, Cohadon F, Massarotti M (eds) Le coma traumatique. Padova: Liviana, Padova, pp 165–185
6. Gentleman SM, Roberts GW, Gennarelli TA et al (1995) Axonal injury: a universal consequence of fatal closed head injury? Acta Neuropathol (Berl) 83:537–543
7. Ommaya AK, Gennarelli TA (1974) Cerebral concussion and traumatic unconsciousness. Correlation of experimental and clinical observations on blunt head injuries. Brain 97:633–654
8. Graham DI, Lawrence AI, Adams JH et al (1981) Pathology of mild head injury. In: Hoff JT, Anderson TE, Cole TM (eds) Mild to moderate head injury. Blackwell, Boston, pp 3–75
9. Povlishock JT (1992) Traumatically induced axonal injury: pathogenesis and pathobiological implications. Brain Pathol 2:1–12
10. Saatman K (1992) Biomechanical observations after tensile loading to the isolated sciatic nerve axon in the rat. PhD thesis, University of Pennsylvania, Philadelphia
11. Thibault LE (1992) Brain injury from the macro to the micro level and back again: what have we learned to date?, International Research Council for the Biomechanics of Impact (IRCOBI). Bryon, France 14:3–25
12. Gennarelli TA, Thibault LE, Tipperman R et al (1989) Axonal injury in the optic nerve: a model simulating diffuse axonal injury in the brain. J Neurosurg 71:244–253
13. Tomei G, Spangnoli D, Ducati A et al (1990) Morphology and neurophysiology of focal axonal injury experimentally induced in the guiena pig optic nerve. Acta Neuropathol (Berl) 80:506–513
14. Maxwell WL, Irvine A, Graham DI, Adams JH, Gennarelli TA (1991) Focal axonal injury: axon response to stretch. J Neurocytol 20:157–164

15. Maxwell WL, Watt C, Graham DI, Gennarelli TA (1993) Ultrastructural evidence of axonal shearing as a result of lateral acceralation of the head in non-human primates. Acta Neuropathol (Berl) 86:136–144
16. Yawo H, Kuno M (1983) How a nerve fiber repairs its cut end: involvement of phospholipase A2. Science 222:1351–1352
17. Fern R (1995) Axon resealing: filling in the holes. Neuroscientist 1:253–254

Discussion

Beathmann:
This was a very nice comprehensive presentation, with a lot of information on calcium. When listening to your talk I wondered whether there are measures to selectively intervene in order to influence the course of events leading to axonal rupture. If this were the case, diffuse axonal injury would meet the requirements of a secondary process, which in principle (by whatever method) can be therapeutically attenuated or even prevented.

Gennarelli:
A very good question. I think the answer is, it does not appear that we conceive of some therapeutic intervention that can decrease the primary calcium entry. If the calcium is, in fact, due to a hole in the membrane we cannot conceive of a mechanism that will keep ions from coming in, so that one then has to look more downstream. Can anything be done that will increase calcium binding within the cell? Can one, perhaps, think about increasing calcium pumping out of the cell? For example, can the calcium adenosine triphosphatase (ATPase) pump the calcium–sodium exchange, or calcium transporter be augmented. Those events we do not know. Theoretically, if you could increase those pumps it could be useful. Probably, it is more likely to go the next step downstream and to try to inhibit the effects of calcium on the activation of various enzymes. There certainly are now more calpain inhibitors that are available and they appear to be more specific than the previous generation of calpain inhibitors. That is an attractive target because complete protease activation and degradation probably takes about 72 h to occur, so that there is a window that exists for intervention. We have preliminary experience of improvement after using a protease inhibitor. Calpain inhibitor does seem to improve outcome and is in fact, protective and that is what is shown as well in the N-methyl-D-asparate (NMDA) type of model as well. And similarly, inhibitors of free radical production that would penetrate the blood–brain barrier may be useful because lipid peroxidation takes hours and days to maximize its deleterious effects. So the answer is, I think there are multiple areas where there are potential therapeutic targets, it is not going to be just one target area in that entire cascade.

Traber:
You had mentioned in the beginning that you had an elaborate slide of possible treatment with lazaroids. Since you brought up the subject of oxygen free radical scavengers, have you tested any of the lazaroids in your studies?

Gennarelli:

We have not tested it specifically in localized models, but based on the work that has been done by Hall, he suggested that of the global effects of the free radical scavengers, some 90%, he estimated, were on the vascular site, so he would not anticipate substantial free radical damage within neurons.

Baethmann:

My point concerns the experimental model of your investigations: You said that axon lesions were studies in vitro by using isolated (?) squid axons. Is it also possible to produce respective graded axonal lesions of stage I, stage II or stage III, etc., in animals in vivo with quantitative assessments of the numbers of axons which eventually disrupt. This would probably provide an excellent basis to investigate methods of therapeutical inhibition.

Gennarelli:

We used a number of models, the purest one is the squid axon, because it has a very large caliber axon.

We tried to move up the complexity scale. We have used the isolated sciatic nerve axon of the frog as a model but that is still not mammalian although this axon is myelinated. The results are virtually the same in that model in terms of immediate calcium flux. We have then jumped from there to evaluate stretching of multiple axons in the guinea pig optic nerve. This is the only mammalian system that we have studied. In this model one can laboriously do morphometric studies to count axons, and it turns out that about 17% of the axons are injured in one way or another. Axotomy occurs in 3% of the axons, thus the numbers are very small to do a treatment study and because of the difficulties using morphometric analysis for treatment response we need a different outcome measurement in order to do treatment studies.

Redl:

You have done your studies in vitro without inflammatory cells present, but wouldn't you think that if there were activated inflammatory cells present there would be another development of the axonal injury?

Gennarelli:

I guess that is true, if you could tell me what activates them.

I am not sure we know that specifically in pure forms of axonal damage where little vascular damage occurs.

Kochanek:

You know that Tracy MacIntosh has actually looked at that relatively recently, I think it was in the December 1995 issue of the Journal of Neurosciences. He used the fluid percussion model and assessed neutrophil infiltration in different regions of brain. and what he found was that in the regions with axonal injury there was no neutrophil influx, whereas in the regions in which there was blood–brain barrier injury there was robust neutrophil influx. I really enjoyed your slide where you compartmentalize the different potential theoretical mechanisms involved in these different types of injury.

I noticed that in your diffuse injury category it was really diffuse axonal injury. I was interested in your thoughts, more global thoughts about diffuse injury, in particular the diffuse swelling phenomenon: What is known about the interaction between diffuse axonal injury and diffuse swelling?

Gennarelli:
I think the easiest answer is that to my knowledge there are several phenomena in brain injury that have not been developed in model form. Brain swelling is probably the most important brain injury that has no model to study at all. So I do not think I know what causes diffuse brain swelling.

Morganti:
There is not only damage of neurons and axons but also astrocyte swelling, and I think it plays a very important role. We have established the model of Marmaroa. We can see that in a diffuse axonal injury model you have also astrocyte swelling and it is known that activation of astrocytes can be a benefit for the injured brain because they synthesize a variety of molecules which are aimed at repairing the damaged nervous system from neurotropic factors to glutamate synthase and so on. But astrocyte swelling is a sort of degenerative change which may impair the beneficial function of astrocytes. On the other hand, activation of microglial cells seems to be more deleterious because they release toxic factors which can cause secondary damage of the injured brain. So it is important to consider the function of glial cells in the processes which lead to axonal injury.

Gennarelli:
I think that is right because new diagnostic techniques such as diffusion weighted magnetic resonance imaging (MRI) show increased intracellular water soon after stroke and traumatic brain injury. Thus, water and swelling may be increased both in neurons and in astrocytes. So the answer is probably its complex in both astrocytes and neurons.

Baethmann:
May I come back to the axonal injury: Is there any evidence whether secondary processes are involved which might be inhibited? Or is the axonal injury you are describing enhanced by systemic disturbances like hypoxia or ischemia? With regard to what you were reporting on cations and an involvement of free radicals, I assume that such events would have an impact.

Gennarelli:
There is no direct evidence that I know of to demonstrate that ischemia worsens traumatic axonal damage. However, ischemia is one of the mechanisms that can produce axonal damage. At one time, the Vienna group of neuropathologists proposed that what we now call diffuse axonal injury is an ischemic injury, not a mechanical injury. For example, in survivors of global ischemia there can be areas without an infarction in the brain where axons are damaged, so there is no question that ischemia can cause axonal damage. We can decrease local membrane metabolism by in vitro freezing of a portion of the axon which may have a mechanism similar

to ischemia and cause all the same types of axonal damage. But I think what we see in axonal damage is one of the very few ways that an axon can respond to any sort of insult whether it is systemic or traumatic. I do not think that the axon has a repertoire that is very sophisticated.

Inflammatory Process in the Pathobiology of Secondary Damage After Traumatic Brain Injury

P.M. KOCHANEK, S.T. DEKOSKY, T. CARLOS, R.S.B. CLARK, and M. WHALEN

Summary

The acute inflammatory process participates in the evolution of secondary damage after traumatic brain injury. Endothelial adhesion molecule upregulation, complement activation, leukocyte adhesion to cerebrovascular endothelium and invasion into brain parenchyma, microglial activation, expression of inducible nitric oxide synthase, and signaling of the neurotrophic response represent some of the components of a cybernetic, highly redundant process orchestrated by cytokines, chemoattractants and other mediators. However, the exact contribution of acute inflammation, its net impact on injury extension or cellular recovery, and the nature of the inflammatory process in specific cell types within brain parenchyma and the cerebral microcirculation all remain to be determined. Evidence supporting the participation of key components of the inflammatory cascade after traumatic brain injury in both experimental models and humans will be presented. Acute inflammation potentially contributes to a wide range of events in the pathobiology of traumatic brain injury, including; posttraumatic cerebrovascular failure, neuronal injury, neuronal protection, and recovery. Finally, the effect of moderate hypothermia on the development of the acute inflammatory response to traumatic brain injury will be discussed. Targeted manipulation of the inflammatory process after traumatic brain injury may produce novel therapeutic opportunities for this difficult but important clinical problem.

Introduction

The acute inflammatory process in the central nervous system (CNS) has been largely neglected by clinicians and neuroscientists. The brain has been considered to be immunologically privileged, and other than an endogenous response of microglia, acute inflammation has not been considered to be either of great importance or a potential therapeutic target. Roots of our understanding of the pathobiology of the acute inflammatory process in traumatic brain injury lie in the study of cerebral ischemia. Hallenbeck (1977) suggested that a "blood damaged tissue interaction" existed in injured brain regions and that although cybernetic and highly complex, this process contributed to the evolution of the injury. Similarly, Giulian (1987) suggested important participation of parenchymal elements, specifically microglia in inflammation-mediated secondary damage after brain injury, and Giulian and Robertson (1990) reported infiltration and participation of circulating mononuclear phagocytes in the pathogenesis of secondary injury after CNS ischemia–reperfusion. Based on recent findings, however, it also appears that the inflammatory process signals important aspects of recovery and repair. Work by our collective investigative groups and by others has begun to provide insight into the specific participants in the acute inflammatory response in traumatically injured brain. A framework outlining these participants is beginning to emerge. Included in the injury response are cytokines, adhesion molecules, complement, blood-borne and parenchymal inflammatory cells, inducible nitric oxide synthase, and neurotrophins. Our current understanding of the nature of the involvement of each of these participants will be discussed in this review. Other inflammatory mediators such as kinins, aracidonic acid metabolites, chemokines, and platelet-acivtating factor may play important roles in the response to traumatic brain injury (Unterberg and Baethmann 1984; Ellis et al. 1989; Lindsberg et al. 1991); however, this review will focus only on those aspects of the inflammatory process under current investigation at our center.

Cytokines

Cytokines are low molecular weight polypeptides that have immunomodulatory effects and can effect cellular growth and proliferation. They signal cascades of events in response to infection or tissue injury, in addition to having important homeostatic effects on normal metabolism (reviewed by Ott et al. 1994). Cytokines, particularly interleukin (IL)-1-β, TNF-α, and IL-8 are key participants in signaling the development of the inflammatory response in response to endotoxin or other infectious agents (Movat 1987). Other cytokines, such as IL-6 and IL-10, appear to attenuate selected aspects of the inflammatory response (Ott et al. 1994). Cytokines are involved in the pathogenesis of CNS infections (Frei et al. 1990; Lieberman et al., Symons et al. 1987), and have recently been shown to be increased in brain in experimental models of stroke (Liu et al. 1994; Yamasaki et al. 1995).

With respect to traumatic brain injury, local increases in IL-1 were first reported by Giulian and Lachman (1985) after cerebral stab wounds in rats. Shohami and Novikov (1994) reported increased brain tissue levels of TNF-α and IL-6 during the initial 8 h and 24 h, respectively, after closed head injury in rats. Goss et al. (1995), and Yakolev and Faden (1995) have reported expression of IL-1β message in rats after traumatic brain injury produced by contemporary injury models such as controlled cortical impact and fluid percussion injury, respectively. The time course of IL-1β message in the lesion penumbra after controlled cortical impact as reported by Goss et al. (1995) is shown in Fig. 1. More recently, expression of IL-1β message has been demonstrated as early as 30 min after injury (Yakolev and Faden 1995). Recent studies also support production of cytokines in human brain after head injury. Marion et al. (1997) reported increased levels of IL-1β in ventricular CSF of adults after severe traumatic brain injury. Similarly, Pinto et al. (1996) recently reported increases in jugular venous levels of IL-1β during the initial 48 h after head injury in children. Both IL-1β and TNF-α produce injury to cerebrovascular endothelium, as demonstrated

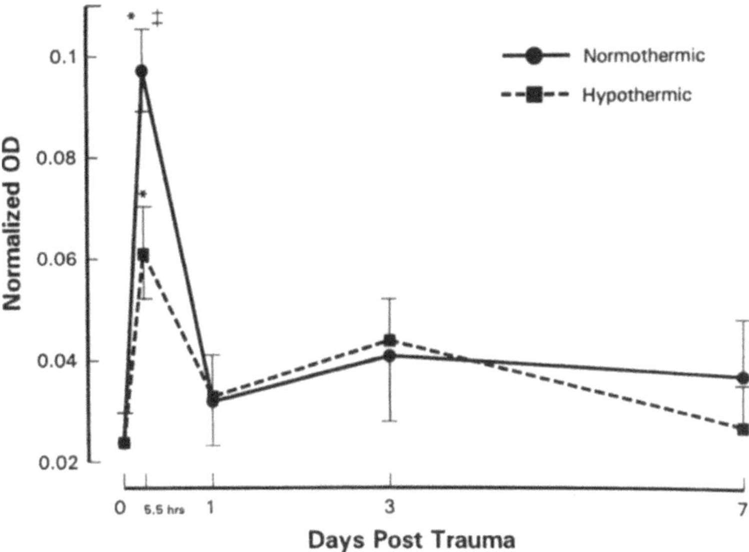
Normalized OD
Normothermic
Hypothermic
0.1
0.08
0.06
0.04
0.02
0
5.5 hrs
1
3
7
Days Post Trauma

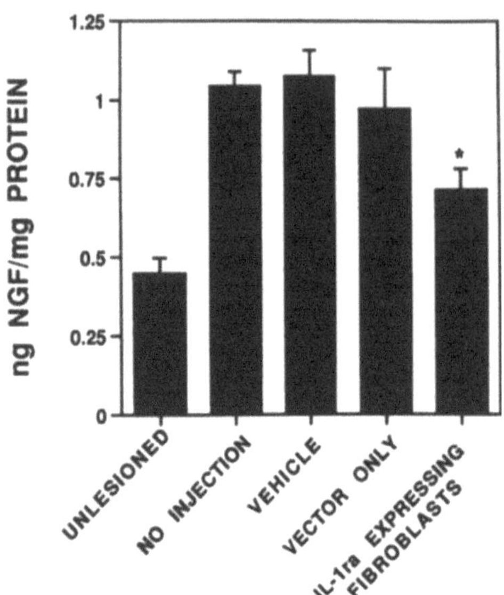

1.25
1
0.75
0.5
0.25
0
ng NGF/mg PROTEIN
UNLESIONED
NO INJECTION
VEHICLE
VECTOR ONLY
IL-1ra EXPRESSING FIBROBLASTS
*

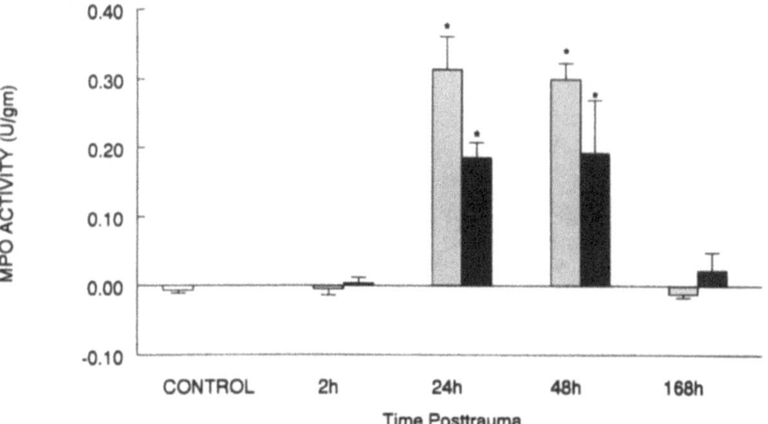

0.40
0.30
0.20
0.10
0.00
-0.10
MPO ACTIVITY (U/gm)
CONTROL
2h
24h
48h
168h
Time Posttrauma

24 h after injury in this model. This again suggests that contusion may be a key factor in determining the participation of circulating acute inflammatory cells in traumatic brain injury. Consistent with this notion, Soares et al. (1995) recently reported significant neutrophil accumulation in areas of blood–brain barrier injury after fluid percussion. In their fluid-percussion model, neutrophils were not seen in brain regions with isolated axonal injury. Several key questions remain to be addressed. Do the accumulated neutrophils contribute to blood–brain barrier injury, edema, hyperemia (specific process associated with cerebral swelling) or other types of secondary damage? Do infiltrating monocytes mediate secondary damage or have other roles during delayed periods after traumatic brain injury?

Inhibition of Posttraumatic Leukocyte Accumulation in Brain

We have begun to define the contribution of several of the leukocyte adhesion pathways to posttraumatic neutrophil accumulation. Curiously, unlike the nearly complete inhibition of leukocyte accumulation by adhesion antagonist therapy in either models of inflammation outside of the CNS, or infection in the CNS (Saez-Llorens et al. 1991; Tuomanen et al. 1989), selective antagonists of either ICAM-1 (TM-8, Athena Neurosciences) or MAC-1 (Repligen), blocked only between 35% and 50% of posttraumatic neutrophil accumulation (Carlos et al. 1995; Clark et al. 1996a). This level of inhibition is similar to that observed with adhesion antagonists in the experimental models of focal cerebral ischemia (Zhang et al. 1994) and suggests the participation or multiple pathways for leukocyte recruitment into contused brain. It also suggests similarities between the mechanisms involved in leukocyte recruitment after cerebral contusion and stroke. It is, however, somewhat disappointing and implies the possible need for multiple agents if a high level of inhibition of infiltration of neutrophils into brain parenchyma is required to produce clinical benefit. Recently Cody et al. (1995) reported a modest improvement in functional outcome in rats treated with an inhibitor of P-selectin after fluid percussion. However, treatment failed to reduce posttraumatic neutrophil accumulation in this model. It is possible that parenchymal actions of adhesion molecules such as MAC-1 or ICAM-1 may mediate important deleterious pro-inflammatory effects, independent of neutrophils. This has been observed for MAC-1 in models of acute lung injury (Mulligan et al. 1995). Further investigation of agents targeting these adhesion molecules are needed in models of traumatic brain injury. To our knowledge, the effect of adhesion molecule antagonists on monocyte adhesion and accumulation have not been investigated in an experimental model of traumatic brain injury.

Leukocytes as Possible Mediators of Secondary Damage After Traumatic Brain Injury

Neutrophils are a key participant in the acute inflammatory process outside of the central nervous system and play and important role in inflammatory processes in brain, such as meningitis (reviewed in Kochanek and Hallenbeck 1992). Their role in ischemic brain injury, however, appears to be strongly model dependent. Neutrophils

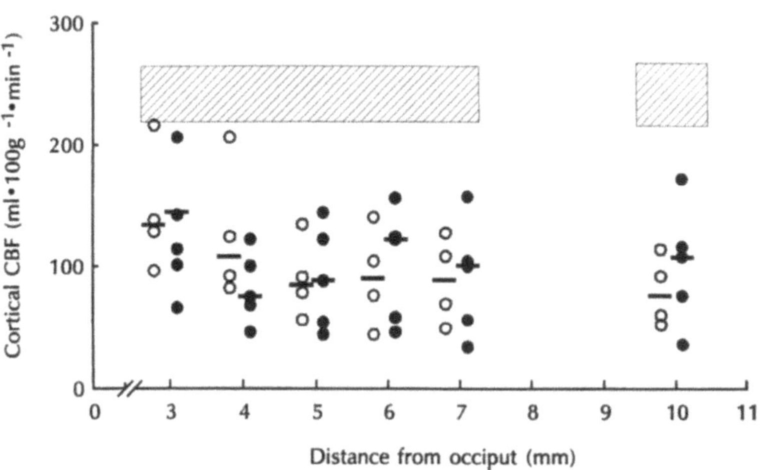

300

Cortical CBF (ml•100g -1•min -1)

200

100

0

0   3   4   5   6   7   8   9   10   11

Distance from occiput (mm)

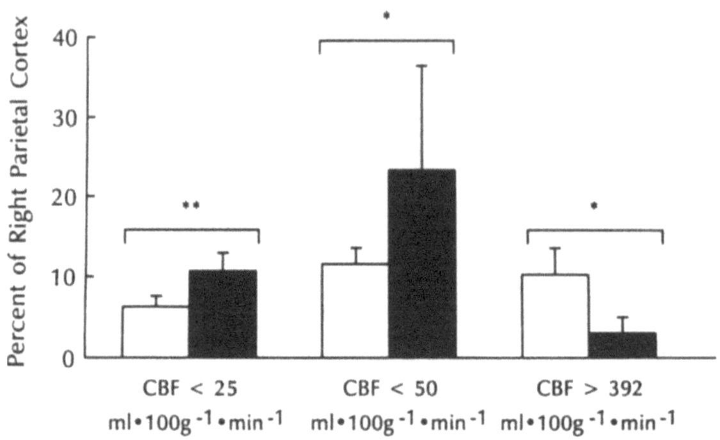
Percent of Right Parietal Cortex
40
30
20
10
0
**
*
*
CBF < 25
ml•100g -1•min -1
CBF < 50
ml•100g -1•min -1
CBF > 392
ml•100g -1•min -1

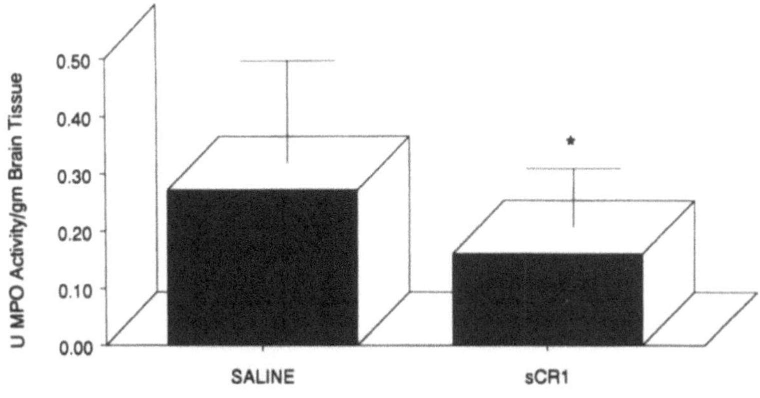

U MPO Activity/gm Brain Tissue
0.50
0.40
0.30
0.20
0.10
0.00
SALINE
sCR1
*

nature of the contribution of iNOS-derived NO in brain injury remains to be determined.

Effect of Hypothermia on the Acute Inflammatory Response to Traumatic Brain Injury

Moderate hypothermia is effective in reducing secondary damage after traumatic brain injury in both experimental models and in humans (Clifton et al. 1991, Clark et al. 1996b; Marion et al. 1993). The mechanism of this protective effect is, however, unclear. For example, Palmer et al. (1993) reported, that hypothermia reduced contusion volume after injury, but failed to attenuate the increase in brain interstitial excitatory amino acid concentration. It has long been known that hypothemia produces marked inhibitory effects on numerous aspects of the acute inflammatory process (Ledingham 1908; Svanes 1964). However, effects of hypothermia on acute inflammation have not been suggested as a possible mechanism for the therapeutic benefit of this therapy. We have begun to examine the influence of brain temperature on the development of acute inflammation after controlled cortical impact (Whalen et al. 1996). In these preliminary studies, mild hypothermia (32°C) or hyperthermia (39°C) almost completely prevented neutrophil accumulation in brain parenchyma at 4 h posttrauma, while mild hyperthermia markedly increased neutrophil accumulation. This suggests that part of the beneficial effect of hypothermia in brain injury may be mediated by effects on acute inflammation. Conversely, hyperthermia may augment brain injury in part via an enhanced inflammatory response.

Finally, it may be essential to realize that not all effects of hypothermia are beneficial to either the injured brain, or the brain injured patient. Bohn et al. (1986) reported that sustained hypothermia can suppress systemic immunity in humans and can be associated with increased infection risk, particularly when hypothermia is used for more than 48 h. Recently, DeKosky et al. (1996) reported that 4 h of moderate hypothermia produced a sustained inhibition of nerve growth factor production in brain after controlled cortical impact injury in rats (Goss et al. 1995). Thus, there appear to be important systemic and local effects of hypothermia on otherwise protective aspects of the inflammation that may require additional therapeutic strategies (such as supplementation of nerve growth factor or other neurotrophins).

Conclusion

Studies in laboratory models of cerebral ischemia and our recent findings in traumatic brain injury (in both experimental models and in humans) clearly demonstrate that key components of the inflammatory process are active in the injured brain. Detrimental and beneficial effects of selected aspects of the inflammatory process are possible. Based on current information, the net effect of the inflammatory process appears to be detrimental and thus represents a novel therapeutic target in traumatic brain injury. Future studies must determine the role of the inflammatory process in the development of specific aspects of secondary brain injury, such as posttraumatic cerebrovascular failure, edema, and neuronal injury, and the potential role of inflammatory intermediates in signaling aspects of neuronal protection and recovery.

References

Albina J, Cui S, Mateo R, Reichner J (1993) Nitric oxide-mediated apoptosis in murine peritoneal macrophages. J Immunol 150:5080–5085

Becker P, Zieger S, Rother U et al (1987) Complement activation following severe head injury. Anaesthesist 36:301–305

Betz A, Yang G-Y, Davidson B (1995) Attenuation of stroke size in rats using an adenoviral vector to induce overexpression of interleukin-1 receptor antagonist in brain. J Cereb Blood Flow Metab 15:547–551

Billiar T, Curran R, Harbrecht B et al (1990) Modulation of nitrogen oxide synthesis in vivo: N^G-monomethyl-L-arginine inhibits endotoxin-induced nitrite/nitrate biosynthesis while promoting hepatic damage. J Leuk Biol 48:565–569

Bohn D, Biggar W, Smith C et al (1986) Influence of hypothermia, barbiturate therapy, and intracranial pressure monitoring on morbidity and mortality after near-drowning. Crit Care Med 14:529

Carlos T, Clark R, Franicola-Higgins D, Schiding JK, Kochanek PM (1995) Expression of endothelial adhesion molecules after traumatic brain injury in rats (Abstr). J Neurotrauma 12:458

Chopp M, Zhang RL, Chen H, Li Y, Jiang N, Rusche JR (1994) Postischemic administration of anti-mac-1 antibody reduces ischemic cell damage after transient middle cerebral artery occlusion. Stroke 25:869–876

Clark R, Schiding JK, Kaczorowski SL, Marion DW, Kochanek PM (1994) Neutrophil accumulation after traumatic brain injury in rats: comparison of weight-drop and controlled cortical impact models. J Neurotrauma 11:499–506

Clark R, Kochanek P, Brookens M et al (1995) Cerebrovascular, inflammatory cell, and neuronal inducible nitric oxide expression after trauma in immature rats. Pediatr Res 37:43A

Clark R, Schiding JK, Carlos T, Bree M, DeKosky S, Kochanek P (1996a) Antibodies against mac-1 attenuate neutrophil accumulation after traumatic brain injury in rats. J Neurotrauma 13:333–341

Clark R, Kochanek P, Marion D et al (1996b) Mild posttraumatic hypothermia reduces mortality after severe controlled cortical impact in rats. J Cereb Blood Flow Metab 16:253–261

Clark R, Kochanek PM, Schwarz MA et al (1996c) Inducible nitric oxide synthase expression in cerebrovascular smooth muscle and neutrophils after traumatic brain injury in immature rats. Pediatr Res 39:784–790

Clark R, Kochanek P, Obrist W et al (1996d) Cerebrospinal fluid and plasma nitrite and nitrate concentrations after head injury in humans. Crit Care Med 24:1243–1251

Clifton G, Jiang J, Lyeth B, Jenkins L, Hamm R, Hayes R (1991) Marked protection by moderate hypothermia after experimental traumatic brain injury. J Cereb Blood Flow Metab 11:114–121

Cody R, Maris D, Seckin H, Sharar S, Grady M (1995) P-selectin blockade after fluid percussion injury: behavioral and anatomic sequelae. J Neurotrauma 12:976

DeKosky ST, Goss JR, Miller PD, Styren SD, Kochanek PM, Marion D (1994) Upregulation of nerve growth factor following cortical trauma. Exp Neurol 130:173–177

DeKosky ST, Styren S, O'Malley M et al (1996) Interleukin-1 receptor antagonist suppresses neurotrophin response in injured rat brain. Ann Neurol 39:123–127

Ellis EF, Chao J, Heizer ML (1989) Brain kininogen following experimental brain injury: evidence for a secondary event. J Neurosurg 71:437–442

Frei K, Nadal D, Fontana A (1990) Intracerebral synthesis of tumor necrosis factor-alpha and interleukin-6 in infectious meningitis. Ann NY Acad Sci 594:326–335

Gallinaro R, Cheadle W, Applegate K et al (1992) The role of the complement system in trauma and infection. Surg Gynecol Obstet 174:435–440

Giulian D (1987) Amebold microglia as effectors of inflammation inthe central nervous system. J Neurosci Res 18:155–171, 132–133

Giulian D, Lachman L (1985) Interleukin-1 stimulation of astroglial proliferation after brain injury. Science 228:497–498

Giulian D, Robertson C (1990) Inhibition of mononuclear phagocytes reduces ischemic injury in the spinal cord. Ann Neurol 27:33–42

Goss J, Styren S, Miller P et al (1995) Hypothermia attenuates the normal increase in interleukin 1β RNA and nerve growth factor following traumatic brain injury in the rat. J Neurotrauma 12:159–167

Hallenbeck J (1977) Prevention of postischemic impairment of microvascular perfusion. Neurology 27:3–10

Hallenbeck JM, Dutka AJ, Tanishima T et al (1986) Polymorphonuclear leukocyte accumulation in regions with low blood flow during the postischemic period. Stroke 17:246–253

Hewett S, Corbett J, McDaniel M, Choi D (1993) Interferon-γ and interleukin-1β induce nitric oxide formation from primary mouse astrocytes. Neurosci Lett 164:229–232

Horner H, Setler P, Fritz L et al (1992) Characterization of leukocyte infiltration in traumatic brain injury in the rat. Soc Neurosci Abstr 18:173

Iadecola C, Zhang F, Xu X (1995) Inhibition of nitric oxide synthase ameliorates cerebral ischemic damage, A. J Physiol 268:R286–R292

Kaczorowski SL, Schiding JK, Toth CA, Kochanek PM (1995) Effect of soluble complement receptor-1 on neutrophil accumulation after traumatic brain injury in rats. J Cereb Blood Flow Metab 15:860–864

Kochanek P, Hallenbeck J (1992) Polymorphonuclear leukocytes and monocytes/macrophages in the pathogenesis of cerebral ischemia and stroke. Stroke 23:1367–1379

Ledingham J (1908) The influence of temperature on phagocytosis. Proc R Soc Lond 80:188–195

Liebermann AP, Pitha PM, Shin HS et al (1989) Production of tumor necrosis factor and other cytokines by astrocytes stimulated with lipopolysaccharide or a neurotropic virus. Proc Natl Acad Sci USA 86:6348–6352

Lindholm D, Heumann R, Hengerer B, Thoenen H (1988) Interleukin-1 increases stability and transcription of mRNA encoding nerve growth factor in cultured rat fibroblasts. J Biol Chem 263:16348–16351

Lindsberg PJ, Hallenbeck JM, Feuerstein G (1991) Platelet-activating factor in stroke and brain injury. Ann Neurol 30:117–129

Liu T, Clark R, McDonnell P et al (1994) Tumor necrosis factor-alpha expression in ischemic neurons. Stroke 25:1481–1488

MacMicking J, Nathan C, Hom G et al (1995) Altered responses to bacterial infection and endotoxic shock in mice lacking inducible nitric oxide synthase. Cell 81:641–650

Mansfield RT, Schiding JK, Hamilton RL, Kochanek PM (1996) Effects of hypothermia on traumatic brain injury in immature rats. J Cereb Blood Flow Metab (in press)

Marion D, Obrist W, Carlier P, Penrod L, Darby J (1993) The use of moderate therapeutic hypothermia for patients with severe head injuries: a preliminary report. J Neurosurg 79:354–362

Marion DW, Penrod LE, Kelsey SF, Obrist WD, Kochanek PM, Palmer AM, Wisniewski SR, DeKosky ST (1997) Treatment of traumatic brain injury with moderate hypothermia. N Engl J Med (in press)

Marmarou A, Abd-Elfattah F, Van Den Brink W, Campbell J, Kita H, Demetriadou K (1994) A new model of diffuse brain injury in rats. J Neurosurg 80:291–300

Matsuo Y, Onodera H, Shiga Y et al (1994) Correlation between myeloperoxidase-quantified neutrophil accumulation and ischemic brain injury in the rat: effects of neutrophil depletion. Stroke 25:1469–1475

Megyeri P, Abraham C, Temesvari P et al (1992) Recombinant human tumor necrosis factor a constricts pial arterioles and increases blood-brain barrier permeability in newborn piglets. Neurosci Lett 148:137–140

Movat H (1987) Tumor necrosis factor and interleukin-1: Role in acute inflammation and microvascular injury. J Lab Clin Med 110:668–681

Mulligan M, Vaporciyan A, Warner R et al (1995) Compartmentalized roles for leukocytic adhesion molecules in lung inflammatory injury. J Immunol 154:1350–1363

Ott L, McClain C, Gillespie M, Young B (1994) Cytokines and metabolic dysfunction after severe head injury. J Neurotrauma 11:447–472

Palmer A, Marion D, Botscheller M, Redd E (1993) Therapeutic hypothermia is cytoprotective without attenuating traumatic brain injury-induced elevations in interstitial concentrations of aspartate and glutamate. J Neurotrauma 10:363–372

Pasinetti G, Johnson S, Rozovsky I et al (1992) Complement C1qB and C4 RNAs response to lesioning in rat brain. Exp Neurol 118

Pastor C, Billiar T (1995) Regulation and functions of nitric oxide in the liver in sepsis and inflammation. New Horiz 3:65–72

Pfister H, Koedel U, Haberi R et al (1990) Microvascular changes during the early phase of experimental bacterial meningitis. J Cereb Blood Flow Metab 10:914–922

Pinto A, Kuluz J, Schleien C (1996) Cerebral production of IL-1β in children with traumatic and anoxic brain injury. Crit Care Med 24 Suppl:A135

Rebhun J, Botvin-Madorsky J, Glovsky M (1991) Proteins of the complement system and acute phase reactants in sera of patients with spinal cord injury. Ann Allergy 66:335–338

Rothwell N, Lawrence C, Loddick S et al (1994) Cytokines and cerebral ischemia. In: Krieglstein J, Oberpichler-Schwenk H (eds) Pharmacology of cerebral ischemia. Wissenschaftliche Verlagsgesellschaft, Stuttgart, pp 419–425

Saez-Llorens X, Jafari H, Severien C et al (1991) Enhanced attenuation of meningeal inflammation and brain edema by concomitant administration of anti-CD18 monoclonal antibodies and dexamethasone in experimental haemophilus meningitis. J Clin Invest 88:2003–2011

Schoettle RJ, Kochanek PM, Magargee MJ, Uhl MW, Nemoto EM (1990) Early polymorphonuclear leukocyte accumulation correlates with the development of posttraumatic cerebral edema in rats. J Neurotrauma 7:207–217

Schürer L, Prugner U, Kempski O, Arfors K-E, Baethmann A (1990) Effects of antineutrophil serum (ANS) on posttraumatic brain oedema in rats. Acta Neurochir (Wien) S51:49–51

Shohami E, Novikov M (1994) Closed head injury triggers early production of TNFα and IL-6 by brain tissue. J Cereb Blood Flow Metab 14:615–619

Soares HD, Hicks RR, Smith D, McIntosh TK (1995) Inflammatory leukocyte recruitment and diffuse neuronal degeneration are separate pathological processes resulting from traumatic brain injury. J Neurosci 15:8223–8233

Spranger M, Lindholm D, Brandtlow C et al (1990) Regulation of nerve growth factor (NGF) synthesis in the rat central nervous system: comparison between the effects of interleukin-1 and various growth factors in astrocyte cultures and in vivo. Eur J Neurosci 2:69–76

Stoclet J, Fleming I, Gray G et al (1993) Nitric oxide and endotoxemia. Circulation 87 Suppl 5:V77–V80

Svanes K (1964) Studies in hypothermia. I. The influence of deep hypothermia on the formation of cellular exudate in acute inflammation in mice. Acta Anaesthesiol Scand 8:143–156

Svensson M, Bellander M, Aldskogius H, von Holst H (1994) Evidence for activation of the complement cascade and increase of the complement regulator sulfated glycoprotein-2 in the vicinity of a cortical contusion injury in the adult rat. Soc Neurosci Abstr 20/1:421

Symons J, Bundick R, Suckling A et al (1987) Cerebrospinal fluid interleukin 1 like activity during chronic relapsing experimental allergic encephalomyelitis. Clin Exp Immunol 68:648–654

Takeshima R, Kirsch J, Koehler R et al (1992) Monoclonal luekocyte antibody does not decrease the injury of transient focal cerebral ischemia in cats. Stroke 23:247–252

Tuomanen E, Saukkonen K, Sande S, Cioffe C, Wright S (1989) Reduction of inflammation, tissue damage, and mortality in bacterial meningitis in rabbits treated with monoclonal antibodies against adhesion-promoting receptors of leukocytes. J Exp Med 170:959–968

Uhl MW, Biagas KV, Grundl PD et al (1994) Effects of neutropenia on edema, histology, and cerebral blood flow after traumatic brain injury in rats. J Neurotrauma 11:303–315

Unterberg A, Baethmann AJ (1984) The kallirein-kinin system as mediator in vasogenic brain edema. J Neurosurg 61:87–96

Whalen MJ, Carlos TM, Kochanek PM et al (1996) Hypothermia reduces acute inflammation after traumatic brain injury in rats (Abstr). Pediatr Res (in press)

Yakolev AG, Faden AI (1995) Molecular strategies in CNS injury. J Neurotrauma 12:767–778

Yamasaki Y, Matsuo Y, Matsuura N, Onodera H, Itoyama Y, Kogure K (1995) Transient increase of cytokine-induced neutrophil chemoattractant, a member of the interleukin-8 family, in ischemic brain areas after focal ischemia in rats. Stroke 26:318–323
Zhang R, Chopp M, Li Y et al (1994) Anti-ICAM-1 antibody reduces ischemic cell damage after transient middle cerebral artery occlusion in the rat. Neurology 44:1747–1751

Discussion

Traber:
Were any of your patients in which you measured nitrite levels infected or septic?

Kochanek:
No, the levels were determined in patients with isolated brain injury without sepsis. We did, however, have one patient who became septic after about 1 week and the CSF nitrite and nitrate level increased probably five to seven times normal in that patient. I think it is extremely interesting because it has long been known that injured patients who become septic are an extremely high risk group of patients. It may be that the brain becomes primed from the initial injury, and either secondary blood–brain barrier permeability or a second inflammatory stimulus like that observed in immunologic priming lead to this marked increase in that patient. Our data from the initial 3 days after head injury, however, did not include any septic or infected patients.

Traber:
I guess you misinterpreted what my question was, and that was: Relationship to iNOS and the hippocampus where you had that staining of the cell, and you said that you had a neuronal NOS antibody that you had tested. Were you showing upregulation of neuronal NOS in trauma as well?

Kochanek:
No, we have not done that. We have only looked at iNOS and we have not looked to see if actually neuronal NOS was induced. I think it may be possible. Several investigators have talked about the concept that the neuronal form of NOS could potentially be induced.

Zornow:
As you know, a lot of us are interested in the use of perioperative hypothermia; Dr. Todd, for example, is trying to start a hypothermia during aneurysm surgery trial, and I think a lot of us are concerned about the possible increased risk of infection. I think some of our colleagues are going to be reticent about allowing us to induce hypothermia in some of these patients. I wonder if you could just comment on the risk of infection in hypothermic patients.

Kochanek:
I have two specific thoughts on that: One is that neither of the feasibility studies in humans showed an important increase in infection rate. This was with either 24 or 48h of hypothermia. The other point to take away from the recent New England

Journal article is that all those patients had colonic surgery. It may be that this is a very specific effect in that group of patients, and that this phenomenon would not be observed in other types of surgery.

Kossmann:
One of the questions is about the adenosine levels you showed in your presentation. What kind of controls did you use? I am asking because the reviewers always give us a hard time to show the difference to the intraventricular measurements. Are your controls from the spine or where do you get them?

Kochanek:
One of the beauties of the ventricular CSF is that this is fluid that is otherwise discarded, and thus is a previously unrecognized resource for new information. However, the control issue is a tricky one. We do have several subsets of patients that we have examined. One of them is patients with brain tumors who have electively placed ventricular catheters. Patients with shunt revisions are another group and lumbar CSF is also used. Obviously, none of these are perfect controls. In addition, this is a similar problem for all of these markers which are measured.

Young:
I enjoyed your paper very much and I think looking at inflammatory mediators is an important contribution. You mentioned, but I do not think looked at the issue, of excitatory amino acids. I think it would be important to assess the relative contribution of inflammatory mediators and excitotoxins separately. I wondered if there were plans to have an experimental animal model where you could, for instance, block the effect of glutamate receptors, to assess the relative roles of inflammation versus cytotoxicity.

Kochanek:
There is a wealth of information on the role of excitotoxicity in brain injury in traumatic brain injury. Tracy McIntosh and others led the way in terms of looking at this area. I would mention, however, that Allen Palmer and Don Marion have measured CSF glutamate levels in the same normothermic and hypothermic patients. The hypothermic humans (maintained hypothermic for 24h after injury) have lower excitatory amino acid levels in CSF. This seemed particularly true in the patients that were Glasgow 5–8 on admission. A gradual and progressive rise in glutamate in human CSF is observed. It may be that this aspect is not modelled well by the rat, since delayed increases are not seen. Claudia Robertson in Houston, Texas, and Ross Bullock at Medical College in Virginia have very elegantly demonstrated with human microdialysis that when intracranial pressure increases, there are intermittent bursts of excitatory amino acid release. Thus, you are correct that this is very likely another important therapeutic target.

Morganti:
First, congratulations on your talk, it was very interesting. And second, some work has shown that injection of IL-1 receptor antagonist decreases the neuronal damage, so that there is a controversy between the deleterious and beneficial effect of cytokines in terms of induction of neurotrophins, NGF and so on. The work on IL-1

receptor antagonist has been done by Nancy Rothwell and collaborators in Manchester, and I would like to hear your opinion on that. In addition, what she has also shown is that probably what plays a role in this dichotomy is the concentration of cytokines. So depending on whether or not you have high or low levels of cytokines you can have more or less deleterious or beneficial effects on the injured brain. In particular, low IL-1 seemed to promote regeneration whereas high IL-1 was associated with increased neuronal death.

Kochanek:
You are probably aware also that Dr. Betz at the University of Michigan, has recently done some studies, manipulating IL-1 receptor production in stroke models, and has shown, as you suggest, by inhibiting IL-1, that infarct size is decreased. I presented the issue of blocking regeneration as a potential downside of hypothermia. It is important that we keep an open mind to the potential risks of what we are doing with hypothermia or other anti-inflammatory strategies. In the brain or maybe in other places we may have a three-edge sword when inhibiting inflammation. This may reduce secondary damage but also could increase infection and inhibit regeneration. Again, I agree, though, that in the models that have been used to study cytokine manipulation, particularly cerebral ischemia models, the general effect has been a beneficial one and not a detrimental one. I hope I did not suggest otherwise.

Baethmann:
My point is concerned with the findings you were presenting on the cerebral influx of neutrophils using neutrophil-specific antibodies in the controlled cortical impact model, and you have shown that it is the area of necrosis where a gradual increase of neutrophils is taking place. The crucial question here is concerned with the cause-effect relationship of the inflammatory response. Looking at your data one might conclude that the necrosing tissue area was attracting the neutrophils, which invade the lesion to scavenge the tissue debris. Our own data have indicated that if you systemically deplete neutrophils the situation may be made even worse, for example the perifocal brain-swelling is markedly enhanced. The other point addresses hypothermia which you were endorsing as a promising method. There are certainly good reasons for that at this moment. Some first clinical experience in head injury patients, however, seems to indicate that the pathophysiological problem of secondary brain damage is literally frozen, preserved if you wish, but not solved. Thus, if these patients are rewarmed again, all the adverse mechanisms are activated again, too. It might be assumed that the rate of warming up is quite important also. Of course, we now may make clever remarks and comments, although we should wait for the results of the hypothermia study conducted in the US in severe head injury.

Kochanek:
As for your first question, I agree. I think that we really do not know anything about causality in acute inflammation and traumatic brain injury. I think that is still up in the air, specifically the neutrophil component; the cytokine component, that is what we are studying right now. And there is, I think, a suggestion in your paper, it may be that neutrophils and platelets are plugging injured vessels. That could even be a beneficial effect. I do not know the answer to that. With regard to the issue of

hypothermia delaying rather than preventing injury, I think that is an extremely interesting area. Certainly Dalton Dietrich in Miami has led the way in this area and some of the results that he has found in global cerebral ischemia suggest delay rather than reduction of injury. However, it is important to note that in the rat models hypothermia is used for only a few hours. The depth of hypothermia, the duration of hypothermia and the onset may all be very important factors. Most of the animal studies that have shown this recrudescence of delayed neuronal death have used very short periods of hypothermia, 2h, 4h. The animal studies have not been performed with 1 day or 2 days of hypothermia. This is something that we are contemplating to try in the rat models. In addition, as you suggest, the rate of rewarming may also be important. For instance, in the animal models we warm over 1 hour. This is faster than the method used to rewarm humans. There is a great deal more to be learned about this.

Kossmann:
Just coming back to the hypothermia patients: One of the things I found we have to look at cautiously is where we are measuring hypothermia. There is a very nice paper published in 1994 in Neurosurgery, showing when you are measuring in the bladder, in the intestine, in the mouth or even in the brain there are substantial differences. So hypothermia does not mean hypothermia in all the patients, since one is thick, one is thin, and so on. I think the term hypothermia has to be defined very accurately. Where do we measure it? The second comment to your presentation is that I was very astonished how the proinflammatory cytokines actually go down in the hypothermia patients. We will show tomorrow some of our results, demonstrating that you need quite a substantial amount of proinflammatory cytokines to induce, for example, NGF. So, I am very much looking forward to your outcome results in these hypothermia patients.

Kochanek:
So are we, everybody is.

Experimental Cerebral Effects of Intravenous Fluid Therapy

M.H. Zornow

Summary

Intracranial hypertension resulting from cerebral edema is a major cause of morbidity and mortality in patients with traumatic brain injury. In the noninjured brain, water movement between the vasculature and the brain parenchyma is determined primarily by osmolar gradients. Administration of hypertonic solutions such as mannitol or concentrated saline solutions produces a brain-to-plasma osmotic gradient favoring the movement of water out of the brain parenchyma and into the vessels. This osmotic gradient can be maintained due to the high reflection coefficients for sodium ions, chloride ions, and mannitol, which effectively prevent them from crossing the blood–brain barrier.

Cryogenic lesions have long been used to model the pathophysiology of traumatic brain injury. These lesions are highly reproducible and it is a simple matter to vary their intensity depending on the goals of the studies. Many of the histologic features of traumatic brain contusions are found in cryogenic lesions, including cytolysis of neurons, petechial hemorrhages, an inflammatory response as evidenced by the accumulation of monocytes and leukocytes, and the appearance of edematous tissue at the periphery of the lesion. Using cryogenic lesions, various investigators have examined the ability of hypertonic solutions to decrease brain edema and control intracranial hypertension. Although most studies have concluded that hypertonic saline is superior to isotonic solutions, there is little or no evidence that it is superior to more conventional therapy with an equiosmolar dose of mannitol.

One of the most promising new techniques for study of cerebral edema is the use of magnetic resonance imaging (MRI). This technology should allow the serial noninvasive measurement of regional brain water content. Additional studies are required to correlate MRI findings with more direct measures of brain water content.

Introduction

Brain injury is a major cause of mortality in the traumatized patient. The presence of a severe brain injury (Glasgow Coma Scale score ≤ 8), increases the risk of death in a trauma patient from 0.9% to more than 30% (Baxt and Moody 1987). Approximately 50 000 patients die each year in the United States of traumatic brain injury and an additional 50 000–100 000 survive, but with significant neurologic deficits (Kurtzke

1982). Cerebral edema is a major cause of much of this excess morbidity and mortality. Uncontrolled intracranial hypertension, due in part to cerebral edema, is the single most common cause of death among head-injured patients who reach the hospital alive (Marshall and Bowers 1985). Many patients who "walk and talk" after their primary brain injury eventually succumb to progressive cerebral edema and intracranial hypertension. This progression is one of the most frustrating and tragic of circumstances to confront neurointensivists.

Many animal models of traumatic brain injury and cerebral edema have been studied over the past several decades in various laboratories around the world. Fluid-percussion injury, weight-drop models, epidural balloons, and cryogenic lesions have all been used by investigators as models of the cerebral edema that develops after traumatic brain injury. We believe that the cryogenic lesion has provided the most useful and reproducible model of the pathophysiology that accompanies traumatic brain injury. For that reason, much of this chapter will focus on investigations that use cryogenic lesions.

Normal Physiology

More than 100 years ago, Starling (1896) described the forces that govern the movement of fluids between the intravascular and interstitial spaces. The mathematical formula that was eventually written to codify his observations is as follows:

$$Q_f = K_f S\{(P_c - P_t) - s(\pi_c - \pi_t)\}$$

where Q_f represents the net amount of fluid that moves between the capillary lumen and the surrounding extracellular space; K_f is the filtration coefficient for the capillary membrane; S is the surface area of the capillary membrane; P_c is the hydrostatic pressure in the capillary lumen; P_t is the hydrostatic pressure (usually negative) in the extracellular space of the surrounding tissue; and s is the coefficient of reflection. This number, which can range from 1 (no movement of the solute across the membrane) to 0 (free diffusion of the solute across the membrane), quantitates the "leakiness" of the capillary and is different for vessels in the brain vs peripheral tissues; π_c is the oncotic pressure of the plasma; π_t is the oncotic pressure of the fluid in the extracellular space (Peters and Hargens 1981).

From his studies, Starling concluded that oncotic pressure produced by plasma proteins in the intravascular space prevented edema formation. It is important to note that Starling's observations pertain only to peripheral tissues (e.g., isolated limb preparations) and not the central nervous system. The brain, unlike peripheral tissues, is isolated from the vasculature by the presence of the blood–brain barrier. This barrier, which is thought to anatomically consist of the tight junctions between adjacent endothelial cells lining the capillaries of the brain and spinal cord, prevents the movement of even very low molecular-weight molecules and ions between the vascular lumen and the brain's interstitial space. The blood–brain barrier acts very much like a semipermeable membrane lining the capillary walls. Movement of water across this barrier is determined by osmolar gradients that may exist between the intravascular and interstitial spaces. The osmotic pressure, which is the driving force for water movement, can be easily calculated using basic physical principles and the following equation:

$$\pi = \Delta CRT$$

where π is the osmotic pressure in atmospheres, ΔC is the difference in osmolality between the intravascular and interstitial spaces, R is the gas constant (0.082061 atm/mol·K) and T is temperature in degrees Kelvin.

Using this equation, it can be calculated that for each milliosmolar difference across the blood–brain barrier, an osmotic pressure gradient of 19.3 mm Hg will be produced. This gradient is a potent force for the movement of water between the brain and the vasculature. The ability of the blood–brain barrier to inhibit the movement of low-molecular-weight particles between the vasculature and the brain makes it possible to manipulate brain water content by the intravenous administration of hypertonic solutions of mannitol or saline. The ability of the blood–brain barrier to prevent the transit of intravascular molecules and ions can be quantified by measuring the reflection coefficient for a given solute. The reflection coefficient may vary between 0 (free movement of the solute across the blood–brain barrier) and 1 (completely excluded). The reported reflection coefficients for both mannitol and sodium chloride are high, ranging between 0.90 and 1.00 (Fenstermacher 1984). The small particles in these solutions can therefore be effectively excluded from the brain's interstitium by the intact blood–brain barrier, creating an osmotic pressure gradient favoring the movement of water from the brain into the intravascular space.

These observations have been substantiated by experimental studies we and others have conducted. Using plasmapheresis to manipulate plasma osmolality and oncotic pressure, it has been found that large decrements in oncotic pressure (from 20 ± 2 to 7 ± 1 mm Hg) had no effect on cortical water content or intracranial pressure in neurologically normal rabbits. In contrast, a 13 mosmol decrease in plasma osmolality resulted in increased cortical water content ($\approx$ 0.5%) as assessed by microgravimetry; there was an associated increase in intracranial pressure (Zornow et al. 1987). Although these studies were acute in nature, more prolonged (8-h) reductions in colloid oncotic pressure have also been without demonstrable effect on brain water content, although, as predicted by the Starling equation, they do result in edema of the peripheral tissues (Kaieda et al. 1989).

The Cryogenic Lesion

Cryogenic or freeze lesions of the brain have long been used to study cerebral pathophysiology. Much of the early work on cryogenic injury was conducted in the 1950s by Clasen, Klatzo, and their colleagues. Klatzo et al. (1955) applied a metal plate, cooled to −50°C by a mixture of dry ice in acetone, directly to the exposed pial surface. The "inevitable sticking" of the plate to the cortex could be released by application of a few drops of a fructose solution. In contrast, Clasen et al. (1953) produced cryogenic injuries by applying isopentone–liquid nitrogen directly to the intact skull. By varying the length of time that the liquid nitrogen was in contact with the skull,

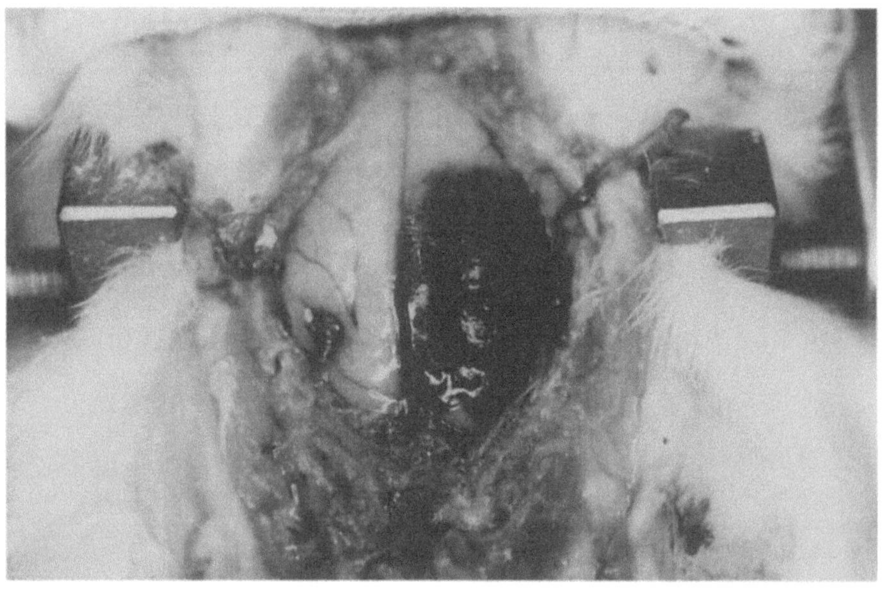

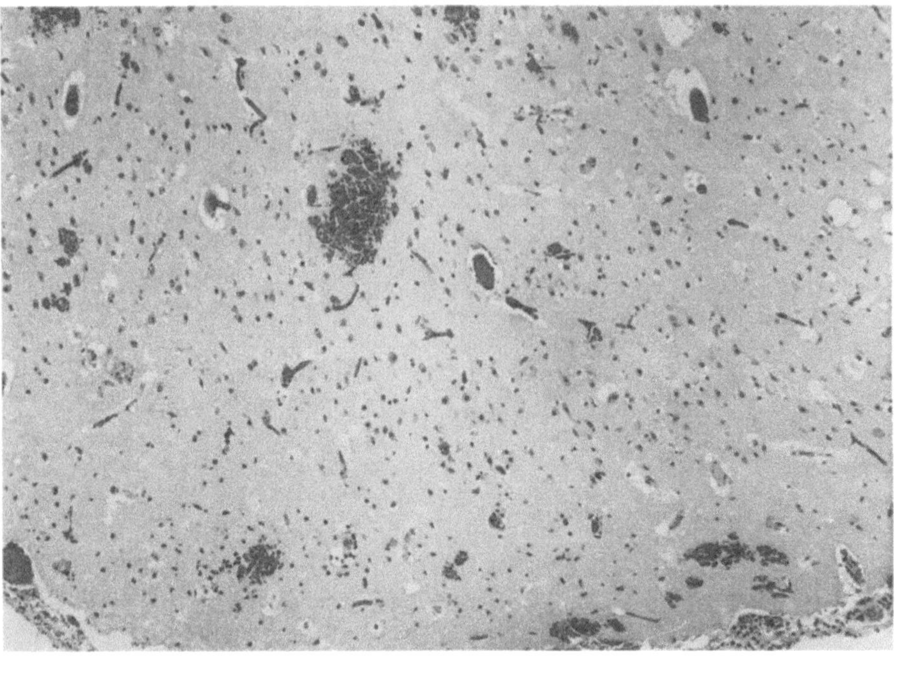

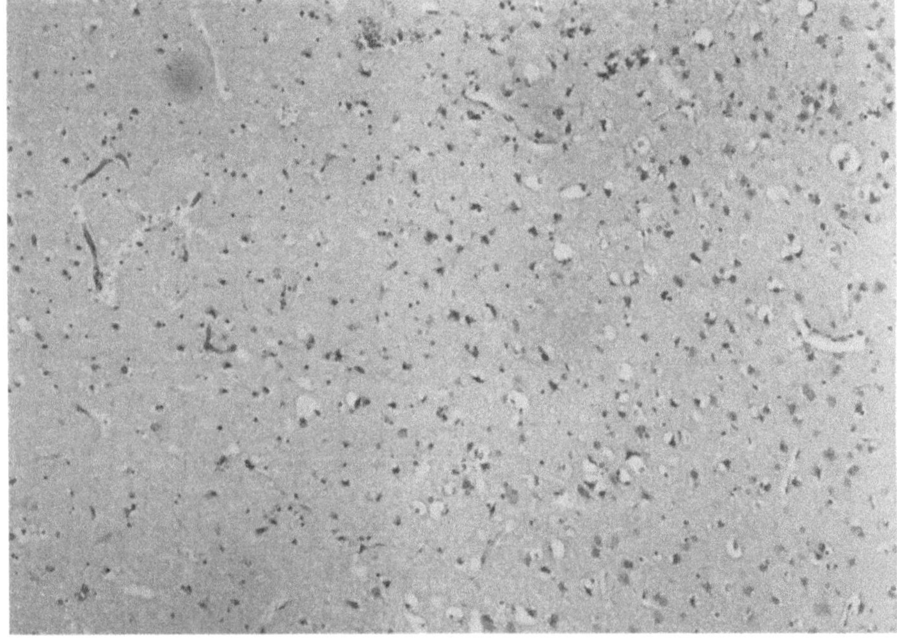

As in traumatic injury, there are elements of both cytotoxic edema and vasogenic edema in cryogenic lesions. Cytotoxic edema is an increase in intracellular water content due to the inability of a cell to volume regulate. This failure may result from a variety of causes, including ischemia, energy failure or exposure to excitatory neurotransmitters. In contrast, vasogenic edema results from a breakdown of the blood–brain barrier and extravasation of plasma proteins and electrolytes into the interstitium of the brain. It is rare to have exclusively one form or another of brain edema. Often a vicious cycle is established in which vasogenic edema compromises regional tissue perfusion, resulting in cellular ischemia. This ischemia causes cellular energy failure, compromising various membrane pumps, resulting in cellular swelling (cytotoxic edema). This swelling, in turn, may further damage the blood–brain barrier, resulting in more vasogenic edema, thereby completing the cycle.

Much of the edema seen on histologic examination after cryogenic injury represents vasogenic edema, as its composition is similar to that of the plasma (Gazendam et al. 1979). This edema fluid tends to propagate into the white matter surrounding the lesion site and eventually drains into the cerebral ventricles by bulk flow (Reulen 1976). Within 72 h of the lesion, the damaged vessels that leaked edema fluid into the interstitial space begin to be repaired, with the repair being completed within 7 days (Orita et al. 1988).

Therapy of Experimental Brain Edema

Clasen et al. (1957) were among the first to investigate the ability of hypertonic solutions to alter brain water content in animal models of brain injury. In 1957 they published their findings on the effects of various hypertonic solutions on intracranial pressure and hemispheric water content. In these studies, brain water content was assayed by lipid extraction and vacuum drying of each cerebral hemisphere to a constant weight. Although the hypertonic (50%) glucose solution did cause a transient decrease in intracranial pressure, there was no corresponding decrease in the water content of the lesioned hemisphere. Administration of 25% albumin was without effect on either water content or intracranial pressure, while 20% dextran exacerbated both intracranial hypertension and cerebral edema. These studies were limited by difficulty in measuring regional water content and the fact that such determinations could not be made in a serial fashion.

Some of the earliest studies on the cerebral effects of hypertonic saline solutions were conducted by Weed and McKibben in 1919. These investigators directly observed the effects of hypertonic saline on the degree of brain protrusion through a craniotomy site, as described in this excerpt from one of their papers:

As the intravenous injection of the salt is continued, the brain falls away from the skull until the surface presented becomes concave. The maximum shrinkage has been observed usually in from 15 to 30 min after the completion of the injection, when the brain lies flaccid, 3–4 mm below the inner table of the skull. (Weed and McKibben 1919)

Although this end point may seem crude by today's standards, their conclusion that hypertonic saline reduces brain volume has not changed. Since these early studies however, only in the last 10–15 years has there been a resurgence in interest in the use of hypertonic saline solutions. Initially, this interest was directed primarily at the use of hypertonic saline for the resuscitation of patients with hemorrhagic shock. Typical of these studies was an investigation conducted by Peters et al. (1986) Using a porcine model of hemorrhage, these investigators compared Ringer's lactate solution (272 mosmol/l) with either a hypertonic saline solution (470 mosmol/l) or a hypertonic mannitol solution (479 mosmol/l) on cardiac output, blood pressure, and mortality. Anesthetized pigs were bled to one-third of their blood volume and maintained in this shock state for 1 h before being resuscitated with one of the study solutions. The investigators found that the hypertonic mannitol solution was associated with a high mortality rate and did not maintain cardiac output as well as the hypertonic saline solutions. The resuscitation with hypertonic saline also required the smallest infused volume of the three solutions.

As the beneficial effects of hypertonic saline solutions in the resuscitation of trauma patients became more apparent, a number of investigators began to examine the effects of these solutions on various cerebral parameters, both in normal and brain-injured animals. Prough et al. (1985) compared the effects of hypertonic saline (2400 mosmol/l, 7.5% solution) with those of lactated Ringer's solution on intracranial pressure in dogs that had sustained 30 min of hypovolemic shock (mean arterial pressure = 50 mm Hg). Blood pressure and cardiac output were returned to baseline values in both groups, but plasma osmolality increased from 285 to 335 mosmol/l in those animals randomized to receive hypertonic saline. Intracranial pressure was the other variable that showed the greatest difference between the two groups in the immediate postresuscitation period. In the animals that received hypertonic saline, the intracranial pressure was 7.1 ± 1.6 mm Hg vs 15.0 ± 3.5 mm Hg in the lactated Ringer's group. These results suggested that hypertonic saline solutions may not only be efficacious for the rapid restoration of circulating blood volume, cardiac output and blood pressure, but may also be useful in neurotrauma patients at risk for intracranial hypertension.

To examine the effects of hypertonic solutions on cerebral variables in an animal model of traumatic brain injury, Zornow et al. compared lactated Ringer's solution (254 mosmol/kg) with a hypertonic lactated Ringer's solution (469 mosmol/kg) in rabbits that had received a hemispheric cryogenic lesion (Zornow et al. 1989). The lesion was produced by applying liquid nitrogen to a 1-cm diameter area of the intact skull for 70 s. The animals were then hemodiluted with either the lactated Ringer's solution or the hypertonic solution for a period of 45 min to simulate ongoing hemorrhage with crystalloid resuscitation. The test solutions were infused at whatever rate was necessary to maintain blood pressure and central venous pressures at baseline values. The animals were then killed and their brains removed for determination of regional water content by microgravimetry and wet–dry weights. Although intracranial pressure increased during hemodilution in both groups, the increase was greatly attenuated in the animals that received the hypertonic solution (1.7 ± 1.5 vs 9.5 ± 2.4 mm Hg). In the hypertonic group, cortical brain water was decreased as assessed by microgravimetry in all regions remote from the lesion. This study suggests that hypertonic solutions may offer benefits in the acute resuscitation of neurotrauma

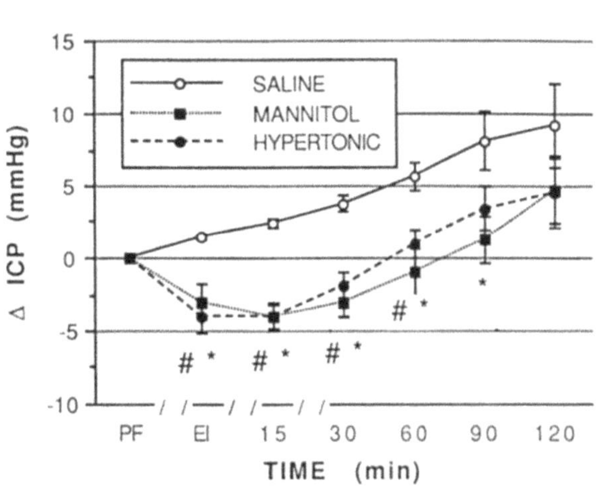

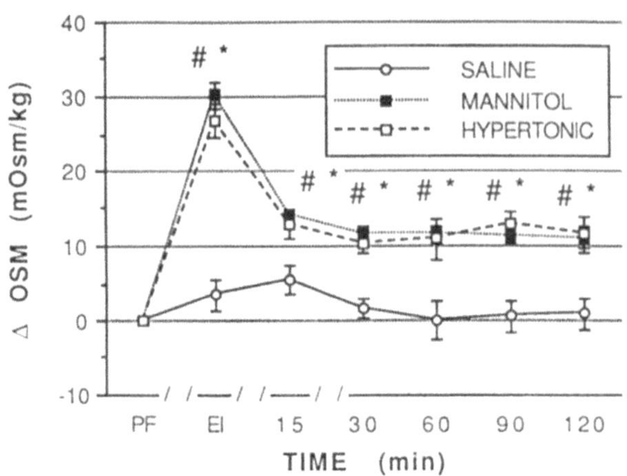

40
30
20
10
0
-10
Δ OSM (mOsm/kg)
*
*
*
*
*
*
SALINE
MANNITOL
HYPERTONIC
PF
EI
15
30
60
90
120
TIME (min)

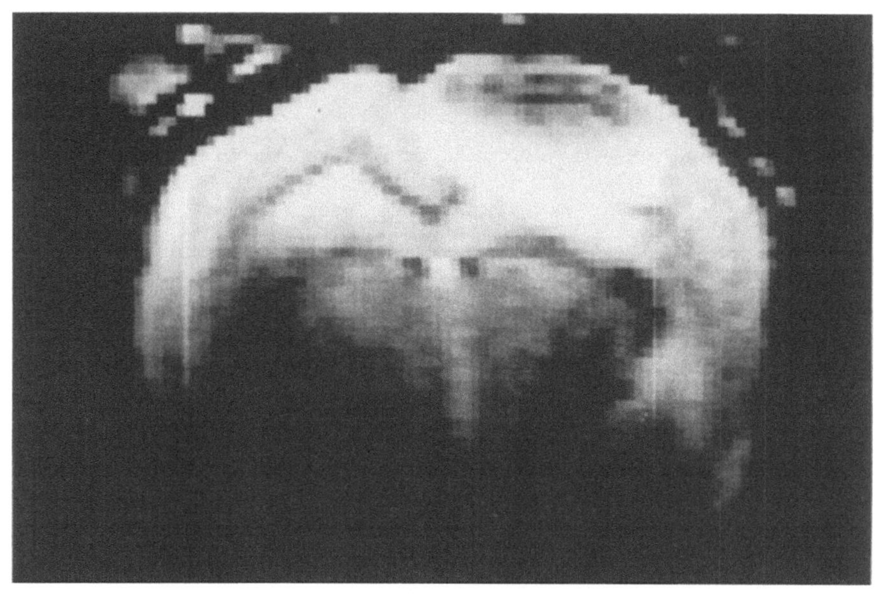

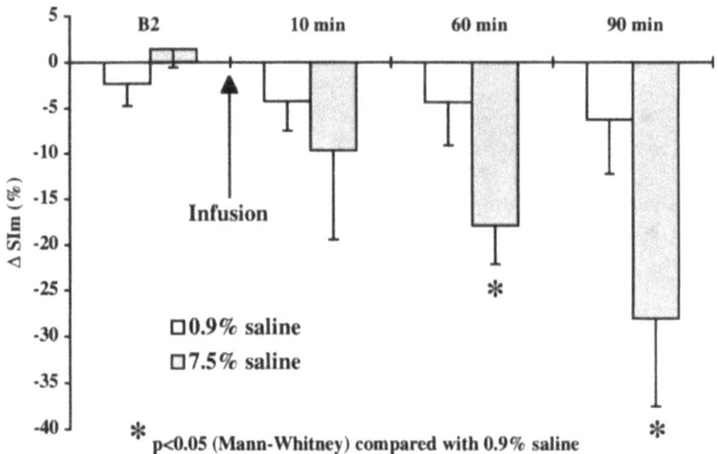

ΔSIm (%)
B2
10 min
60 min
90 min
Infusion
5
0
-5
-10
-15
-20
-25
-30
-35
-40
□ 0.9% saline
□ 7.5% saline
*
*
* p<0.05 (Mann-Whitney) compared with 0.9% saline

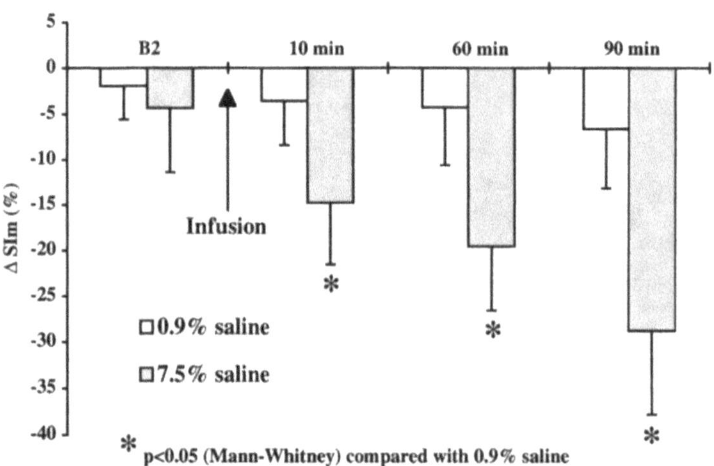

ΔSIm (%)
B2
10 min
60 min
90 min
Infusion
5
0
-5
-10
-15
-20
-25
-30
-35
-40
□ 0.9% saline
□ 7.5% saline
*
*
*
* p<0.05 (Mann-Whitney) compared with 0.9% saline

References

Baxt WG, Moody P (1987) The differential survival of trauma patients. J Trauma 27:602–606

Cascino T, Baglivo J, Szewczykowski J, Posner JB, Rottenberg DA (1983) Quantitative CT assessment of furosemide- and mannitol- induced changes in brain water content. Neurology (Cleve) 33:898–903

Clasen RA, Brown DVL, Leavitt S, Hass GM (1953) The production by liquid nitrogen of acute closed cerebral lesions. Surg Gynecol Obstet 96:605–616

Clasen RA, Prouty RR, Bingham WG, Martin FA, Hass GM (1957) Treatment of experimental cerebral edema with intravenous hypertonic glucose, albumin, and dextran. Surg Gynecol Obstet 104:591–606

Fenstermacher JD (1984) Volume regulation of the central nervous system. In: Staub NC, Taylor AE (eds) Edema. Raven, New York

Gazendam J, Go KG, van Zanten AK (1979) Composition of isolated edema fluid in cold-induced brain edema. J Neurosurg 51:70–77

Kaieda R, Todd MM, Warner DS (1989) Prolonged reduction in colloid oncotic pressure does not increase brain edema following cryogenic injury in rabbits. Anesthesiology 71:554–560

Klatzo I, Piraux A, Laskowski EJ (1955) The relationship between edema, blood-brain barrier and tissue elements in a local brain injury. J Neuropathol Exp Neurol 17:548–564

Kurtzke JF (1982) The current neurologic burden of illness and injury in the United States. Neurology (NY) 32:1207–1214

Marshall LF, Bowers SA (1985) Medical management of head injury. Clin Neurosurg 29:312–325

Mintorovitch J, Yang GY, Shimizu H, Kucharczyk J, Chan PH, Weinstein PR (1994) Diffusion-weighted magnetic resonance imaging of acute focal cerebral ischemia: comparison of signal intensity with changes in brain water and Na^+, K^+-ATPase activity. J Cereb Blood Flow Metab 14:332–336

Orita T, Nishizaki T, Kamiryo T, Harada K, Aoki H (1988) Cerebral microvascular architecture following experimental cold injury. J Neurosurg 68:608–612

Peters RM, Hargens AR (1981) Protein vs electrolytes and all of the Starling forces. Arch Surg 116:1293–1298

Peters RM, Shackford SR, Hogan JS, Cologne JB (1986) Comparison of isotonic and hypertonic fluids in resuscitation from hypovolemic shock. Surg Gynecol Obstet 163:219–224

Prough DS, Johnson JC, Poole GV, Stullken EH, Johnston WE, Royster R (1985) Effects on intracranial pressure of resuscitation from hemorrhagic shock with hypertonic saline versus lactated Ringer's solution. Crit Care Med 13:407–411

Reulen HJ (1976) Vasogenic brain oedema. Br J Anaesth 48:741–751

Scheller MS, Zornow MH, Oh YS (1991) A comparison of the cerebral and hemodynamic effects of mannitol and hypertonic saline in a rabbit model of acute cryogenic brain injury. J Neurosurg Anesth 3:291–296

Schmoker J, Zhuang J, Shackford S (1991) Hypertonic fluid resuscitation improves cerebral oxygen delivery and reduces intracranial pressure after hemorrhagic shock. J Trauma 31:1607–1613

Starling EH (1896) On the absorption of fluids from the connective tissue spaces. J Physiol (Lond) 19:312–326

Walsh JC, Zhuang J, Shackford SR (1991) A comparison of hypertonic to isotonic fluid in the resuscitation of brain injury and hemorrhagic shock. J Surg Res 50:284–292

Weed LH, McKibben PS (1919) Experimental alteration of brain bulk. Am J Physiol 48:531–555

Zornow MH, Todd M, Moore S (1987) The acute cerebral effects of changes in plasma osmolality and oncotic pressure. Anesthesiology 67:936–941

Zornow MH, Scheller MS, Shackford SR (1989) Effect of a hypertonic lactated Ringer's solution on intracranial pressure and cerebral water content in a model of traumatic brain injury. J Trauma 29:484–488

Discussion

Shackford:
First, Mark, I wanted to compliment you on a very fine presentation; you are just as thoughtful as ever. I do, however, have a recommendation for you, and that is don't spend any more time trying to understand those T2 spin-weighted images. You have got to accept that like electricity and television. Just accept it on faith and leave it at that. Regarding the efficacy of mannitol, when you and I were collaborating I remember when you were talking about this work and I suffered from one of the vulnerabilities of every experimenter and that is, I had a bias that hypertonic saline was better than mannitol. Back in the 1960s, mannitol was shown to have a hypotensive effect, which was very transient. At that time there was no work on the use of mannitol in hemorrhagic shock combined with brain injury. And right about the time that you were doing this work, Israel and a group from Denver General published a very nice study on the use of mannitol in a model of epidural balloon in hemorrhagic shock and showed that the transient hypotension did not occur, hemodynamics were well maintained over the 3-h period of the study, and it appeared that mannitol was a good drug to give to brain-injured, shocked patients. To my knowledge, there have not been any further studies, so I would think that mannitol and hypertonic saline are probably equivalent drugs.

Kochanek:
I enjoyed your paper. This work and your studies over the years have certainly educated me in terms of the issues of fluid management and brain injury. I would disagree with Dr. Shackford and suggest that we try to learn as much as possible about ADC, DWI, and the other techniques that are being used to assess edema in MRI. I do, however, have a concern about the freeze lesion. It appears to behave less like a contusion or what is produced by fluid percussion, and rather more like a stroke. Faden et al. used the fluid percussion model using DWI and they were very hard-pressed in the early time period after the injury to find any diffusion-weighted signal. It appears to me that the freeze lesion looks more like a stroke or compression ischemia model from an epidural or subdural hematoma (post evacuation). In support of the concept that the freeze injury is very much different from trauma you observe CA1 not CA3 cell death in the hippocampus. In both the fluid percussion and the controlled cortical impact model, CA3, the dentate and the hilus are injured, whereas CA1 is generally spared, even though CA1 is right underneath the impact. Do you consider your model more like a stroke model rather than actually a trauma model?

Zornow:
I really do not have much experience with other models of TBI. Maybe I am emphasizing the similarities that I want to see. Certainly, the histology correlates with the MRI findings. And when I make the specific gravity measurements at the periphery of the lesion and from the core of the lesion, it looks like there is increased water content that gets more marked as you move in towards the lesion. If you are trying to model a direct contusion to the brain, say a depressed skull fracture perhaps, this is a good

model. If you try to model the type of brain injury that occurs from acceleration-deceleration injuries, it is probably not.

Kochanek:
I was not directly knocking the model. In terms of producing edema and manipulating edema it is an excellent tool. It does appear to take much more time in the contusion model for cerebral edema to develop.

Baethmann:
I would like to come back to the problem of the rebound effect after administration of hypertonic fluid, in particular of hypertonic saline under these circumstances. I wonder whether you have studied later periods after infusion of the hypertonic saline, whether a rebound occurs when, let's say, the hyperosmolar bolus in the intravascular compartment is dissipated or diluted. During infusion of hypertonic fluid and shortly thereafter, there is the possibility of an efflux of hypertonic plasma into the brain at the lesion site with an open blood–brain barrier. When the plasma osmolality has normalized there could be a movement of fluid into the opposite direction, i.e., into the brain. As you have available MRI imaging as a non-invasive method to follow up animals for longer periods, I wonder whether you have studied a later phase when rebound might have occurred.

Zornow:
As I said, we are just beginning these MRI imaging studies; what you have seen is what we have done. In terms of earlier studies we were looking at brain water content or ICPs, most of these studies were of an acute nature, and that is one of their failings – I mean they really are acute, short-term studies. The chronic studies that I alluded to were our circulatory arrest model in monkeys, that required a tremendous amount of effort but had nothing to do with brain water content or hypertonic solutions.

Young:
I think this is a very nice model. I wanted to ask about the relative changes in brain water content near the lesion and away from the lesion in the lesioned hemisphere.

Zornow:
Well, the maximum increase in our measurement of brain water content by specific gravity was in the core of the lesion. The core of the lesion was most edematous. And then as you moved away from the lesion, water content progressively decreased until at the sampling site from the frontal cortex it was about the same on the contralateral hemisphere.

Young:
But then, after you gave the hyperosmolar saline, what part of the lesioned hemisphere was most affected?

Zornow:
As you got closer to the damaged area of the brain, the specific gravity measurements became more and more variable, and the standard deviations were very large. So, we could no longer statistically demonstrate a difference between the hypertonic and the isotonic groups. There are two possibilities to explain this: One is that there is a

difference, but because of the large standard deviations you cannot statistically demonstrate it. The other possibility, which I tend to believe, is that hypertonic solutions, be they mannitol or hypertonic saline, work on normal brain, but they do not work on areas of injured brain where the blood–brain barrier has been disrupted.

Young:
I suppose there is a critical lesion size in which you really will not affect very much the swelling in the lesioned hemisphere. You can remove the fluid out of the non-lesioned hemisphere, but if the lesion is really massive, you probably will not change things very much in the affected hemisphere.

Zornow:
Yes, I think that is true. If you have a massive breakdown of the blood–brain barrier, say somebody with sustained cardiac arrest, there is widespread structural breakdown of the blood–brain barrier. In that case you may not see any benefit with the administration of any kind of hypertonic solution. Similarly, in patients who have severe brain injury and major depression of cerebral metabolic rate, if you give pentabarbitol to those patients, you may not see a decrease in ICP because the metabolic rate is already suppressed. So you really cannot gain anything by giving barbiturate. So, you are correct. The effect really depends on the size of the lesion.

Prough:
Mark, in looking at the images of the cryogenic injury and the edema spreading along the convexity, it looked similar to data that, I think, Hoff produced, probably 15 years ago, describing the spread of cerebral edema once it had produced in an area of blood–brain barrier disruption. One way to look at your findings might be that the hypertonic solution cleared the edema out of the area in which it had collected, but in which the blood–brain barrier was not damaged. However, the area of the core in which the blood–brain barrier was damaged was just as densely edematous as before.

Zornow:
We would like to do a more regional analysis of the signal intensity in the future. Our original expectation was that we would not see a change in signal intensity right around the lesion itself, but we have not got quite to that level of analysis yet.

Shackford:
Just one other point. It is interesting, Mark, in all of your data and our data and Don Prough's data that osmolar effect in improving intracranial compliance is transient. Like any medical therapy for ICP, this is not a definitive therapy. It is basically to improve intracranial compliance for a short period of time until the patient can have more definitive treatment. Hypertonic saline is not the be all and end all.

Zornow:
I think that is very true. Basically, you are buying some time, and that is about it. You can only buy a limited amount of time.

Pathophysiology, Management and Outcome After Multiple Trauma

G. Regel, U. Lehmann, E. Rickels, T. Pohlemann,
H.C. Pape, and H. Tscherne

Introduction

Severe head injury is the most frequent cause of permanent disability after trauma in our society. It is often associated with multiple trauma (69% in our own patient population) and additionally the most frequent injury combination in association with extremity injuries (63%) (Regel et al. 1995) (Fig. 1).

The mortality rate in these patients is high at 12%–20% (Gennarelli et al. 1989; Regel et al. 1995). Trauma causes about 150000 deaths per year in the USA, almost half due to severe head injuries. Head injury is the most limiting factor in these patients in the early phase after trauma (Fig. 2).

Early studies demonstrated that posttraumatic brain damage is not only the result of events at the time of injury (primary damage), but rather occurs subsequently, and in this case even may be preventable (secondary damage) (Anderson et al. 1988). The anatomical basis of primary brain damage is mechanical disruption of neurons and disturbance of the cerebral microcirculation at the time of injury. Even today little can be done to prevent this direct brain damage.

Intermittent improvement of neurologic status in the posttraumatic course was demonstrated in some cases, proving that late death is not always a consequence of overwhelming primary brain damage (Reilly et al. 1975). Postmortem studies showed that 90% of these patients had evidence of raised intercranial pressure (ICP). Next to evacuation of intracranial hematoma the therapeutic failure to correct systemic hypoxia and hypotension was shown to contribute to death in these patients (Rose et al. 1977; Jennett and Carlin 1978).

The common denominator among the causes of secondary brain damage is now known to be a reduction in cerebral tissue perfusion and oxygenation, often associated with a rise in the ICP (Miller and Becker 1982). It has been shown experimentally that mechanically injured neurons have increased susceptibility to hypoxic–ischemic damage (Eisenberg et al. 1983; Ishige et al. 1987).

Thus the clinical challenge is to minimize these secondary disturbances to the brain through optimal organization of prehospital and early hospital management of these patients. This is very much dependent on a better understanding of the underlying pathomechanisms.

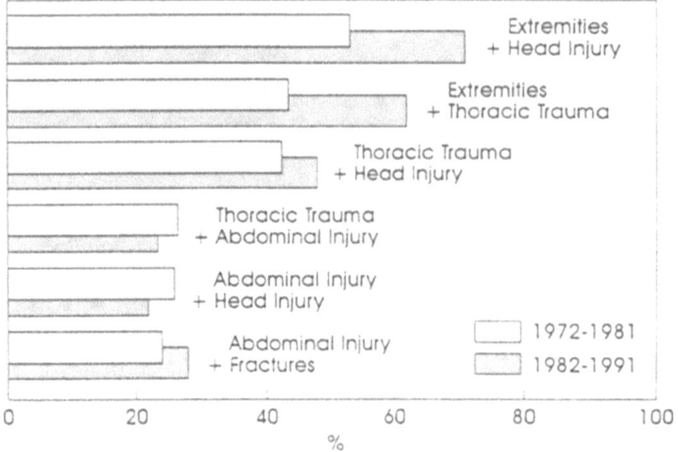

Fig. 1. Most frequent injury combinations in association with extremity injuries (Regel et al. 1995)

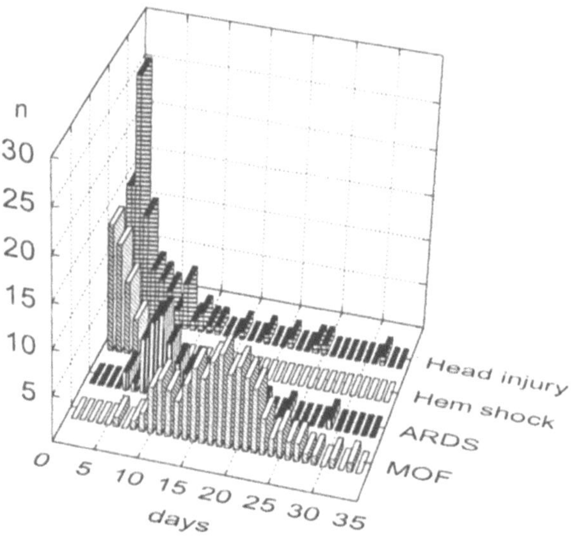

Fig. 2. Distribution and etiology of trauma death in multiple trauma patients ($n = 826$). Notice the frequency of death due to severe head injury in the early posttraumatic course (Regel 1996). *ARDS*, acute respiratory distress syndrome; *MOF*, multiple organ failure

Pathophysiology

The primary lesion after initial trauma is associated with vascular disruption as well as contusion and axonary injury (Fig. 3). The extent ranges diagnostically from a layer of superficial blood to involvement of the whole depth of the brain. Abnormal vascular and autoregulatory responses lead to the formation of endothelial lesions. Abnormalities of vascular smooth muscle and of the blood–brain barrier ensue. Accelerated vesicular transport of protein leads to extensive extravasation of protein into the vessel wall and perivascular compartmental pressure increase. This in most cases leads again to a disturbance of the autoregulation mechanisms, and thereby to an increase of cerebral blood flow (CBF) and consequently to a primary increase of ICP, *at first independent* of prehospital treatment (Fig. 4).

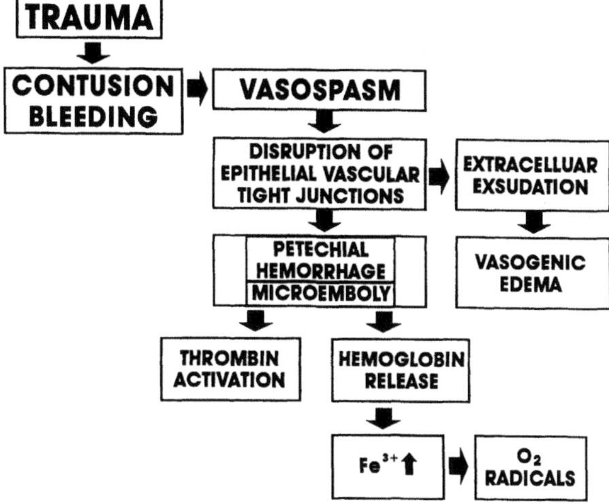

Fig. 3. Vascular disruption leads to abnormal vascular and autoregulatory responses and the formation of endothelial lesions. Abnormalities of vascular smooth muscle and of the blood–brain barrier ensue. Accelerated vesicular transport of protein leads to extensive extravasation of protein and the developement of vasogenic edema. With hemoglobin release oxygen free radicals develop

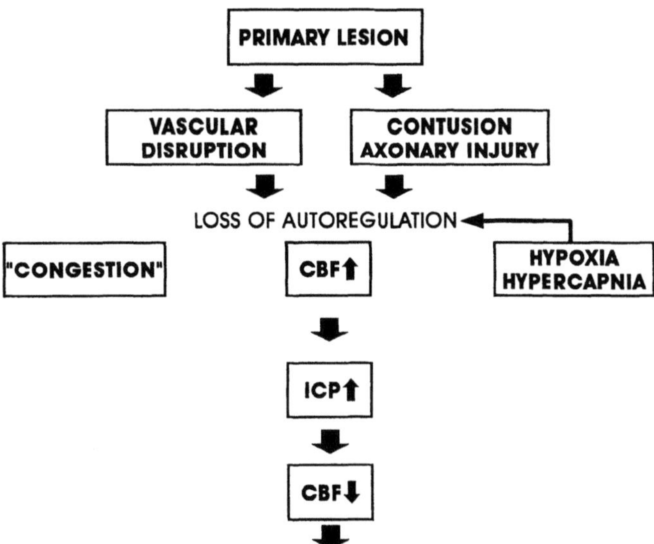

Fig. 4. The primary lesion after initial trauma is associated with vascular disruption as well as contusion and axonary injury. The increase of intracranial pressure (*ICP*) in a second stage leads to a reduction of cerebral blood flow (*CBF*) and thereby to hypoxic brain tissue damage

The ultimate causes of the secondary lesion are hypoxia and ischemia. This process involves a complex interplay of mechanisms. The reduction of perfusion causes a lack of glucose and oxygen. The result is a shortage of ATP, forcing the cell to use the anaerobic glycolysis, causing lactate acidosis with a decrease of pH. A depolarization occurs at this time causing an intracellular calcium overload, and an excessive release of the excitatory aminoacid neurotransmitters glutamate and aspartate (Fig. 5).

Calcium overload then initiates the activation of the arachnoid acid cascade and the introduction of oxygen free radicals induced by lipid peroxidation. The release of these toxic metabolites results in the developement of the so-called cytotoxic edema with an increase of vascular permeability, and consequently to an increase of cerebral edema (Fig. 6.) In the following the main mechanisms will be discussed in detail:

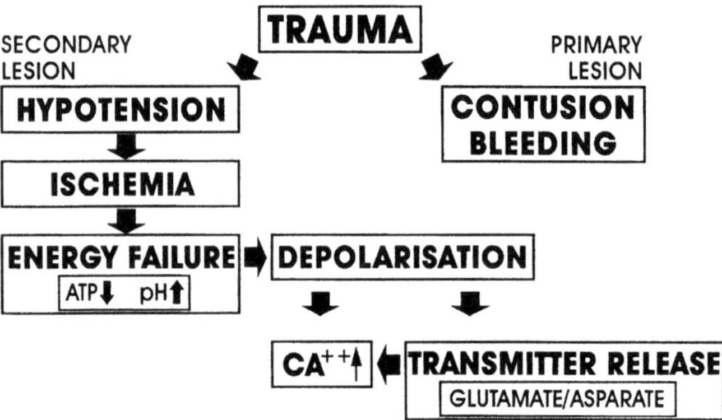

Fig. 5. A depolarization occurs at this time causing an intracellular calcium overload, and an excessive release of the excitatory aminoacid neurotransmitters glutamate and aspartate

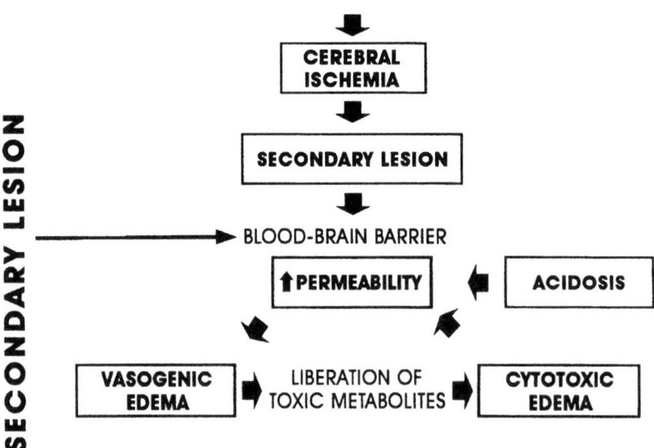

Fig. 6. The further increase of intracranial pressure in the second stage leads to a reduction of cerebral blood flow and thereby to ischemic brain tissue damage, mechanisms resulting in the so-called cytotoxic edema with an increase of vascular permeability and consequently an increase of cerebral edema

Cerebral Blood Flow

CBF is normally dependant on the cerebral perfusion pressure (CPP), the vascular threshold and the mean arterial pressure (MAP). The CPP is thereby calculated as the difference between the MAP and the ICP: CPP = MAP − ICP (mm Hg). With normal brain function the autoregulation mechanism guarantees a constant CBF even with an alteration of MAP in a range between 60 and 100 mm Hg. This results from contraction or dilatation of the cerebral vasculature (Obrist et al. 1984).

Reduction of CPP below 20 ml/100 g brain tissue per minute will cause a depletion of the EEG and evoked potentials. Below 12 ml/100 g per minute this will result in a destruction of the cell membrane and consequently to cell death. That means that cells where perfusion ranks between 12 and 20 ml/100 g per minute are not able to perform their normal cell function but still survive. The area in this stage is called "penumbra" (Table 1).

On the other hand the CBF correlates with the consumption of oxygen and glucose and therefore is also an index for the cerebral metabolism (Rosner and Coley 1986; Cruz et al. 1995). Under physiologic conditions the CBF increases with the decrease of the glucose concentration or the oxygen saturation in a direct proportional relation. In association with trauma the resucitation time of brain tissue is less than 10 min due to the minimal storage of energy supplying glucose and the short inefficient anaerobic glycolysis (Lassen 1974). All efforts of resuscitation are therefore aiming to get the cells away from the penumbra status to a higher perfusion level as soon as possible.

Hypoxia emphasizes the loss of autoregulation, with an initial increase of cerebral blood volume and a further increase of ICP. This is called the vasodilatory cascade (Rosner and Daughton 1990; Rosner et al. 1995) (Fig. 7). Similarly hypercapnia results in a vasodilatation and thereby similarly to an increase of intracerebral blood flow and ICP (Paulson et al. 1972; Donegan et al. 1985). This vasoparalysis directly after trauma and the acute increase of intracerebral blood volume is called "congestion". It has to be distinguished from the pathophysiology of the different types of posttraumatic edema (Table 2).

The further increase of ICP in the second stage then leads to a reduction of CBF and thereby to ischemic brain tissue damage (Fig. 4). Ischemia is the most common mechanism in more than 80% of fatal head injuries. Clinical symptoms correlate with the degree of hypoxemia and the decrease of oxygen saturation (Table 2). With hypoxia the increase of anaerobic metabolism leads to a high lactate concentration

Table 1. Reduction of cerebral perfusion pressure (CPP) below 20 ml/100 g brain tissue per minute causes a depletion of the EEG and evoked potentials

CPP = MAP − ICP (mm Hg)

CPP < 20 ml/100 g brain tissue per minute alterations of EEG and SEP

CPP 12 and 20 ml/100 g per minute → reduced cell function, but still survive → "penumbra"

CPP < 12 ml/100 g brain tissue per minute destruction of the cell membrane → cell death

MAP, mean arterial pressure; ICP, intracranial pressure; SEP, somatosensory evoked potential.

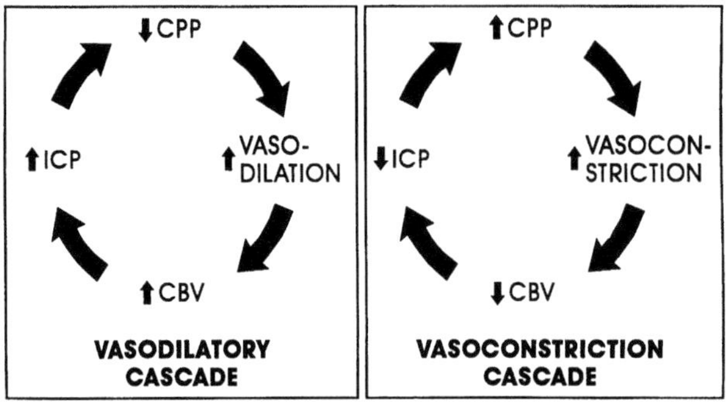

Fig. 7. Hypoxia emphasizes the loss of autoregulation, with an initial increase of cerebral blood volume (*CBV*) and a further increase of intracranial pressure (*CIP*). This is called the vasodilatory cascade (Rosner and Daughton 1990). *CPP*, cerebral perfusion pressure

Table 2. Clinical symptoms correlate to the degree of hypoxemia (PaO_2 in mm Hg) and the decrease of oxygen saturation (pvO_2 in mm Hg) in the cerebral system (Jennett and Teasdale 1989)

HYPOXIA			
PaO_2 (mm Hg)	Cerebral pvO_2 (mm Hg)	Biochemical changes	Clinical symptoms
<50	<35	glycolysis/Lactate ↑ ATP = /neurotrans- mitter ↓	EEG minimal changes
<35	<25	↑lactate (phosphate)	EEG significant changes
<20–25	<10–15	ATP ↓ ECP ↑ NADH/NAD +↑	Coma/EEG Slow nerves
<5–10	tissue O_2 < 2	Irreversible damage of the neurones	†Hypoxia Hearf failure

ECP, eosinophil cationic protein; NADH, nicotinamide adenine dinucleotide, reduced; NAD, nicotinamide adenine dinucleotide.

and acidosis and thereby to secondary brain damage (DeSalles et al. 1986). The pathomechanisms include changes of:

Tissue Acidocis and Ionhomeostasis

Stores of glucose in brain tissue can maintain normal energy consumption for only a few seconds. When circulation is interrupted phosphocreatine and ATP levels approach a minimum within 2 min. After anoxia active transport or biosynthesis utilize stores of phosphocreatine and ATP formed through anaerobic glycolysis, which yields two molecules of ATP, two of lactate and two protons (H^+) and thus leads to an intracellular and extracellular acidosis. Intracellular pH falls as a function of lactate concentration reaching its minimum very fast.

The ATP depletion causes a failure of energy consuming antiporter systems (H^+/ Na^+ pump; Ca^{2+} pump and others) at the cell membrane, leading to a depolarization (Fig. 8).

These systems are necessary to keep the gradient between the extracellular space and the inner cell milieu. For example, the potassium concentration in the cell in 40 times higher than outside the cell and the gradient of concentration of calcium between inner and outer cell in 1:10000 (Branston et al. 1977). The cell tries to compensate the increase of H^+ and decrease of pH by activation of the Na^+/H^+ antiporter system. The exchange of H^+ against sodium causes a passive influx of water with the consequence of a cell edema.

Glutamate- and Aspartate-Induced Excitoxicity

Glutamate and aspartate are normally elicit postsynaptic responses mainly at dentritic sites. In the context of secondary posttraumatic injury the subtypes of *N*-methyl-D-aspartate (NMDA) and β-amino-3-hydroxy-5-methyl-isooxazole-4-

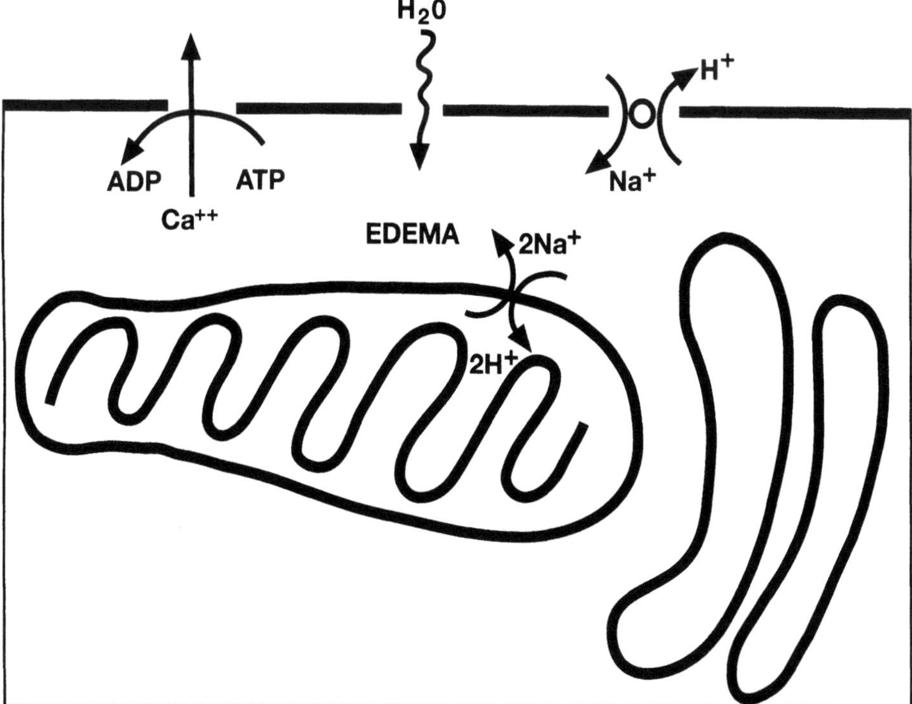

Fig. 8. The ATP depletion causes a failure of energy consuming antiporter systems (H^+/Na^+-pump; Ca^{2+} pump and others) at the cell membrane, leading to a depolarization. The efflux of Ca^{2+} is mainly dependent on ATP-driven and electrogenic sodium–calcium systems. Calcium can be stored inside the endo-plasmatic reticulum and in the mitochondria

propionic acid (AMPA) receptors appear to be pathophysiologically important (Faden et al. 1989).

When excessive amounts of aspartate or glutamate are released, or their uptake is compromised excitotoxic neuronal injury occurs (Fig. 5). The interaction of glutamate and glutamate recognition sites leads to an activation of inward calcium and sodium currents. The glycin recognition, polyamine, and phoshorylation sites, when acted upon by selective agonists, each serve to enhance the effects of glutamate receptor activation.

The NMDA receptor controls a postsynaptic voltage-dependent slow calcium channel. The sudden changes in Na, Cl, and Ca are tied to the depolarization and sudden release of excitatory amino acids, with an ensuing stimulation of receptor operated channels. The voltage dependence requires physiologic concentrations of Mg which blocks the NMDA channel at normal membrane potentials by binding it in the channel. When the membrane is depolarizied Mg no longer prevents calcium from entering the cell through the channel. In addition to ionotropic receptors glutamate activates a metabotropic receptor coupled through G proteins to inositol phospate or adenosine 3':'5-monophosphate formation.

Calcium Intracellular Overload

Calcium is an important messenger in cell-to-cell communication as well as a messenger inside the cell. The cell has many possibilities to store and eliminate this messenger. The efflux off the cell is mainly dependent on ATP-driven and electrogenic sodium–calcium systems. Calcium can be stored inside the endoplasmatic reticulum and in the mitochondria (Fig. 8). These mechanism of Ca^{2+} homeostasis is important since a non-physiological increase of calcium initiates different mechanisms of cell destruction.

Calcium rise will encompass proteolysis with enzyme conversion and breakdown of the cytoskeleton. It is very important that calcium is an activator of the phosphorlipases A and C. In particular, the Ca-dependent phosphorlipase C initiates cell membrane damage by splitting phosphatidyl-inositol, producing diacylglycerol and via a lipase-producing arachidonic acid (Fig. 9). The arachidonic acid is modified by the help of a cyclooxygenase to prostaglandine G_2 or via a lipoxygenase to leukotrienes. Prostaglandine G_2 is modified to other vasoactive substances as for instance prostaglandines or thromboxanes. Thromboxane A_2, for example, is the most powerful known vasoconstrictor to cerebral vessels. The production of another arachidonic metabolite is a free radical generating process.

Oxygen Free Radicals and Lipid Peroxidation

A free radical is an atom or molecule that possesses an unpaired electron in its outer orbit, a characteristic that makes the free radical highly reactive as it seeks a molecule from which it can attract an electron.

In a biological context the free radicals attempt to extract an electron from DNA,

RNA, proteins or lipids. The main target of free radicals during secondary brain damage is the polyunsaturated fatty acids of the cell membrane phospholipids (Chan et al. 1982) (Fig. 10).

Normally every intracellular system has some coping mechanisms like the cytochrome oxidase, Vitamine E and A, superoxide dismutase, cysteine.

In the injured nervous system a possible source of free radical production in-

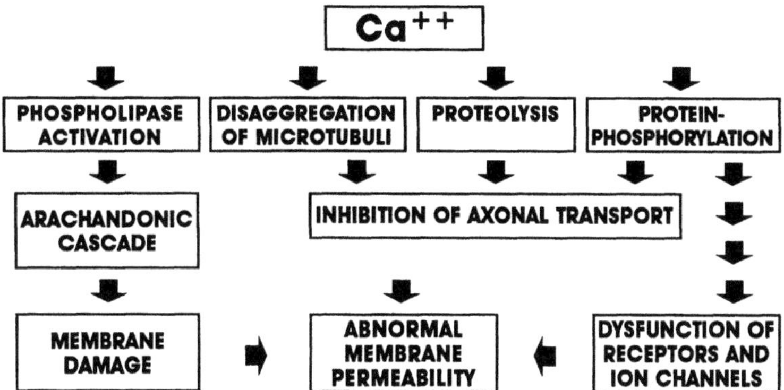

Fig. 9. It is very important that calcium is an activator of the phospholipases A and C. In particular, the Ca-dependent phosphorlipase C initiates cell membrane damage by splitting phosphatidyl

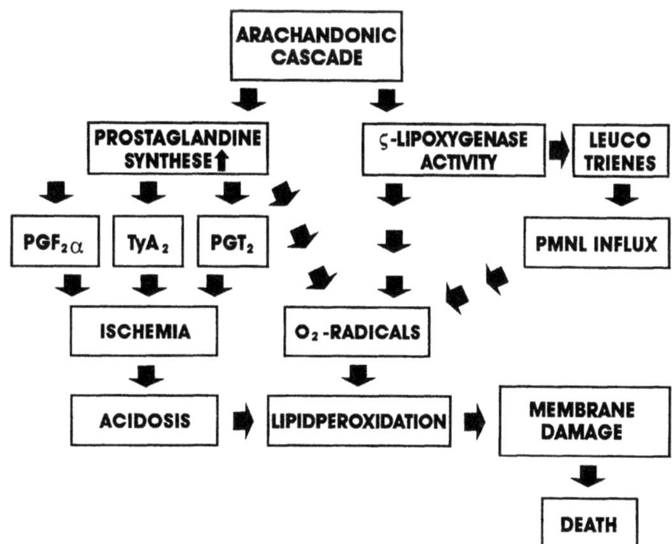

Fig. 10. The arachidonic acid is modified by the help of a cyclooxygenase to prostaglandin G_2 (PGG_2) or via a lipoxygenase to leukotrienes. Prostaglandin G_2 is modified to other vasoactive substances such as, for instance, prostaglandins or thromboxanes. Thromboxane A_2, for example, (TxA_2) is the most powerful known vasoconstrictor to cerebral vessels. The production of different arachidonic metabolites is a free radical generating process. The main target of free radicals during secondary brain damage is the polyunsaturated fatty acids of the cell membrane phospholipids. PGI_2, prostaglandin I_2; $PMNL$, polymorpho-nuclear leukocytes

cludes the arachidonic acid cascade, catecholamine oxidation, mitochondrial leaks, oxidation of extravasted hemoglobin, oxidation of xanthine by xanthine oxidase, and infiltrating activated neutrophils.

In addition to its role in the formation of hydroxyl radicals ferryl ion and other iron–oxygen complexes are considered.

Initiation of lipid peroxidation occurs when a radical species attacks and removes an allylic hydrogen from an unsaturated fatty acid resulting in a chain reaction.

Pathomechanisms of Edema Formation

Parallel to these changes an increase of capillary permeability is seen, and with the exsudation of proteins into the parenchyma the formation of a vasogenic edema is initialized (Table 3). This secondarily leads to the liberation of kinine, serotonine, as well as the production of other toxic metabolites (oxygen radicals and proteases) (Fig. 6).

Vasogenic edema is believed to result from an impairment at the blood–brain barrier, permitting the passage of water, sodium and protein into the interstitial space. The edema is formed largely in the gray matter but accumulates in the more compliant white matter. The rate of formation of edema is increased by hypercapnia, arterial hypotension, and an elevation of the body temperature. It has to be distinguished from the so called hydrostatic edema, which is most often the consequence of a mass lesion after intercranial bleeding.

The so-called cytotoxic edema is closely related to the critical threshold levels of reduced cerebral blood flow. With the liberation of toxic metabolites a disturbance at the cell membrane is seen (Fig. 6). Toxic damage to the astrocytes and glia substance then leads to a loss of electrical activity, when cerebral blood flow falls below 40% of base line and increases over time when blood flow falls to 20% of normal and the membrane ion pump mechanisms fail. As the ischemic process proceeds, potassium accumulates in the extracellular space, and calcium influx to the cell begins, setting off a cascade of reactions, which lead from membrane dysfunction to irreversible damage of the cell membrane.

In the pathogeneses of cytotoxic focal edema the polymorphonuclear leukocyte (PMN) is an important factor since these accumulate in the area of cerebral injury and lead consequently to capillary injury. Arachidonic acid metabolites and oxygen radicals seem to be responsible for this capillary injury (Chan et al. 1982; Hayashi et al. 1988).

The strict classification distinguishing between vasogenic and cytotoxic edema is, however, hypothetical since the isolated form is never seen in the clinical setting.

Posttraumatic brain edema results both from hypotension in association with hemorrhagic shock and hypoxia a consequence of reduced oxygenation. This could be demonstrated in experimental models on traumatic brain edema (Chesnut et al. 1993). Especially in multiple trauma patients with a traumatic head injury a prolonged hypoxia can lead to secondary brain damage. Hypoxia often results also from thoracic injury. The influence of decreased oxygen distribution to the brain

Table 3. Pathophysiology of the different types of posttraumatic edema; cerebral congestion and brain edema: occurence, types and features

Type of brain edema	Morphology	Pathogenetic mechanism	Reason/occurrence
Cerebral congestion (hyperemia)	Rapid increase in cerebral blood volume	No brain edema Precapillary vasodilation/ vasomotor paralysis or compression of cerebral veins	Initial (before brain edema) Brain injury, hypertensive crisis Inflammation, terminal: ischemia, hypoxia hypothermia (terminal pressure decompression, vasomotor paralysis), hydrocephalus, inflammation (meningoencephalitis)
Vasogenic edema (primary vasogenic, secondary cytotoxic)	Increasing water content of white matter (higher outlet resistance in grey matter hindering the spread of the cortical edema) ↓ Secondary hydrops of astrocytes (cytogenic type; swelling of the neuroglia)	Increasing permeability of the blood–brain barrier ⇒ influx of plasmatic exudate in the extracellular brain tissue ⇒ liberation of biogenic amines (kinin, 5-HT, bradycinin), prostaglandin UFA, free radicals, amino acid and lysosomal enzymes. The extent depends on T and CPP (transmural pressure gradient of extra- and intracellular compartment)	Brain injury, hypertensive encephalopathy, cerebral hemorrhage, brain tumor, abcess, encephalitis (primary); cerebral infarction, brain ischemia (secondary), vasculitis, severe acidosis, brain surgery, ARDS, severe hypoxia and hypercarbia
Cytotoxic brain edema (primary cytotoxic, secondary vasogenic)	Primary hydrops of astrocytes; 4–6 h later secondary vasogenic (decreasing barrier function) ⇒ increasing extent of the extracellular compartment	No primary damage to the blood–brain barrier (basal membrane and endothelium are intact). Toxic neuroglia damage with ion pump dysfunction: increasing influx of sodium chloride and water with K outflow	Primary: ischemia, hypoxia, hypothermia. Toxic: lead, mercury, organic solution, radiation damage. Secondary: brain injury, inflammation, brain tumor, brain surgery

UFA, unesterified fatty acids; T, temperature; CPP, cerebral perfusion pressure; ARDS, acute respiratory distress syndrome.

on secondary head injury could be demonstrated in both clinical (Miller 1985; Rhee et al. 1990; Pfenninger and Lindner 1991) and experimental models (Ishige et al. 1987).

An important therapeutic aspect of this issue is the problem related to the expansion of intracranial volume. The bony skull has a consistent volume and cerebral spinal fluid (CSF), blood, and cerebral tissue normally have a consistent volume in relation to each other. With the alteration of one compartment a decrease in volume of the other compartment has to result. An increase of intracranial volume in association with severe head injury can result primarily from intra- or extracerebral bleeding or can result secondarily from cerebral edema. At the beginning this intracranial volume, and therefore pressure increase, can be compensated since 10% of the intracranial volume can be shifted by distributing the fluid in the spinal fluid compartment and by increasing the resorption of CSF. When, however, these compensation mechanisms are reached, the intracranial pressure increases fulminantly. When the swelling is focal rather than diffusely distributed, the process will be complicated by the development of brain shift and eventually by brain herniation leading to death (Miller et al. 1978).

Initial Management of the Multiply Injured with Severe Head Injury

Understanding the complex relationship between brain swelling, edema, raised ICP, reduced cerebral perfusion pressure, brain shift and cerebral ischemia remain crucial for the optimal management of the patient with severe head injury. Especially in the multiple trauma patient these interactions are hard to calculate. For this close monitoring of ICP, CPP and oxygen saturation have to be considered.

Monitoring After Severe Head Injury

If the computed tomography (CT) scan confirms a severe head injury the patient will receive additional cerebral monitoring (Table 4). In these cases we monitor the ICP, the venous saturation in the jugular bulb (Sv jO$_2$), and the oxygen tissue pressure in the brain in an area next to the lesion (p$_{bt}$O$_2$).

There are different systems of ICP monitoring commercially available. The main problem of all industrial by manufactried ICP monitoring systems is the reliability of the measurement. If the ICP probe is positioned in or on the brain you can not gauge the real zero mm Hg of the ICP, which is important to verify the reliability of the measurement. The choice of system mainly depends on cost. Besides these epidural systems there is a tendency at the moment to use systems of direct ventricular puncture and to measure the ICP via CSF pressure transducer (Fig. 11). In this case we have to monitor early since with increasing ICP the lateral ventricles will be compromised and it becomes difficult to install the catheter. The ICP monitoring system should be connected to the hemodynamic monitoring system of the patient. The increase of ICP causes a reduction of CBF. Since the ICP on its own gives no real impression of the CBF we calculate the CPP by CPP = MAP − ICP. It is necessary to realize that the reference point for the MAP for calulating brain perfusion is the

Table 4. If the CT scan confirms a severe head injury the patient will receive additional cerebral monitoring (Fig. 11)

Cerebral Monitoring
Invasive arterial pressure monitoring (MAP)
Epidural or intraventricular measurement of intracranial pressure (ICP)
Venous saturation in the jugular bulb (SvjO$_2$)
Oxygen tissue pressure in the brain in an area next to the lesion (p$_{bt}$O$_2$)

MAP, mean arterial pressure.

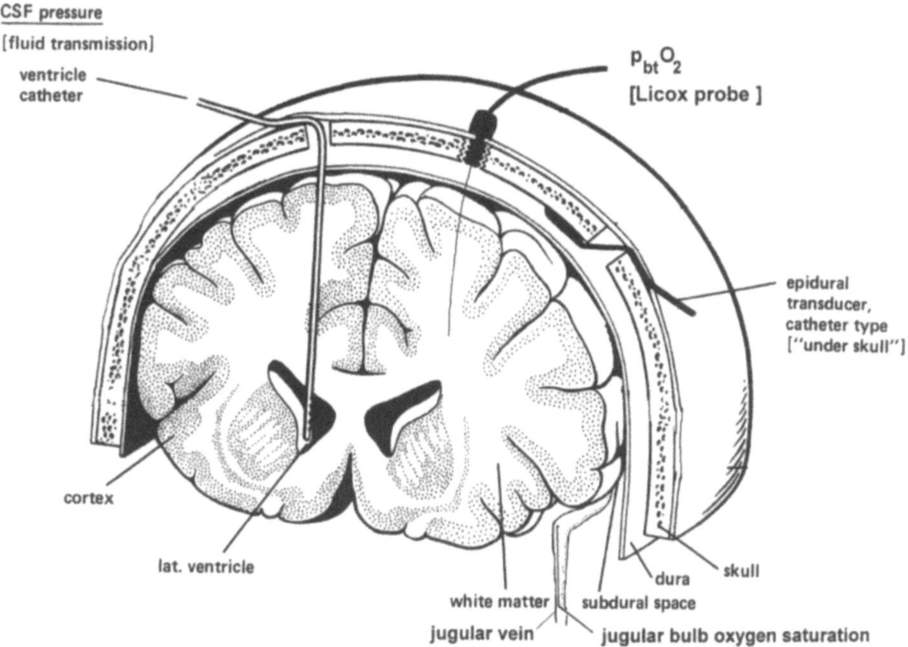

Fig. 11. Documenting intracranial pressure (*ICP*): at present, systems of direct ventricular puncture and ICP measurement via CSF pressure transducer are preferred. Additionally, the venous saturation in the jugular bulb ($SvjO_2$) and the oxygen tissue pressure in the brain in an area next to the lesion ($p_{bt}O_2$) are monitored

cranial basis. Even when the head is elevated you have to subtract from the MAP with reference to the heart. In this case it is easier to put the blood pressure transducer on the cranial basis level. It is important to make a trend analysis and document the CPP continuously on the patients chart.

The measurement of jugular bulb oxygen saturation gives an impression of the oxygen consumption of the brain (Souter and Andrews 1996). The hypothesis for measuring in the jugular vein is the fact that it is the only important outlet of cerebral blood and that at the level of the jugular bulb there is no inflow from extracranial veins. Knowing the saturation of the arterial blood entering the brain a reduction of the saturation of outcoming venous blood indicates the oxygen consumption. A reduction of $SvjO_2$ below 60% is considered to be harzardous. The main problem of this parameter is the reliability of the measurement (Souter and Andrews 1996). The loose fixation of the catheter to the neck and ongoing manipulation of the head forces frequent recalibration in the postraumatic course. In addition, the tip of the probe is prone to clot with blood, making the measurement uncertain.

The measurement of tissue oxgenation in the brain ($p_{bt}O_2$) is a new method. A very small probe is placed via a 3-mm borehole in the white matter of the brain next to the lesion. The measurement is very reliable and the catheter can remain in position for weeks without risk of infection. Fixation with a titanium screw in the bone prevents motion artefacts. PO_2 changes are documented extremly fast, although representing oxygen saturation only in a very small area. Although there is still scientific discussion, values of $PO_2 < 10\,mm\,Hg$ are regarded as very dangerous for survival of the brain tissue (Fig. 12).

All three systems have some technical problems making their handling difficult. The reason for measuring with all systems parallel is that it enables one to verify the plausibility of changes. Changes in one measurement system can be due to a technical defect; changes in all three systems indicate a definite change in oxygen consumption and thereby a new metabolic state.

Initial Management

The growing interest in auditing and improving the results of trauma management has initiated new interest in the need to prevent hypoxia and hypotension after head injury (Gildenberg and Makela 1985; Talucci et al. 1988; Gentleman 1990). Certain complications in serious head injury are well known to carry a high risk in the primary phase. On the other hand, a great deal relies on early management strategies, where significant errors can definitely support the developement of secondary brain damage.

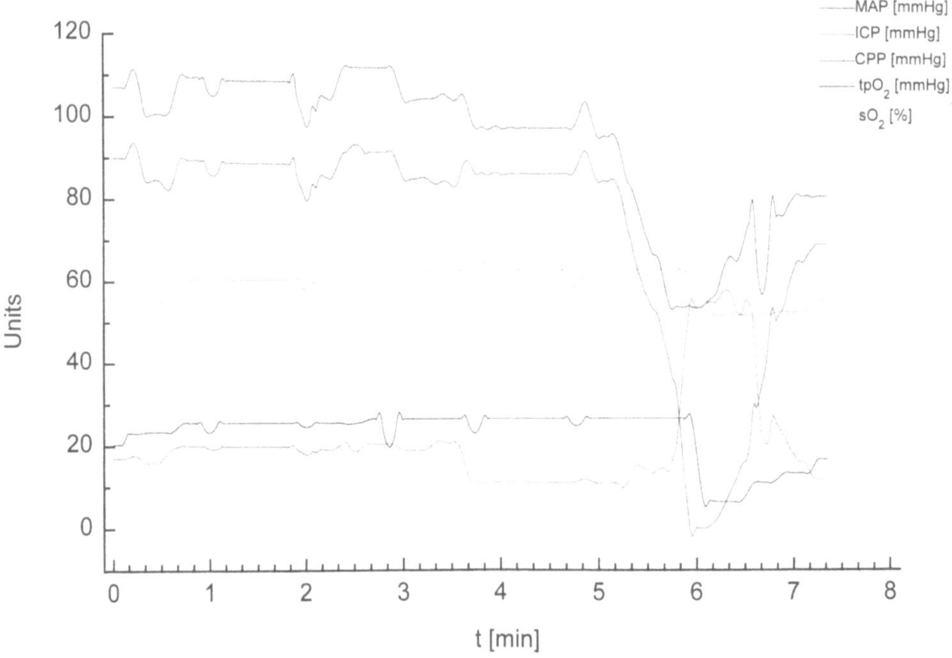

Fig. 12. The measurement of tissue oxygenation in the brain ($p_{bt}O_2$) is a new method. PO_2 changes are documented extremely fast, although representing oxygen saturation (sO_2) only in a very small area. *MAP*, mean arterial pressure; *ICP*, intracranial pressure; *CPP*, cerebral perfusion pressure

General Aspects

To reduce these disturbances early prehospital and hospital management should include skilled aid, bringing doctors or paramedics to the scene of the accident and initiating immediate sufficient airway care and shock therapy. Rapid transportation to the hospital it then essential and optimally to a designated trauma center (Trunkey 1991).

At the time of admission the patient with known or suspected trauma and additionally abnormal mental status presents a variety of complex management issues. When caring for a patient with an apparently isolated head injury, the neurosurgeon must be particularly alerted to the possibility of other significant but clinically inapparent injuries.

When caring for the patient with evidence of multiple injuries, the neurosurgeon must work closely with the emergency and trauma specialists in initial diagnostics, evaluation and management. In particular, the underestimation of major extracranial injuries and, most of all, serious mass bleeding can aggrevate the developement of secondary brain damage (Kohi et al. 1984). This requires a systematic approach to assessment, thorough clinical examination, and appropriate emergency investigations (X-ray, ultrasound of the abdomen). In respect to the continuing danger of hypoxia and hypotension in this phase long transport or transfer routes for diagnostics should be avoided (Gentleman 1990). The decision, however, the bypass a assessment CT and proceed directly to the operating room with a trauma victim who is exsanguinating from a thoracic or abdominal injury requires close cooperation between the disciplines and possibly a multidisciplinary, simultaneous approach to these patients. Thus, for instance, epidural bleeding with progressive neurologic symptoms can be evacuated parallel to the management of intraabdominal mass bleeding.

On the other hand patients with first priority severe head injury should not be rushed to the intensive care unit without basic resuscitation and exclusion of ongoing, underestimated apparently minor blood loss.

Influence of Hypoxia During Primary Treatment

Approximately 35% of neurologic deficits noted in trauma patients are ultimately attributed to hypoxia and hypotension (Gildenberg and Makela 1985; Chesnut et al. 1993); a higher rate shows unsatisfying oxygen saturation on admission. A correlation between inadequate airway control and poor outcome has been shown in epidemiologic studies of head-injured patients (Jennett and Carlin 1978). Hypoxia and hypercarbia result in an immediate increase in CBF and predispose the injured brain to an elevation in ICP (Heffner and Sahn 1983). Thus the clinical threshold for intubation of the significantly head-injured patient should be low. The decision to intubate should address four issues:

1. Protection of patient's airway from aspiration
2. Maintenance of adequate ventilation and oxygenation delivery

3. Anticipation of possible neurologic deterioration during transport or investigative studies, when optimum personnel and equipment for emergency airway management are not available
4. Anticipation of progressive structure compromise from hematoma of the neck or pharynx.

There are, however, several factors that limit intubation techniques for the patient with head injury:

1. The risk of associated cervical spine injury
2. Significant associated neck maxillofacial injury or CSF rhinorrhea
3. Stimulation of tracheal reflexes may precipitate acute rises in blood pressure and ICP which can lead to neurologic deterioration.

The choice of intubation technique is dictated by the above noted considerations and the urgency of the need for airway control. The patient who is apneic or has significant airway obstruction requires immediate intubation, either via the orotracheal route with inline stabilization of the cervical spine, or via surgical tricothyroidotomy. Although there is still a debate over the safety of orotracheal intubation in the patient with potential cervical spine injury, no studies have demonstrated adverse consequences when the neck is carefully maintained in the neutral position during intubation (Rhee et al. 1990; Talucci et al. 1988). Surgical tricothyroidotomy is associated with a number of complications and is therefore recognized as a ultima ratio treatment.

Since hypoxia is one main pathomechnism leading to secondary brain injury adequate airway management is obligatory. The results of a literature review by Chesnut et al. (1993) suggests that the most important and effective therapy in head injuries is to accomplish sufficient oxygenation ($SaO_2 > 96\%$) as soon as possible. Therefore, every isolated head injury with a Glasgow Coma Score (GCS) below 9, or a head trauma with a pupil difference should be intubated and ventilated. Patients with a GCS between 12 and 9 should be intubated according to suspected problems with transport or management (Tables 5, 6).

The situation in multiple trauma is more complicated. Thus, for instance, with associated thoracic trauma, reversible airway obstruction can result from aspiration of vomitus, blood, or loose teeth, or from fractures of the maxilla and mandible. Patients with blunt or penetrating injuries to the neck or oropharynx may have

Table 5. Indications for intubation and ventilation in severe head injury

Sufficient oxygenation ($SaO_2 > 96\%$)
Isolated head trauma with a GCS less than 9
Head trauma with a pupil difference → immediate intubation and ventilation
Multiple trauma (ISS > 30) with a GCS between 9 and 12

GCS, Glasgow Coma Score; ISS, Injury Severity Score.

Table 6. Ventilatory settings adjusted to the guidelines of the European Brain Injury Consortium (EBIC)

Ventilatory settings
Guidelines of the European Brain Injury Consortium (EBIC)
Intermittent Positive Pressure Ventilation (IPPV)
Mild to moderate hyperventilation ($PaCO_2$ 30–35 mm Hg)
$PaO_2 > 75$ mm Hg and oxygen saturation at 96%

rapidly expanding hematomas which compromise pedancy and necessitate urgent or prophylactic intubation.

Causes of ventilatory inadequacy include flail injuries to the chest wall, hemothorax, pneumothorax, as well as pulmonary contusion. Additionally, patients with underlying cardiopulmonary disorders are at higher risk of respiratory compromise following trauma.

All patients should initially receive 100% oxygen and should have continuous pulse-oximetry monitoring during resuscitation, subsequent transportation, and radiologic procedures on admission.

A widely advocated method to lower ICP is the institution of hyperventilation to achieve a PCO_2 of 25–30 mm Hg, which results in respiratory alkalosis and a desired induction of cerebral vesoconstriction (Heffner and Sahn 1983; Paulson et al. 1972). ICP decreases during hyperventilation because the cerebral vasoconstriction produced by hypocarbia results in lower intracranial blood flow. The success of this intervention depends on the capacity of the vessels in the injured brain to respond to changes in CO_2. The use of hyperventilation does not benefit all patients. A "reverse steal" effect has been described leading to a paradox hyperperfusion and an increased vasogenic edema of the injured side (Darby et al. 1988). Increased arterial venous O_2 ($avDO_2$) differences suggesting ischemia have been shown to occur in some head-injured patients with normal CO_2 responsiveness who received hyperventilation (Obrist et al. 1984). The responsiveness is said to have a short-term effect.

Influence of Hypotension (Traumatic Hemorrhagic Shock) During Primary Treatment

The presence of shock is associated with a poorer outcome in the head-injured patient (Jennett and Carlin 1978; Chesnut et al. 1993). Treatment of shock improves CPP and enhances delivery of oxygen to the brain, which results in a decreased autoregulatory dilatation of the cerebral vessels (Rosner and Coley 1986). During this loss of autoregulation that occurs with head injury, CBF is directly reflective of systemic arterial pressure, with poor maintenance of CPP and uncoupling of CBF from the cerebral metabolic rate for oxygen ($CMRO_2$) (Fig. 4). Therefore, despite the benefits of aggressive prehospital airway treatment, it can be powerfully neutralized if concommittant hypotension is not reversed (Chesnut et al. 1993).

It was shown in other studies that rapid and adequate resuscitation could reduce the biochemical effects of inadequate perfusion (lactic acidosis and net base deficit).

Brain-injured multiple trauma patients in whom there is a more adequate control of blood loss in the immediate 24-h postinjury period appear to return to a level of function consistent with home discharge and an improved outcome (Siegel et al. 1991).

The maintenance or reestablishment of adequate, but not excessive, intravascular volume is more important than concern regarding exacerbation of vasogenic edema due to the administration of fluid. Standard treatment of hypovolemic shock at the scene requires initial adminisitration of 2 l of normal saline or lactated Ringer's solution. Hypovolemic shock in the trauma patient unresponsive to 2 l of normal saline should be transferred immediately to the emergency department since here a significant mass bleeding is occuring.

Recent studies of hypertonic saline resuscitation in animal models of shock with freezeinduced brain injuries (Battistella and Wisner 1991) and mass lesions (Gunnar et al. 1988) have demonstrated significant acute decreases in ICP when compared with animals resuscitated with Ringer's lactate or normal saline. In these models, however, only the acute effects of hypertonic saline were studied. The long-term effects on ICP and the rate of equilibration of sodium across the blood–brain barrier were not determined.

Anothr approach to maintain adequate cerebral perfusion and thereby to reduce ICP is the administration of systemic vasopressors (Rosner and Daughton 1990). The CPP is thereby used as a "vasoconstrictor" (Fig. 6). The method which has found practical application is to hold the CPP directly above the critical threshold, where the ICP increases. Rosner and Daughton (1990) report threshold values at about 70 mm Hg. However, in multiple trauma patients, CPP values of 90–100 mm Hg were sometimes required to stabilize ICP. These values were far higher than the traditionally quoted values of 50 mm Hg which have been viewed in some centers as adequate. These low values, however, were recently shown to potentiate an ICP-induced cycle of continuously decreasing CPP leading to generalized brain edema, ischemia, and death.

Series could demonstrate that with the above-mentioned method CPP could be artificially elevated without deleterious ICP and systemic effects. Rosner and Daughton (1990) describe how many of his patients, however, did not require vasopressors at all and CPP could be successfully managed for an average of 2–3 weeks with only careful adjustment of fluid therapy, transfusion, vascular expansion, and the avoidance of overhydration (Gunnar et al. 1988; Batistella and Wisner 1991).

In order to prevent overhydration with excessive increase in total body water, concentrated albumin has been used (25–50 gm/day). On the other hand, red cell transfusion has been shown to have the best vascular expander effect and the ability to mobilize extravascular water into the vascular space. Lasix has only been used in those cases where an increase in total body sodium was found.

Influence of Osmotherapy in Multiple Trauma Patients

There are different therapeutic possibilities to treat a reduction in CPP. Best known is mannitol 20%. It has to be given in a bolus or short infusion of 125 ml. The effect is due to an osmotic gradient (Muizelaar et al. 1984; Rosner and Coley 1987). With an osmolarity >355 osmol mannitol shows no effect. Therefore, it is necessary to measure the osmolarity of the patient every day. If the CPP can not be maintained with mannitol we use trometamol (TRIS/THAM); 250 ml of 8.4% THAM are added to 750 ml G5 solution and 125 ml of this mixture is given to the patient per infusion. As TRIS is a buffer and mannitol can cause an acidosis it is helpful to use mannitol and TRIS alternately.

If this medication is not effective we also use sorbitol 40% at 125 ml per infusion. In rare cases we have to extend this therapy with 100 ml glycerin 80% via a gastric tube. Although there are some non-responders to this approach in most cases it is very helpful.

If none of these procedures is effective we use barbiturates, although the scientific basis for a reduction of the metabolic rate in the cell is very doubtful at the moment.

Influence of Analgesia and Sedation in Multiple Trauma with Associated Head Injury

Sedation is mostly accomplished with short-acting barbiturates. Barbiturates are said to decrease cerebral metabolism and demonstrate a cerebroprotective effect in most cases of cerebral ischemia (Bleyaert et al. 1978; Donegan et al. 1985). They have also been shown to acutely decrease ICP (Shapiro et al. 1973). These beneficial effects on ICP and oxygen utilization appear to depend on intact cerebral autoregulation (Nordstrom et al. 1988). As previously noted, the major disadvantage in using barbiturates during intubation of the multiple injured patient lies in their cardiovascular depressant effect, which may precipitate significant hypotension, particularly in the presense of hypovolemia. Therefore, maximal intravenous administration of fluids in these volume-depleted patients should occur. The administration of 20 mg/kg of thiopental to patients with ICP < 40 mm Hg resulted in a fall of 18% in MAP and a concomittant 50% decrease in ICP (Hayashi et al. 1988).

Other Therapeutic Aspects

Some secondary brain insults will prove untreatable or unpreventable. It is these insults that highlight the need to develop new methods for preventing or diminishing their negative impact. There is, however, no scientific reason for the administration of steroids in brain edema. Free radical scavengers have also failed to improve outcome. The role of agents such as specific inhibitors of free radicals, or alteration of aminoacid toxicity, as well as the possibility of employing agents such as nerve growth factor, thyrotropin releasing factor, opioid antagonists or others, need to be investigated in a search for possible pharmacologic antagonism of secondary brain insults.

In those cases where the reason for ICP increase is a malignant brain swelling a decompressive craniotomy should be considered.

In respect to a possible therapeutic approach, the prevention of systemic
hypotension and also hypoxemia seem to be the most important factors since others
were shown to have either no effect or are still at an experimental stage.

Patient Outcome After Severe Brain Damage in Relation to Injury Severity and the Posttraumatic Course

In order to show the effect of early treatment regimens on the development of
secondary brain damage we performed a retrospective analysis of our multiple
trauma patients, looking especially at parameters characterizing systemic hypoxemia
and hypotension, and additionally at possible therapeutic regimens influencing these
criteria.

Methods

A total of 207 multiple trauma patients Injury Severity Score (ISS) >20 with associated
head injury (according to the initial GCS) were analyzed. A group classification for the
severity of head injury was performed according to the criteria of Miller, distinguishing three groups (Table 7) (Miller and Becker 1982; Miller and Janes 1985).

Patient outcome was related to the Glasgow Outcome Scale (GOS). Death in
group 5 was *in all cases* related to primary or secondary brain damage (Jennett and
Carlin 1978).

All measured parameters were documented in the first 48 h after trauma. Similarly, treatment regimens are noted for this time period.

For statistical analysis we used the univariate analysis of variance (ANOVA). A p
< 0.05 was considered significant; post hoc comparison was verified with the so-called
LSD test. All data are presented as mean ± standard error of mean (SEM).

Results

The influence of systemic hypotension was measured in relation to the posttraumatic
data for systemic arterial blood proessure (SABP), substitution of fluid and packed
red blood cells (PRBC), and the application of catecholamines.

Systemic Blood Pressure. In the preclinical phase no significant differences in SABP
could be demonstrated in the five GOS groups (Fig. 13). On admission all patients had
stable hemodynamics, whereas in the early intensive care phase SABP was significantly worse in groups 4 and 5, demonstrating the influence of systemic blood pressure in this issue.

Fluid resuscitation showed significant differences, with a higher fluid demand in
the patients that died of brain damage in the further time course (GOS 5). Similar
results are seen for blood substitution (PRBC); however, these are not statistically

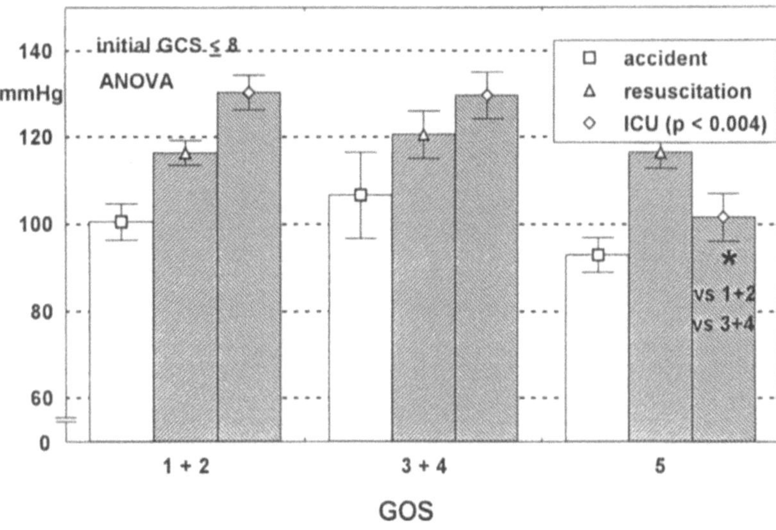

Fig. 13. In the preclinical phase no significant differences in systemic arterial blood pressure (SABP) could be demonstrated in the five GOS groups. On admission all patients had stable hemodynamics, whereas in the early intensive care phase SABP was significantly worse in groups 4 and 5, demonstrating the influence of systemic blood pressure in this issue. *GCS*, Glasgow Coma Score; *GOS*, Goasgow outcome scale; *ICU*, intensive care unit

significant. This must be a consequence of severe brain damage, since the overall injury severity, excluding the head injury, were similar in the different GOS groups.

Vasopressor agents were applied more often in the patients with the worst outcome (GOS 4–5), demonstrating higher demand, but obviously still an insufficient substitution in this patient population (Fig. 14).

Systemic Hypoxemia was measured by means of the so-called Horovitz quotient (PaO_2/FiO_2). We could not find a significant difference in this parameter in the preclinical or early clinical phase. Oxygen saturation was constant in the majority of cases, while decreased values were only demonstrated in patients with associated thoracic trauma; however, these were not significant. Obviously, aggressive preclinical intubation and ventilation in our patient population with a FiO_2 of 1.0 lead to a satisfying oxygenation in this primary phase.

Discussion

The influence of systemic hypotension and also hypoxemia on patient outcome has been demonstrated by different authors in the past. Additionally, a direct correlation of systemic hypotension and also of hypoxemia with the GOS was shown by Siegel et al. (1991) looking for early predictors of outcome after severe head injury in multiple trauma patients. He found that the best correlation was next to GCS, associated with 24-h volume of blood replacement and the base excess. These predominators of

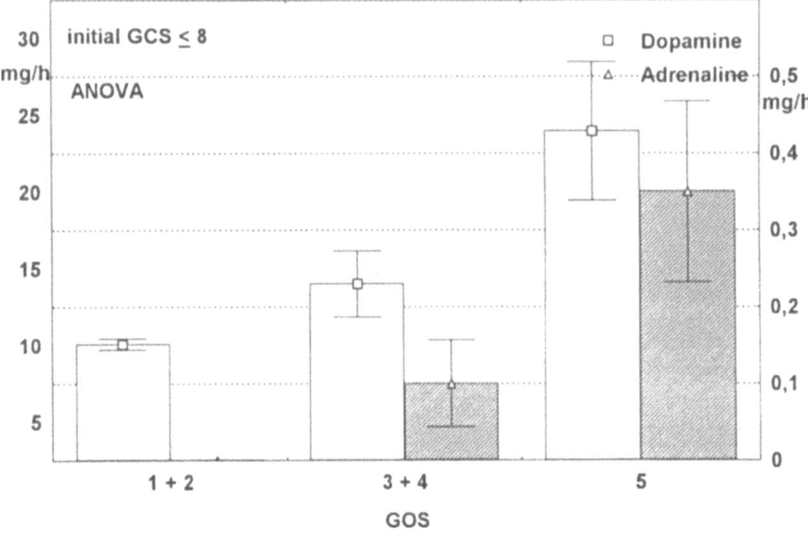

Fig. 14. Catecholamine, first day. Vasopressor agents were applied more often in the patients with the worst outcome [Glasgow Outcome Scale (*GOS*) 4–5], demonstrating higher demand, but obviousoly still an insufficient substitution in this patient population. *GCS*, Glasgow Coma Score

traumatic hemorrhagic shock were shown to be closely related to mortality in these cases, which is possibly an expression of the influence of these factors on secondary brain damage (Siegel et al. 1991). Statistical significance for base excess was not found in our patient population since bicarbonate was administered frequently in the preclinical settings.

Eisenberg et al. (1983) similarly were able to demonstrate the interrelation between hypoxia, as well as shock and patient outcome.

Braakman (1992) compared 23 possible prognostic indicators in a patient group admitted with severe head injury. He used the GOS at 12 months posttrauma as an outcome parameter. He found, besides other parameters, a high correlation between initial PO_2 and also systolic blood pressure.

Waxman (1991) was able to show in patients with an initial GCS score <10, a significant relation between initial systolic blood pressure (<60 mm Hg) and patient outcome using the GOS. He demonstrated, however, that in this group an overall consideration of blood pressure, ventilatory status, injury severity, and age in a multivariance analysis resulted only in a cumulative prediction of 0.61. Hence, more than one third of the variability of outcome could not be predicted with initial evaluation. He therefore favored neurologic reassessment at 6h after trauma, comparing initial GCS to the 6-h value and an aggressive initial treatment protocol for resuscitation and ventilation.

Dacey (1991) proved the relation of neurophysiological outcome (GOS) to both the severity of brain injury, and also to overall systemic injury severity (ISS) depending on the duration of coma (> and <24h). He felt that the assessment of late neurologic outcome in these patients is effected by multiple systems injury and should definitely be taken into account. A more detailed analysis of neurophysiological and psychosocial functioning should, however occur, since significant changes in GOS assessment alone is seen even in trauma patients without head injury. This was something we also found in our patient population. So we initiated a prospective study in patients with severe head injury to analyze the detailed outcome perspective in respect to functional disability and also neurophysiological and psychosocial functioning.

Detailed Analysis of Neurophysiological and Psychosocial Function After Severe Head Injury in Multiple Trauma Patients

Since many authors have been able to show that the evaluation of patient outcome using the GOS is not sensitive enough, we performed an analysis in multiple trauma patients with severe head injury using a great variety of outcome parameters that are known to allow an exact differentiation of neurophysiological and psychosocial functioning. We were also able to show the correlation between different intensive care measures, including factors related to cardiopulmonary status and these outcome function parameters.

Methods

Multiple trauma patients with an ISS greater than 20 were included in this study if the initial GCS was <8 and the age ranged between 16 and 60. All patients were primarily admitted to our trauma center and early rehabilitation was performed in a specialized center (Hessisch Oldendorf, Dr. W. Gobiet). We retrospectively documented all epidemiological data of these patients, the exact treatment periods, and the professional, social, and medical restitution.

In a follow-up study extremity function, including the range of extremity motion (ROM), was documented. In addition a variety of psychological tests were performed.

Results

A total of 58 patients were included in this study with a mean age of 27 years, the youngest being 16, the oldest 52. Their accidents had occured between 1985 and 1992. The average follow-up time was 5.8 years after trauma. The mean injury severity was an ISS of 34, the initial GCS was 6.3.

The duration of coma was 15 days, the ventilation period included 7 days of weaning and 20 days of controlled or assisted ventilation. The intensive care period was in average 33 days. Most of the patients were transferred for early rehabilitation program to the above-mentioned rehabilitation center.

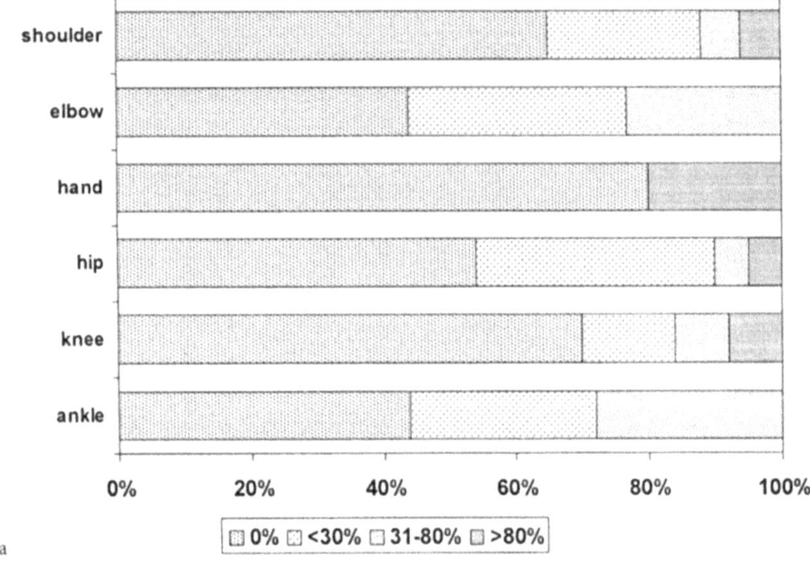

shoulder
elbow
hand
hip
knee
ankle
0%
20%
40%
60%
80%
100%
0% <30% 31-80% >80%
a

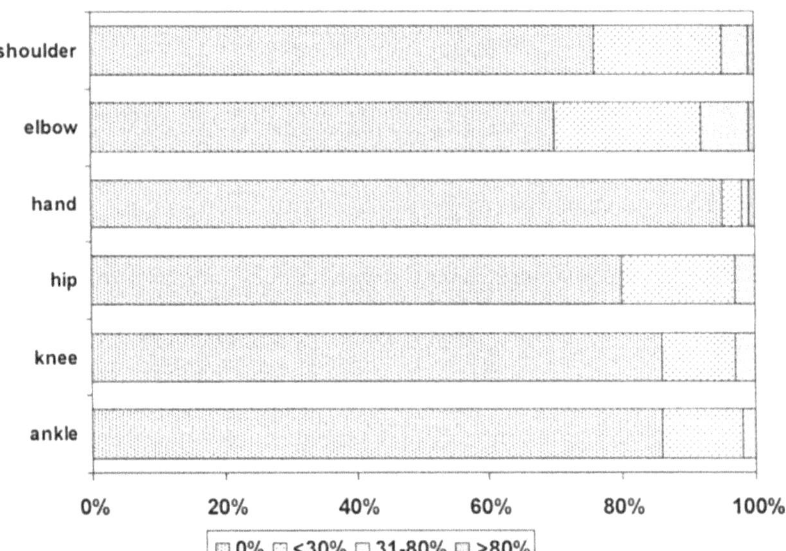

shoulder
elbow
hand
hip
knee
ankle
0%
20%
40%
60%
80%
100%
0% <30% 31-80% >80%
b

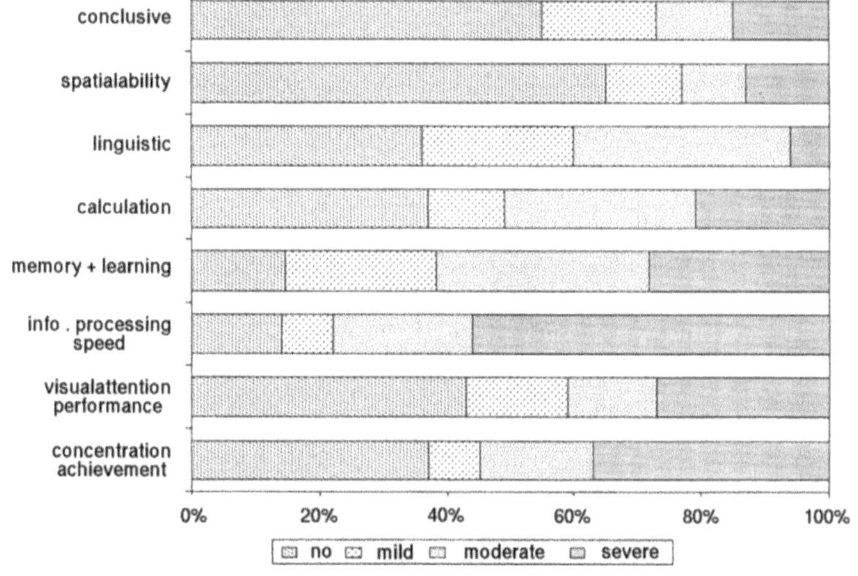

conclusive
spatialability
linguistic
calculation
memory + learning
info . processing speed
visualattention performance
concentration achievement
0%
20%
40%
60%
80%
100%
no
mild
moderate
severe

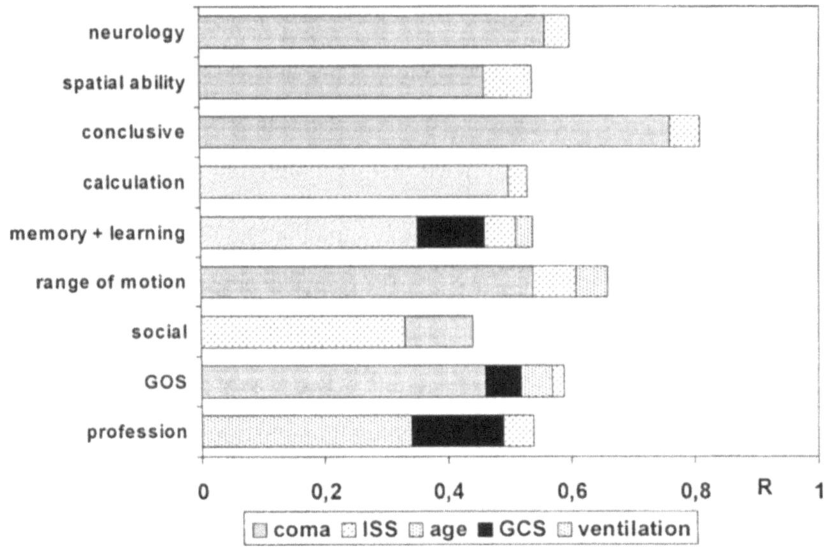

neurology
spatial ability
conclusive
calculation
memory + learning
range of motion
social
GOS
profession
0
0,2
0,4
0,6
0,8
R
1
coma
ISS
age
GCS
ventilation

Dacey R, Dikmen S, Temkin N, Mclean A, Armsder G, Winn HR (1991) Relative effects of brain and non-brain injuries on neuropsyclological and psychosocial outcome. J Trauma 31(2):217

Darby JM, Yonas H, Marion DW, Latchaw RE (1988) Local "inverse steal" induced by hyperventilation in head injury. Neurosurgery 23:84–88

DeSalles AA, Kontos HA, Becker DP, Yang MS, Ward JD, Moulton R, Gruemer HD, Lutz H, Maset AL, Jenkins L et al (1986) Prognostic significance of ventricular CSF lactic acidosis in severe head injury. J Neurosurg 65:615–624

Donegan JH, Traystman RJ, Koehler RC, Jones MD Jr, Rogers MC (1985) Cerebrovascular hypoxic and autoregulatory responses during reduced brain metabolism. Am J Physiol 249:H421–H429

Eisenberg HM, Cayard C, Papanicolaou AC et al (1983) The effects of three potentially preventable complications of outcome after severe closed head injury. In: Ischii S, Nagai H, Brock M (eds) Intracranial pressure vol 5, Springer, New York, pp 549–553

Faden AI, Demediuk P, Panter SS, Vink R (1989) The role of excitatory amino acids and NMDA receptors in traumatic brain injury. Science 244:798–800

Gennarelli TA, Champion HR, Sacco WJ, Copes WS, Alves WM (1989) Mortality of patients with head injury and extracranial injury treated in trauma centers. J Trauma 29:1193–1201

Gentleman D (1990) Preventing secondary brain damage after head injury: a multidisciplinary challenge. Injury 21:305–308

Gildenberg PL, Makela M (1985) Effect of early intubation and ventilation on outcome following head injury. In: Dacy RG (ed) Trauma of the nervous system. Raven, New York, pp 70–90

Gunnar W, Jonasson O, Merlotti G, Stone J, Barrett J (1988) Head injury and hemorrhagic shcok: studies of the blood brain barrier and intracranial pressure after resuscitation with normal saline solution, 3% saline solution, and dextran-40. Surgery 103:398–407

Haysahi M, Kobayashi H, Kawano H, Handa Y, Hirose S (1988) Treatment of systemic hypertension and intracranial hypertension in cases of brain hemorrhage. Stroke 19:314–321

Heffner JE, Sahn SA (1983) Controlled hyperventilation in patients with intracranial hypertension. Application and management. Arch Intern Med 143:765–769

Ishige N, Pitts LH, Hashimoto T, Nishimura MC, Bartkowski HM (1987) Effect of hypoxia on traumatic brain injury in rats. I. Changes in neurological function, electroencephalograms, and histopathology. Neurosurgery 20:848–853

Jennett B, Bond M (1975) Assessment of outcome after severe brain damage. Lancet 1:480–484

Jennett B, Carlin J (1978) Preventable mortality and morbidity after head injury. Injury 10:31–39

Jennett B, Teasdale G (1981) Management of head injuries. Davis, Philadelphia

Kohi YM, Mendelow AD, Teasdale GM, Allardice GM (1984) Extracranial insults and outcome in patients with acute head injury–relationship to the Glasgow Coma Scale. Injury 16:25–29

Lassen NA (1974) Control of cerebral circulation in health and disease. Circ Res 34:749–760

Miller JD (1985) Head injury and brain ischaemia–implications for therapy. Br J Anaesth 57:120–130

Miller JD, Becker DP (1982) Secondary insults to the injured brain. JR Coll Surg Edinb 27:292–298

Miller JD, Jones PA (1985) The work of a regional head injury service. Lancet 1:1141–1144

Miller JD, Sweet RC, Narayan R, Becker DP (1978) Early insults to the injured brain. JAMA 240:439–442

Muizelaar JP, Lutz HA III, Becker DP (1984) Effect of mannitol on ICP and CBF and correlation with pressure autoregulation in severely head-injured patients. J Neurosurg 61:700–706

Nordstrom CH, Messeter K, Sundbarg G, Schalen W, Werner M, Ryding E (1988) Cerebral blood flow, vasoreactivity, and oxygen consumption during barbiturate therapy in severe traumatic brain lesions. J Neurosurg 68:424–431

Obrist WD, Langfitt TW, Jaggi JL, Cruz J, Gennarelli TA (1984) Cerebral blood flow and metabolism in comatose patients with acute head injury. Relationship to intracranial hypertension. J Neurosurg 61:241–253

Overgaard J, Hvid Hansen O, Land AM, Pedersen KK, Christensen S, Haase J, Hein O, Tweed WA (1973) Prognosis after head injury based on early clinical examination. Lancet 2:631–635

Paulson OB, Olesen J, Christensen MS (1972) Restoration of autoregulation of cerebral blood flow by hypocapnia. Neurology (Minneap) 22:286–293

Pfenninger EG, Lindner KH (1991) Arterial blood gases in patients with acute head injury at the accident site and upon hospital admission. Acta Anaesthesiol Scand 35:148–152

Regel G, Lobenhoffer P, Grotz M, Pape HC, Lehmann U, Tscherne H (1995) Treatment results of patients with multiple trauma: an analysis of 3406 cases treated between 1972 and 1991 at a German Level I Trauma Center. J Trauma 38:70–78

Regel G, Grote M, Weltner T, Sturm JA, Tscherne H (1996) Pattern of organ failure following severe trauma, World J Surg 20:422–429

Reilly PL, Graham DI, Adams JH, Jennett B (1975) Patients with head injury who talk and die. Lancet 2:375–377

Rhee KJ, Green W, Holcroft JW, Mangili JA (1990) Oral intubation in the multiply injured patient: the risk of exacerbating spinal cord damage [see comments]. Ann Emerg Med 19:511–514

Rose J, Valtonen S, Jennett B (1977) Avoidable factors contributing to death after head injury. Br Med J 2:615–618

Rosner MJ, Coley IB (1986) Cerebral perfusion pressure, intracranial pressure, and head elevation. J Neurosurg 65:636–641

Rosner MJ, Coley IB (1987) Cerebral perfusion pressure: a hemodynamic mechanism of mannitol and the postmannitol hemogram. Neurosurgery 21:147–156

Rosner MJ, Daughton S (1990) Cerebral pefusion pressure management in head injury. J Trauma 30:933–940

Rosner MJ, Rosner SD, Johnson AH (1995) Cerebral perfusion pressure: management protocol and clinical results. J Neurosurg 83:949–962

Shapiro HM, Galindo A, Wyte SR, Harris AB (1973) Rapid intraoperative reduction of intracranial pressure with thiopentone. Br J Anaesth 45:1057–1062

Siegel JH, Gens DR, Mamantov T, Geisler FH, Goodarzi S, MacKenzie EJ (1991) Effect of associated injuries and blood volume replacement on death, rehabilitation needs, and disability in blunt traumatic brain injury. Crit Care Med 19:1252–1265

Souter MJ, Andrews PJD (1996) A review of jugular venous oximetry. Intensive Care World 13:32–38

Talucci RC, Shaikh KA, Schwab CW (1988) Rapid sequence induction with oral endotracheal intubation in the multiply injured patient. Am Surg 54:185–187

Trunkey D (1991) Initial treatment of patients with extensive trauma. N Engl J Med 324:1259–1263

Waxman K, Sundine MJ, Lysung RF (1991) Is early prediction of outcome in severe head injury possible? Arch Surg 126:1237

Discussion

Traber:
I did not catch how you created the head injury in the animals.

Lehmann:
Cold lesion method described by Klatzo.

Schlag:
You mention the unreamed nail. Do you already have results in your experimental set-up?

Lehmann:
We have measured some patients with ICP monitoring which were stabilized with an unreamed nail and we saw no increase of the ICP.

Schlag:
You see an increase of the ICP?

Lehmann:
No, no difference.

Regel:
We have not done the unreamed nail.

Schlag:
I thought you did it only with a reamed nail in the experimental study? But when did you do the experimental study?

Lehmann:
2 years ago.

Schlag:
So you did not repeat the study with an unreamed nail?

Regel:
Not yet, but this would be the next approach.

Schlag:
We did it in baboons and just finished this study. And we see that the inflammatory response with the reamed nail is much stronger than with the unreamed nail. Of course fat embolism is much higher, we even have a death of fat embolism, which is very seldom with a reamed nail.

Regel:
What would be interesting to look at, he mentioned that we see the capillary permeability change to see which pathomechanisms really lead to it. Is it a fat embolus mechanism or is it the influx of granulocytes which we have not looked at yet.

Schlag:
I think the granulocytes, not the fat.

Prough:
Dr. Regel, I enjoyed your talk very much. It was a nice overall summary. I have a question: It looked to me as if your data on the correlation between the GOS and fluid and blood administration and between the GOS and catecholamine administration ran counter to what one would expect, i.e., that more fluid and more catecholamines would be necessary in patients who are more severely injured systemically. One thing that I was curious about was whether the groups of patients with different GOSs were comparable in terms of baseline GCSs?

Regel:
Yes, the initial GCS was below 8, but was in all groups on average the same. And the same is with the ISS. Because we thought initially that maybe if the patients are

differently severely injured in the groups, then this would have an effect too. But they were all between 20 and 30 ISS. So both the severity of the head injury, as well as the overall injury severity were the same. However, it has the disadvantage of a retrospective study. We would not have this proof if we had just looked at the last 2–3 years, because we have been using catecholamines in this phase all the time, which we have not done before. So the disadvantage is somehow also that the first phase of this retrospective study includes the patients that did not have catecholamines, and the phase now in the last 2 or 3 years includes those that got catecholamines. So it is not the same type of period.

Baethmann:
My point would be similar to Dr. Prough's. I would have expected jusy the opposite: Those who had more blood obviously need no blood and thus had a poorer outcome. You just showed the opposite, and I wonder, since you include a kind of time span in this collective group of patients, whether important management changes had occurred during this observation period. In other words, had you in the later part of your analysis or of patients which were recruited for analysis, a more generous indication to provide fluid and blood than in the former times and thereby might have improved outcome, thus including more general management measures which had improved the outcome, and thus producing your result, which I think is striking, because it would mean, if these patients who had been infused with a low volume of blood or fluid, could have been saved if they had received more, which probably is not your conclusion. And the other thing is concerned with your presentation, where you indicate in the final concept slide that nailing of the femur induces some pulmonary problems with pulmonary arterial hypertension; I wonder whether this shows up in your experimental data? In other words, if you have that, of course you might affect the intracranial compliance and even ICP. Is there any data to show that you have a compromised pulmonary situation under these circumstances?

Regel:
Maybe I can respond to the first question: You are completely right. At the moment you take patients that have a wide spreading ISS where you do not have this narrow group of injury severity, then you show that these patients get more blood and more fluid with the bad prediction, with the bad GOS. But this is not due to the injury or to the secondary brain damage any more, but to the overall injury severity. So that was the same as Segal showed in his work.

Kossmann:
Just one clarification about the blood replacement: This was only during the first 24 h, right? Did you look at the overall need when the patient is there for 10 or 14 days? Did you calculate how many blood products a patient needed? Because I see in the clinic that sometimes there are patients later on who need large amounts of fluids and also blood.

Regel:
To be honest, we have not looked at it yet, but we should. We were looking at secondary brain damage, as I understand this is something that happens in the first

few days after trauma. So we have to look at what happens with management in the first 24–48 h.

Kossmann:
I agree with this, but there is some confusion; why does this patient need just a different amount of blood than we expected? I think that you have to look at the overall need for blood of these patients.

Zarkovic:
I was wondering whether you would mind if I presented some data on patients with traumatic brain injury and bone fractures, and the effects on bone healing?

Kochanek:
I really like the system that you have, it seems to be a very opportune one for treatment trials because you have a large patient population which seems to be managed very homogeneously, and you have an advantage that I think is very important and that I think has been downplayed quite a bit, except very recently, and that is: Many of the head injury treatment trials for which results are coming back are failing – the excitotoxicity CGS 1977 trial, the Peg SOD trial, and others. One of the problems, I think, could be that people are not getting the therapy on board fast enough. Having the physician–helicopter system and a very homogeneous treatment and outcome assessment, I think would be a pretty outstanding setting to try an early treatment approach. That is what I would encourage.

Regel:
The only problem we have with this is that these multiple trauma patients have that amount of volume and blood in the first 24 h that the whole system is very unstable. So I would ask you: When do you think we should start with these trials?

Kochanek:
From the standpoint of systemic effect, most of these treatments have not been shown to produce hypotension or other side effects; there may be central nervous system side effects, but they are dwarfed by the hemodynamic problems you encounter. I would think those types of therapies could be integrated very early without a terribly great amount of concern for the other multiple trauma effects. The only thing in your data that I did not see that I think would be potentially important is a stratification of the types of brain injury. Is it diffuse injury, a focal injury, etc? I think that would be very important to integrate into your presentation of outcome, rather than these are all head injury patients.

Baethmann:
Dr. Kochanek, I think the latter point you are addressing is probably more the problem: That you have in the head injury, which is certainly not a homogenous disorder, responsive lesions versus resistent lesions, and this is probably the case with glutamide antagonists, corticosteroids, or others. I would like to come back to your organizational system which was also addressed by Dr. Kochanek: We heard yesterday about the problem of prehospital fluid resuscitation in unstable shock conditions, that it could actually worsen the outcome, according to the Picker study and other

studies which were mentioned here. How do you manage this problem with unstable circulatory conditions and prehospital fluid resuscitation?

Regel:
We were discussing this point actually concerning the prehospital fluid. The study by Picker showed that that was only penetrating trauma and this is a little bit different from multiple trauma from pathophysiological understanding. We do a maximal fluid resuscitation in these patients. The only thing that we were already discussing is, if there are patients with isolated trunk injury who already show at the scene that they have mass bleeding, then we leave them alone. But that is, I would honestly say, a consequence of the Picker study. If we see at the scene that the abdomen gets tense and that they are bleeding significantly, then we leave them alone and do not give them any further fluid. But all other cases where they have massive extremity and soft tissue injury, then you have to do a mass infusion in these patients, otherwise you kill them.

I did not mention the point with the hypertonic saline, where we do not have any experience, but I think this is a very good approach, especially in the brain-injured patients, that we would have to look at.

Kossmann:
I agree with Dr. Kochanek, that we have to find common standards in the treatment protocol for patients with traumatic brain injury (TBI). I would like to present our treatment protocol, and Prof. Redl was kind enough to put it on the computer.

Basic Treatment. The points of basic treatment are:

- Early intubation (if possible at the site of the accident) and artificial ventilation; goals: (a) $PO_2 \geq 13\,kPa$, (b) normocapnia, and (c) no prophylactic hyperventilation (risk of ischemia).
- Sufficient analgesia, sedation and relaxation.
- Maintenance of normal body temperature, prevention of hyperthermia and hyperglycemia.
- Aggressive circulatory stabilization by means of volume–fluid replacement and catecholamines if necessary; goals: (a) MAP > 80 mm HG, (b) normovolemia, (c) hematocrit > 30, (d) no antihypertensive drugs up to MAP = 130 mm Hg (range of autoregulation) if patient is adequately sedated (demand hypertension), and (e) maintenance of a CPP $\geq$ 70 mm Hg.
- No routinely performed head elevation (lowers CPP, increases volume sequestration)
- Surgical intervention if necessary (CT)
- Continuous ICP monitoring (ventricular drainage catheter if posssible, subdural Wilkinson cup catheter, camino catheter)
- Administration of nimodipin in cases with Doppler sonographic signs of vasospasm.

ICP Increases. In the case of increases in ICP (threshold ICP > 15 mm HG > 5 min) the following are recommended:

- Deepening of sedation, analgesia, muscle relaxation
- CSF drainage if possible
- Insertion of a fiberoptic jugular bulb catheter
- Hyperventilation as long as: (a) $Sv_jO_2 > 60\%$, (b) a-jDL < 0.2 mmol/l, and (c) ICP lowering by means of decrease in $PaCO_2$ is possible.
- Osmotherapy: mannitol IV 25–50–100 ml (slowly; risk of rebound) as long as serum osmolarity is <315 mosmol/l
- Moderate hypothermia ($\pm$ 34°C)
- Barbiturate coma under continuous EEG registration; goal: (a) burst suppression pattern, < six burst/min, and (b) burst suppression relation 1:1. (Start with thiopental 10 mg/kg per minute this therapy may lead to hemodynamic deterioration and requires close monitoring and cardiocirculatory support, guided by the use of a pulmonary artery catheter.)
- Increase of MAP to meet a CPP > 70 mm Hg. (If cause of ICP increase is unknown: CT.)

Wake-Up. The wake-up procedure includes stopping sedation and muscle relaxation. The ventilator settings are changed as soon as possible to an assisted ventilation mode.

The first wake-up is performed only if the following conditions are met:

- No ICP increase above 15 mm Hg within 24 h under normothermia and normoventilation without treatment
- PVI > 18 ml
- Amount of CSF drainage below 50 ml/24 h
- No signs of intracranial hypertension on CT
- Sv_jO_2 and a-jDL within normal range.

The wake-up is stopped and treatment resumed if ICP increases above the threshold for more than 5 min.

Discontinuation of ICP Monitoring. ICP monitoring is discontinued as soon as a neurological assessment is possible, and no therapeutic interventions have been necessary over the previous 24 h.

Shackford:
I think that these are excellent management protocols; I do, however, want to caution you about the use of pressors in individuals who are not normovolemic. What will happen is that you will get intense splanchnic vasoconstriction, and you may be improving the cerebral perfusion pressure, but the gut will die. The patient will still die, but he will not die with head injury, he will, in fact, die from multiple organ failure, because his gut is dead. So I think the most important thing is to get the patients normovolemic before you apply pressors. If I were to choose a pressor to use I would probably choose phenylephrine rather than norepinephrine. One last thing, I noticed that you are aggressive with catecholamines, but you are tentative with the osmotherapy. A 315 mmol/l is not really that high. I went out and ran up and down this hill this morning and I can tell you, when I got up here at the end, my osmolarity

was probably 320, because Mother Nature resuscitates you by allowing you to extract water from cells, because you sweat hypotonic fluid and your osmolarity goes up. Olympic swimmers at the end of a 100 m swim have osmolarities routinely at 360 or 370. I would submit that the exercise physiologists have known for years that a hyperosmotic state is not necessarily bad. Finally, dealing again with the hyperosmolar issue, we have seen patients come in and clearly they are in coma after hyperosmolar nonketonic diabetic coma, who survive without any CNS or renal problems with admission osmolarities of 450. I would submit that you might be able to go higher than 315 on your osmotherapy.

Kossmann:
Thank you very much for these comments. There is a historical reason why we did this, actually: We had some problems, people were just putting in Mannitol uncontrolled, and then we had some bad experiences with this. That is why in our protocol this is like a safety feature.

Regel:
I have to respond to the first issue, the one with the catecholamines. You saw that this was only the third step in the proocol from us, so we are aware of the complications that can arise and what we do know is that we do not combine it with dopamine, but with dopexamine, which has a better feature on the gut circulation, and we feel that it has some better effect. We cannot prove that at the moment.

Shackfore:
You are volume resuscitating, in other words; pressor is not your first therapy?

Regel:
It is the third stage.

Analysis of Immune Mediator Production
Following Traumatic Brain Injury

T. Kossmann, V.H.J. Hans, P.M. Lenzlinger, E. Csuka,
P.F. Stahel, O. Trentz, and M.C. Morganti-Kossmann

Introduction

Patients with severe head injury still carry a high risk of mortality and morbidity despite progress in clinical management (Frankowski et al. 1985; Alberico et al. 1987). Major causes of mortality in these patients are untreatable elevated intracranial pressure (ICP) in the early phase and septic–infectious complications during the later phase (Shackford et al. 1989). The importance of inflammatory events following head trauma even in the absence of systemic injuries has been recognized. Within a short period of time after hospitalization these patients show a depressed T-cell function, an anergy to delayed-type hypersensitivity skin testing, a decrease in the expression of interleukin-2 receptors on T-cells and, furthermore, a diminished in vitro interleukin-2 and γ-interferon production of T-cells as well as suppressed cell cytotoxicity (Quattrocchi et al. 1991; Hoyt et al. 1990). However, the depression of the peripheral immune system may be of a secondary nature and may be regulated by immunological events initiated as a result of the traumatic injury within the brain. In particular cytokines produced and released in the central nervous system (CNS) may play important roles in the pathophysiological events following brain trauma.

The production of cytokines within the CNS has been demonstrated in several diseases of the CNS, such as bacterial and viral meningitis, multiple sclerosis, acquired immunodeficiency syndrome dementia complex and Alzheimer's disease (Morganti-Kossmann et al. 1992a; Morganti-Kossmann and Kossmann 1995). Cytokines are fundamental mediators in the inflammatory response and their effects may be beneficial as well as deleterious. They are produced by a variety of different cell types after activation regulating cell functions such as migration, proliferation and production of other cytokines. Since they are released as soluble factors they act on the cell surface of their target cell, but may display opposite effects depending on the cell type they interact with. A functional redundancy of different cytokines is due to the presence of common receptor subunits for numerous cytokines, activating the same signal transduction pathway. To initiate a biological response only low concentrations of a certain cytokine are necessary due to the presence of high affinity receptors.

Astrocytes, which are the major cell type represented in the brain, and microglia, the resident macrophages of the CNS, are the source as well as the target of cytokines. Numerous in vitro studies on these cells as well as animal studies have driven a new concept on the definition of the brain as an immune-competent organ, which actively participates in its own defense against injury, autoimmune and infectious diseases.

In the following studies the injured brain has been regarded as the center of many immunological reactions initiated after the traumatic impact. This is a new concept, since the CNS has always been regarded as an immunologically privileged site due to its separation from the circulation by the blood–brain barrier (BBB) (Fabry et al. 1994). The interest in cytokines as important mediators in the immune reaction following brain trauma originates from the fact that tumor necrosis factor alpha (TNF-α), interleukin-1 (IL-1) and interleukin-6 (IL-6) have been found in significant amounts within the injured brain using a variety of animal models (Giulian and Lachman 1985; Nieto-Sampedro and Berman 1987; Woodroofe et al. 1991; Taupin et al. 1993). However, the inflammatory events occurring after human brain injury in humans still remain to be elucidated.

Research efforts were divided into a clinical and an experimental section aimed at clarifying the sequelae of cytokine production and whether cytokines produced in the CNS may trigger regenerative processes as well as systemic reactions. Furthermore, the activation of various cell types following a diffuse axonal injury was characterized using an animal model.

The clinical study focused on the monitoring of pro- and antiinflammatory cytokines released into CSF and serum. For this purpose patients with isolated severe traumatic brain injury (TBI) were included after the insertion of indwelling ventricular catheters (IVC) for monitoring and treatment of elevated ICP. This therapeutical approach allowed measurements of TNF-α, IL-1, IL-6, IL-8 and transforming growth factor-beta (TGF-β) in the CSF and serum. In parallel, the alteration of the BBB was analyzed in order to elucidate whether or not these cytokines are produced intrathecally or penetrate the CNS through a leaking BBB.

TNF-α is a cytokine which has been detected in several diseases of the CNS such as meningitis and human immunodeficiency virus-infection. A particular role for TNF-α was demonstrated in autoimmune diseases such as multiple sclerosis (Morganti-Kossmann and Kossmann 1995). In fact, evidence has shown that TNF-α is toxic to oligodendrocytes and causes demyelinization (Selmaj et al. 1991). An experimental brain injury model has demonstrated that early after brain injury TNF-α is produced in the damaged tissue (Taupin et al. 1993). In brain trauma, production of TNF-α has been found to be associated with adherence of neutrophils to endothelial cells, and may lead to increased permeability of the BBB and synthesis of adhesion molecules (Frohman et al. 1989; Bowes et al. 1993). Therefore, this cytokine seems to play an important role in the processes which regulate BBB function and infiltration of cells from the periphery. These events, if uncontrolled, may be responsible for secondary injury since activated cells may produce neurotoxic factors.

IL-6 seems to play an important role in the inflammatory events initiated by TBI, which resemble those described in other CNS pathologies. In experimental head trauma considerable amounts of this cytokine are produced in the CNS following injury (Woodroofe et al. 1991; Taupin et al. 1993). Intrathecal production of IL-6 is predominantly attributed to activated astrocytes and microglia as well as to macrophages invading the CNS (Morganti-Kossmann et al. 1992a). As a multifunctional cytokine (for review see van Snick 1990), IL-6 has the ability to promote regenerative processes by inducing neurotrophic factors and is considered the major regulator of the acute-phase response (Baumann and Gauldie 1994). This response is characterized by fever, neutrophilia, decreased albumin synthesis, depressed serum levels of iron and zinc, increased serum copper levels and augmented synthesis of acute-phase proteins (Akira and Kishimoto 1992; Castell et al. 1988; Kushner and Mackiewicz 1987). The acute-phase response has been described previously in head trauma patients (Young et al. 1988; Feldman et al. 1993); however, its relation to cytokines produced in the CNS was only speculative.

Another pro-inflammatory cytokine monitored in the clinical study was IL-8, a protein with potent chemotactic and activating effects on neutrophils. IL-8 is predominantly released by monocytes–macrophages, but also by a variety of other cell types such as endothelial cells and neutrophils following stimulation with IL-1 and TNF-α (Baggiolini et al. 1989, 1992; Dinarello 1991; Bazzoni et al. 1991). Astrocytes produce IL-8 in response to IL-1 and TNF-α challenge, whereas constitutive expression of IL-8 was demonstrated in transformed astrocytes (Aloisi et al. 1992; Nitta et al. 1992). In addition to its properties shown toward neutrophils, IL-8 displays neurotrophic activity on hippocampal neurons (Araujo and Cotman 1993). Moreover, the expression of the IL-8 receptor on glial cells suggests that this factor may regulate other activities in these cells (Lacy et al. 1995). IL-8 was found in a variety of diseases of the CNS such as bacterial meningitis, meningoencephalitis (Handa 1992; van Meir et al. 1992; Seki et al. 1993; Halstensen et al. 1993; Mastroianni et al. 1994) and malignant brain neoplasms (Nitta et al. 1992; van Meir et al. 1992; Morita et al. 1993; Tada et al. 1993). However, the role of IL-8 in TBI has not yet been elucidated.

TGF-β is regarded as a mediator with immunosuppressive properties (for review see Wahl 1994). TGF-β seems to favor the healing process of the injured brain since it has the ability to modulate matrix deposition, to reduce the action of pro-inflammatory cytokines which can become neurotoxic (e.g., TNF), as well as edema formation (Frei et al. 1990, 1993). In addition, TGF-β was shown to be produced in the injured brain and to trigger the synthesis of nerve growth factor (NGF) in astrocytes, thus also promoting regenerative processes (Lindholm et al. 1990, 1992). It is spontaneously secreted by human glioma cell lines and inhibits the proliferation of lymph node cells specifically activated against myelin basic protein, reducing the severity of experimental allergic encephalomyelitis (Bodmer et al. 1989; Racke et al. 1991). The mechanisms of TGF-β induction by glial cells are not yet fully understood. IL-1, a cytokine usually released in the initial phase of the immune response, was shown to promote TGF-β production by astrocytes, microglia and oligodendrocytes (da Cuhna et al. 1993). An association between IL-6 and TGF-β was already established in thermally injured, immunosuppressed patients (Zhou et al. 1991). Elevated serum-IL-6 was shown to inhibit T-cell mediated immune functions. This impairment seemed to depend on macrophage activities and to be the result of an IL-6 induced increase of TGF-β synthesis or activation.

The clinical study presented several limitations in the understanding of the functional relationship between different cytokines, therefore experiments on primary cultures of astrocytes and microglia were performed. The use of astrocytes in in vitro studies was established in order to elucidate the relationship between cytokines and neurotrophic factors. These cells play a fundamental role in the brain by providing an insulating framework for neurons, and by releasing metabolic intermediates and trophic factors necessary for maintaining the homeostasis of the neuronal environment. After a traumatic impact to the brain, or under other pathological conditions, astrocytes become activated displaying a variety of functions normally attributed to blood-derived macrophages (Table 1).

Following activation, astrocytes show a more intense glial fibrillar acidic protein (GFAP) immunoreactivity, increased growth, migration and production of cytokines as well as of factors which promote regeneration and axonal re-growth (for review see Eddleston and Mucke 1992). It appears that functions displayed by activated astrocytes are more beneficial and directed to restore a normal physiology of the lesioned brain, whereas microglia may likely contribute to the events occurring in secondary brain damage (Morganti-Kossmann and Kossmann 1995). Furthermore, lymphocytes infiltrating the brain tissue initiate and perpetuate the inflammatory processes, acting in a close functional relationship with glial cells.

The major cell type involved in the immune surveillance of the brain are the microglial cells, the resident macrophages of the CNS. They comprise only 20% of the glial cell population, forming a homogenous network throughout the tissue and are activated rapidly in neuropathology (Banati et al. 1993). Microglial cells can be distinguished from astrocytes due to their morphological and metabolic characteristics (Table 1). They show a phagocytic shape and produce a variety of mediators such as cytokines, complement proteins, proteases and reactive oxygen intermediates which are potentially harmful factors for the CNS. They also express major histocompatibility complex (MHC) antigens and adhesion molecules. Clusters of activated microglia have been observed in areas of axonal damage (Clark 1974). The role played by these cells in the injured brain is still poorly understood; however, due to their multiple functions they may regulate several pathological events which take place in the lesioned brain tissue.

In order to extend the results obtained in the clinical study an experimental model of diffuse axonal injury was established (Marmarou et al. 1994). Compared to

Table 1. Activation of glial cells in the injured brain

	Microglia	Astrocytes
Morphology	Ramified → ameboid	GFAP expression increased; scarring, ECM deposition
Migration	Yes	Yes
Proliferation	Yes	Yes
Phagocytosis	Myelin, cell debris	Myelin, cell debris
MHC expression	Class I and II	Class I and II
Cytokine production	IL-1, IL-6, IL-8, TNF-α, TGF-β	IL-1, IL-6, IL-8, TNF-α, TGF-β
Neurotoxic components	Release (glutamate, ORI, NO, proteases)	Metabolism (glutamate, ORI)

GFAP, glial fibrillary acidic protein; ECM, extracellular matrix; MHC, major histocompatibility complex; ORI, oxygen radical intermediates; NO, nitric oxide; IL, interleukin; TNF-α, tumor necrosis factor-alpha; TGF-β, transforming growth factor-beta.

other animal models, this one seems to resemble more closely the injury patterns frequently found in patients following severe head trauma. In fact, in multicenter studies it has been demonstrated that 43%–55% of patients with severe brain trauma suffer from a diffuse type of injury (Gennarelli et al. 1982; Marshall et al. 1991). The activation of glial cells was analyzed following diffuse axonal injury on rat brain tissue. An acceleration impact was applied to the protected skull of rats avoiding depression fractures which cause focal injuries or direct trauma to the dura mater as shown in the fluid percussion model (Foda and Marmarou 1994; Dixon et al. 1988). There are many reports of focal injuries to the brain in numerous animal models; however, diffuse axonal injuries have not been well defined yet and need more experimental elucidation.

Methods

Patients

Patients with a diagnosis of severe isolated traumatic brain injury (TBI), admitted to the Division of Trauma Surgery at the University Hospital of Zürich, Switzerland, were included in the study. All patients had a Glasgow Coma Score (GCS) <9 (Teasdale and Jennett 1974) on admission and alterations in the computed tomography (CT). After clinical and CT evaluation the patients received an indwelling ventricular catheter for ICP monitoring and therapeutic drainage of CSF within 2–4 h of admission. Whenever necessary craniotomy was performed for evacuation of hematomas. All patients were transferred to the intensive care unit (ICU) after surgery. In accordance with a standardized protocol (Stocker et al. 1995) CSF was drained when ICP exceeded 15 mm Hg. Intraventricular catheters were removed after the ICP remained stable (<15 mm Hg) for at least 24 h. Patients with significant extracranial injuries were excluded from the study. The patients were evaluated between 3 and 6 months after the traumatic event by the Glasgow Outcome Score (GOS) (Jennett and Bond 1975). CSF from patients without traumatic head injuries or any other neuropathologies were used as controls following either lumbar diagnostic puncture or ventriculo-peritoneal shunt. (The study protocol was approved by the University Hospital Medical Ethics Board, Zürich, Switzerland. The studies were supported by grants from the Swiss National Foundation, Nos. 31-37375.92 and 31-42490.94.)

Analysis of Cytokines and NGF

Drained CSF and serum were collected from the enrolled patients every 24 h, centrifuged at 1000 rpm for 10 min at 4°C, aliquoted and frozen at −70°C until analyzed. The concentrations of TNF-α, IL-1, IL-6 (R&D Systems, Minneapolis, MN, USA) and TGF-β (Genzyme, Cambridge, MA, USA) were analyzed by sandwich enzyme-linked immunosorbent assays (ELISA) according to the protocols of the manufacturers or as described for NGF and for IL-8 (Kossmann et al. 1996; Halstensen et al. 1993). A microplate reader (Dynatech Laboratories Inc., Alexandria, MD, USA) was used for measuring the absorbance.

Blood–Brain Barrier

According to Reiber and Felgenhauer (1987), the ratio of CSF–serum albumin (Q_A) is considered as a sensitive parameter for monitoring the function of the BBB and was calculated daily during the entire study period. The disturbance of the BBB was assessed as follows: Q_A values below 0.007 were regarded as normal, between 0.007 and 0.01 as a sign of a mild dysfunction, values between 0.01 and 0.02 of a moderate dysfunction, and above 0.02 of a severe BBB dysfunction. Albumin levels were measured by automatized laser photometry (BNA Automat, Behring Werke, Marburg a.L., Germany).

Astrocyte Stimulation with Human CSF or Recombinant IL-6 or IL-8

Primary glial cell cultures were established from neonatal mouse brain as described previously (Morganti et al. 1990). Prior to stimulation, cells were incubated overnight with DMEM containing 1% FCS. Confluent astrocytes were incubated with CSF of brain-injured patients containing different concentrations of IL-6 or IL-8 in the presence or absence of neutralizing anti-IL-6 or anti-IL-8 antibodies (R & D Systems), with control CSF from patients without neurotrauma or with medium alone for 3 days, respectively. Culture supernatants were collected, centrifuged at 1000 rpm for 10 min at 4°C and frozen until assayed for NGF. CSF samples were assayed for NGF before performing the coculture with the CSF of patients.

In parallel experiments astrocytes were exposed to recombinant human IL-6 or IL-8 (Genzyme and R&D System, respectively) for 3 days at different concentrations. Thereafter cell-free supernatants were harvested and assayed for NGF.

Measurements of Acute Phase Proteins

Acute phase proteins were measured daily in serum of brain-injured patients. C-reactive protein (CRP) levels were measured by automatized photometry (Hitachi 747 autoanalyzer, Boehringer Mannheim GmbH, Mannheim, Germany), α1-antitrypsin (α1-AT) and albumin levels were measured by automatized laser photometry (BNA Automat, Behring Werke, Marburg a.L., Germany) and fibrinogen concentrations were determined using an automatized coagulometer (KC 40, Amelung, Lemgo, Germany).

Hematology

Blood differential counts were performed by an automatized cell counter (Technicon H*l, Bayer Diagnostics GmbH, München, Germany).

Animal Model of Diffuse Axonal Injury

The experimental head trauma model causes a diffuse brain injury as described previously (Marmarou et al. 1994). Briefly, the skulls of adult male SIV rats were prepared under anesthesia and a metal disk was fixed with dental acrylic to allow a homogenous distribution of the impact forces. The animals were then placed in a prone position on a foam bed and the injury was delivered by dropping a weight of 250 g on the skull from a hight of 2 m through a vertical tube. After removal of the disk, the scalp was sutured. Rats were sacrificed at different time points, ranging from 1 h up to 2 weeks for trauma, or 2 and 24 h for sham operated animals (control), as listed in Table 2. The brains were frozen at −70°C until analyzed for histology and immunohistochemistry. CSF and serum were also collected for cytokine assays. The animal protocols were reviewed and approved by the Kantonales Veterinäramt Zürich, No. 138/93.

IL-6 Bioassay

IL-6 concentrations in rat serum and CSF were determined using the 7TD1 cell line (kindly provided by Dr. K. Frei, University of Zürich, Switzerland), an IL-6 dependent murine hybridoma cell line (van Damme et al. 1987). Cell proliferation was quantitated following the incorporation of 3-[4,5-dimethylthiazol-2-yl]-2,5-diphenyltetrazoliumbromide as described elsewhere (Mosmann 1983). The absorbance was measured at 550 nm with a microplate reader (Dynatech Laboratories Inc.). The concentrations of IL-6 were calculated by comparing the absorption of the samples with those of a standard curve obtained with recombinant mouse IL-6 (Genzyme). The detection limit of this assay is 7 pg/ml.

Immunohistochemistry

Immunohistochemical staining was performed on frozen sections from rat brain using the horseradish-peroxidase-labeled avidin-biotin procedure (ABC Vecta Stain Kit, Vector Laboratories Inc., Burlingame, CA). Antibodies directed against specific cell markers such as GFAP (Boehringer Mannheim) for astrocytes; OX-42 (Serotec LTD, Oxford, UK) as a marker for microglia–macrophages; OX-6 (Serotec) as a

Table 2. Scheme of the experimental brain injury model

Group	Animals per group	Total number of animals
1, 2, 4*, 8, 16 h	5/4*	24
1, 2, 4, 7, 14 days	5	25
Sham operated: 2 and 24 h	3	6
Death due to trauma	4	4
Total		59

*The 4-h group consisted of only four rats, not five.

marker for cell activation directed against major histocompatibility complex (MHC) class II were utilized as already described (Wahl et al. 1991).

Analysis of Data

Statistical analysis was performed on commercially available software (StatView 4.0, Abacus Concepts Inc., Berkeley, California, USA) using appropriate tests as indicated. The corresponding values in serum and CSF were compared for each day with a paired t-test. A modified Bonferroni correction was applied to correct for the repeated measurements error (Cross and Chaffin 1982). A statistical probabilitiy of two-sided $p < 0.05$ was considered significant. Unless indicated otherwise, means are expressed with the corresponding standard error of the mean.

Results and Discussion of the Clinical Study

IL-6 in CSF and Serum of Patients with Traumatic Brain Injury

The production of IL-6 was monitored in the CSF and serum of 20 patients (14 men, 6 women, 38.3 ± 18.9 years). A total of 17 patients had closed traumatic brain injury to a various extent, and three patients suffered from an open head trauma. Five patients died within 2 weeks after injury due to untreatable intracranial pressure and one patient died after a 103-day period of continuous vegetative state. IL-6 concentrations were found to be dramatically elevated in all patients in the early days after trauma (Fig. 1). At the following time points the cytokine levels decreased; however IL-6 could be detected in almost all samples up to the end of the study period. The highest peaks were found on day 1 and 2. Maximal IL-6 concentrations reached 31 300 pg/ml in CSF and 1100 pg/ml in serum.

As clearly shown in Fig. 1 the amounts of IL-6 measured in serum samples remained significantly lower as compared to those in CSF ($p = 0.01$, paired t-test, Bonferroni correction). However, the kinetics of IL-6 in serum showed a pattern similar to that in CSF and IL-6 levels in serum never reached the levels observed in CSF.

The integrity of the BBB was determined daily in order to clarify whether and at which time points a possible leakage could allow the passage of IL-6 from the CNS into the periphery. In 12 patients a moderate to severe disturbance of the BBB was evident over several days. A restoration to a normal BBB function was observed within 2–3 days after the traumatic impact in five patients. Seven patients showed a BBB disturbance persisting for more than 6 days and in eight patients the BBB remained intact over the whole study period with $Q_A \leq 0.007$.

The relationship between IL-6 levels in CSF and serum was analyzed and compared to the albumin quotient on each day. IL-6 values in CSF and serum were grouped according to their corresponding Q_A (Fig. 2). In cases with a Q_A above 0.020 a correlation between IL-6 in CSF and serum was evident ($r = 0.637$; $p = 0.001$) (Fig.

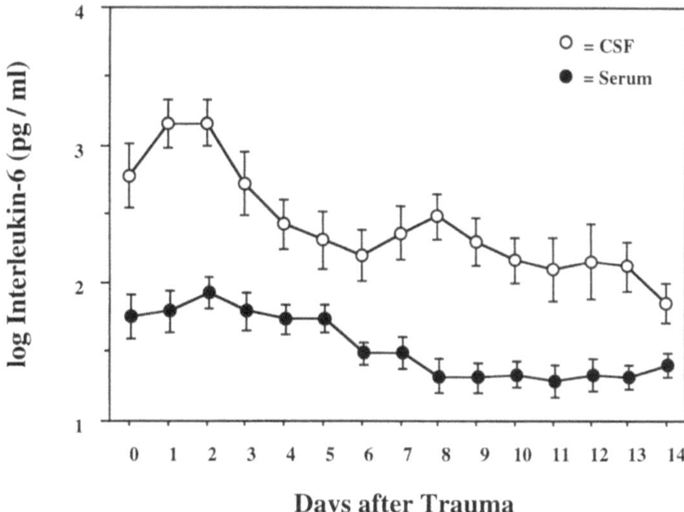

4
3
2
1
log Interleukin-6 (pg / ml)
O = CSF
● = Serum
0 1 2 3 4 5 6 7 8 9 10 11 12 13 14
Days after Trauma

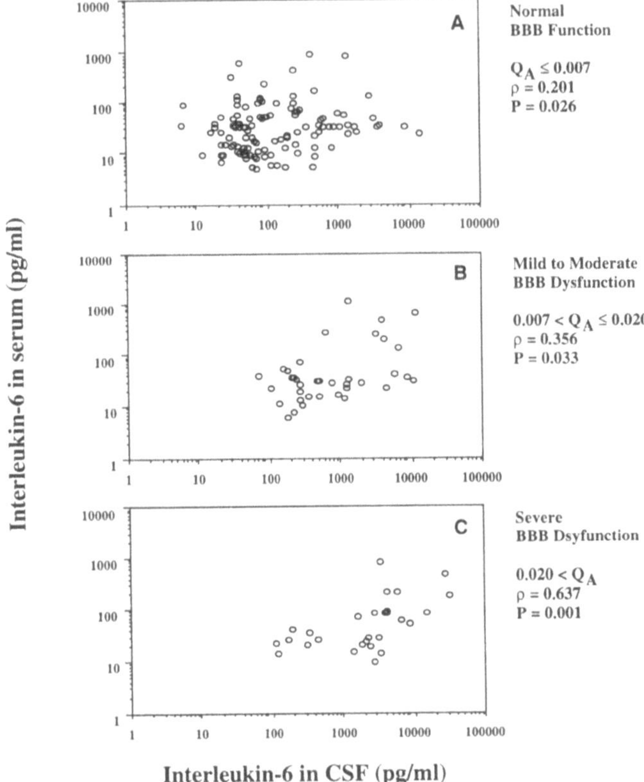

Fig. 2A–C. Serum and CSF interleukin (IL)-6 correlate when the blood–brain barrier (BBB) is altered. IL-6 concentrations in serum and CSF of 20 patients with isolated traumatic brain injury were grouped according to their corresponding albumin ratio (Q_A). A correlation (Spearman rank correlation r for paired values) was only apparent during severe disturbance of the BBB (**C**). No significant correlation was found when the BBB showed either moderate or no dysfunction (**A,B**). (From Kossmann et al. 1995)

Table 3. Serum IL-6 correlates with acute-phase proteins

	CRP	Fibrinogen	α1-AT
IL-6 in serum	$r = 0.605$	$r = 0.455$	$r = 0.719$
	$p = 0.004$	$p = 0.066$	$p = 0.0002$
IL-6 in CSF	$r = 0.216$	$r = 0.145$	$r = 0.027$
	$p = 0.365$	$p = 0.585$	$p = 0.911$

Pearson's correlation coefficient for maximal concentrations of acute phase proteins [c-reactive protein (CRP), fibrinogen, alpha 1-antitrypsin (α1-AT)] in serum to maximal interleukin (IL)-6 concentrations in serum and CSF of 20 patients with head injury. (From Kossmann et al. 1995.)

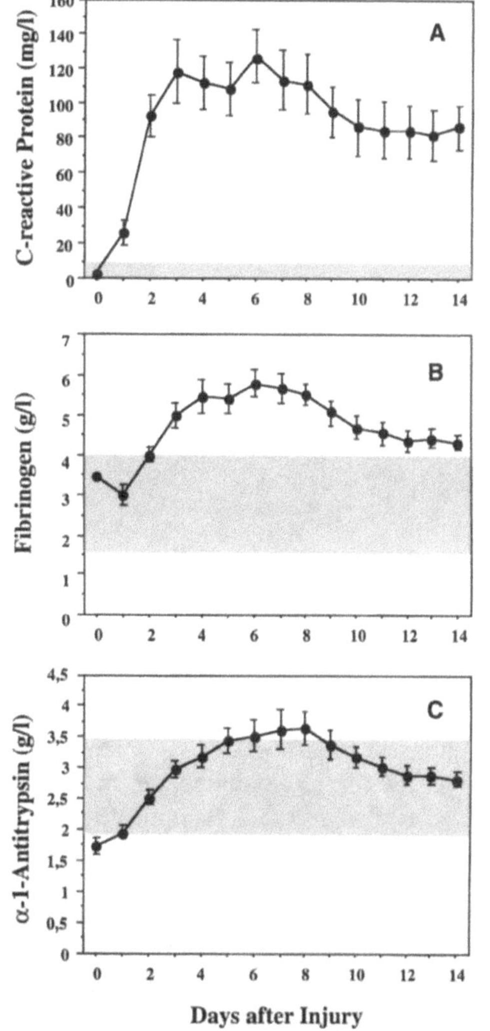

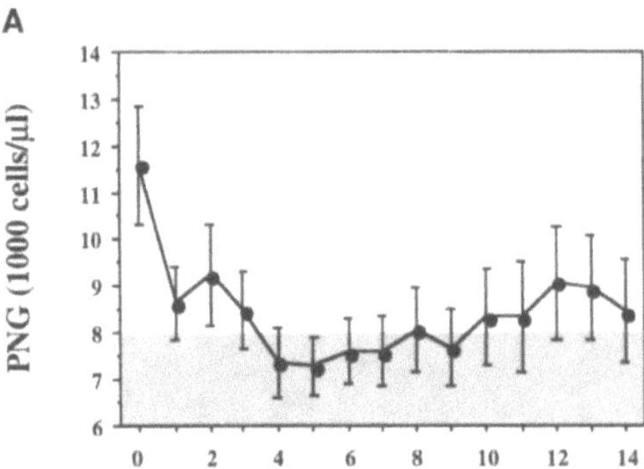

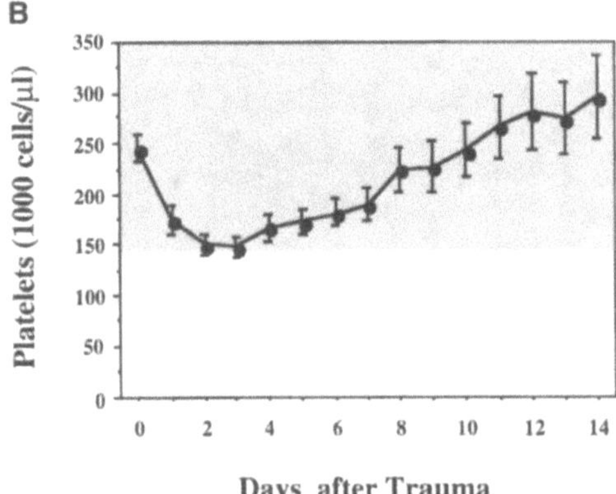

Fig. 4A,B. Differential blood cell counts from 20 patients with isolated head injury. The variation in the number (mean ± SEM) of polymorphonuclear granulocytes (*PNG*) (**A**) and platelets (**B**) was evaluated during the entire study period at each day. Normal ranges are indicated by *gray fields*. (From Kossmann et al. 1995)

evident thrombocytosis over 500 000/ml in three patients. No correlation was noticed between any of the fluctuations in blood cell counts and corresponding IL-6 serum levels.

IL-6 Induces NGF

The presence of NGF was monitored in 22 head trauma patients and was detected in the CSF of 14 patients which contained relevant IL-6 concentrations over the study period. Comparing the kinetics of IL-6 and NGF production, NGF peaks were found either simultaneously with or following the highest IL-6 levels (Fig. 5).

The role of IL-6 in the induction of NGF was analyzed to elucidate the possible regenerative mechanisms initiated after brain injury. Table 4 shows NGF levels obtained after incubation of astrocytes with CSF from eight patients with different levels of IL-6. NGF production was induced by all samples. Control cultures were grown with medium alone and showed only low basal NGF production. Furthermore, coculture of CSF from control patients (ventricular or lumbar CSF) showed either no or slightly elevated NGF levels.

In order to show the specificity of NGF synthesis induced by IL-6, the same CSF samples were preincubated with anti-IL-6 antibodies in neutralizing concentrations

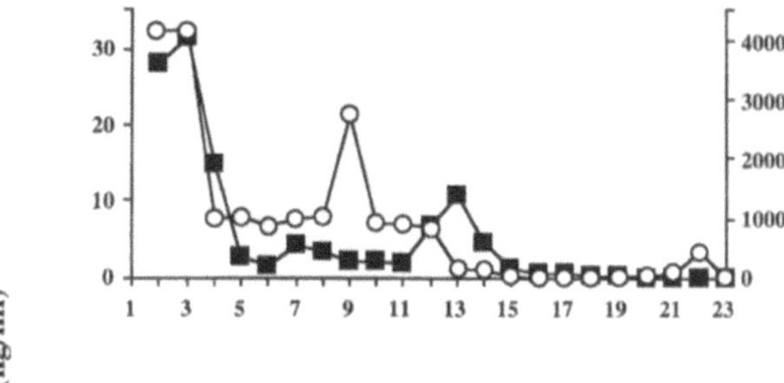

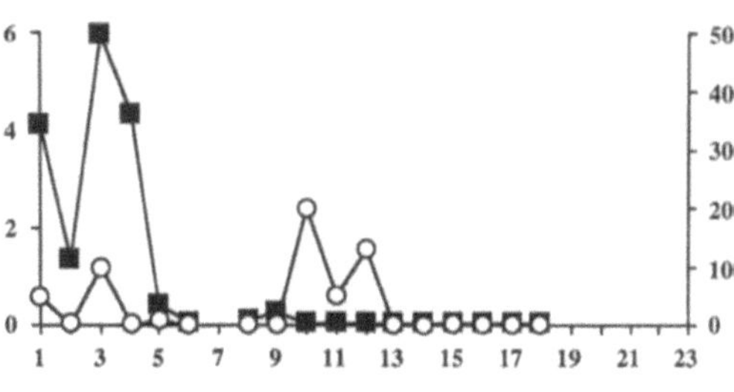

IL-6 (ng/ml)
NGF (pg/ml)
Days after Trauma

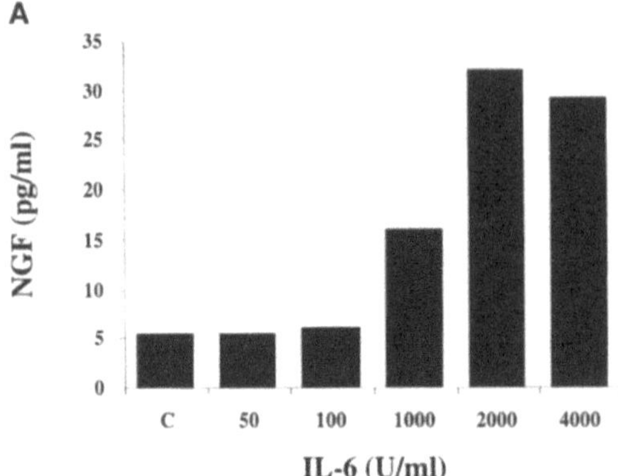

A
NGF (pg/ml)
35
30
25
20
15
10
5
0
C
50
100
1000
2000
4000
IL-6 (U/ml)

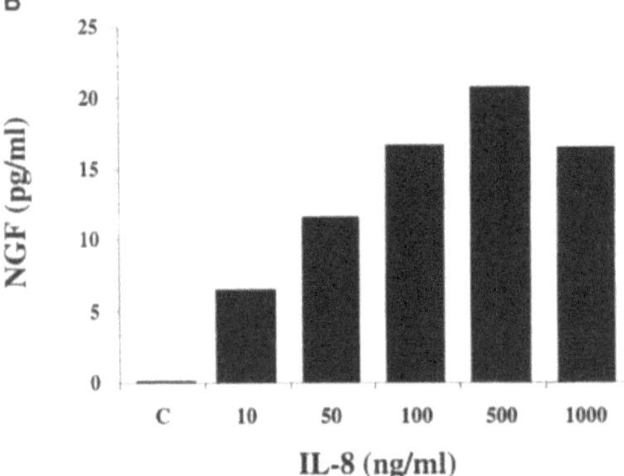

B
NGF (pg/ml)
25
20
15
10
5
0
C
10
50
100
500
1000
IL-8 (ng/ml)

CSF of head trauma patients was exclusively demonstrated at a single time point (McClain et al. 1991), in our analysis we demonstrated that IL-6 remained elevated in the CSF for several days following injury to the brain.

The intracerebral source of IL-6 was attributed to T-cells and monocytes invading the brain tissue (Taupin et al. 1993), since these cells are considered the main source of IL-6 (Okada et al. 1983; Hirano et al. 1985; Aarden et al. 1987; van Snick 1990). However, a wide range of cells is also capable of producing IL-6, such as fibroblasts, endothelial cells, and cells of the nervous tissue like astrocytes and microglia (Frei et al. 1989; Woodroofe et al. 1991; Morganti-Kossmann et al. 1992a). Since IL-6 was detected in the CSF of these patients immediately after the traumatic injury, remaining elevated for several days, and since CSF IL-6 concentrations were significantly higher than in the systemic circulation, we assume that IL-6 production might be also of astrocytic and microglial origin. We cannot exclude, however, that invading cells of the leucocytic lineage are contributing to the high levels of intrathecal IL-6. Such a mechanism has been discussed in experimental traumatic brain injury (Cortez et al. 1989; Taupin et al. 1993). The increase of IL-6 production was also attributed to short-living polymorphonuclear cells since it has been already shown that these cells have the ability to produce several cytokines (Dubravec et al. 1990; Marucha et al. 1990; Terebuh et al. 1992).

The difference in IL-6 levels measured within the CSF of brain-injured patients may derive from the activation of several cell types following the traumatic impact and explain the concentration difference between CSF and serum IL-6. IL-6 levels in both fluids correlated with each other when the BBB was severly disturbed. Therefore IL-6 may leak into the systemic circulation during a severe BBB dysfunction. In fact, a severe dysfunction of the BBB was found in the first posttraumatic days. However, this may not be the only mechanism how IL-6 reaches the systemic circulation. A loss of correlation between the IL-6 levels in CSF and serum appeared following the restoration of BBB function. Since substantial levels of IL-6 can be measured in both compartments also later on, other transport mechanisms may play a role. IL-6 may cross the intact BBB by diffusion (Fabry et al. 1994) or by an active transport (Banks et al. 1995). The low levels of IL-6 detected in the systemic circulation may be explained by a rapid metabolism of the cytokine in the liver (Castell et al. 1988).

Since IL-6 is the major regulator of acute phase protein synthesis (Castell et al. 1989) it was hypothesized that this cytokine may promote the acute phase response in these patients as already described (Young et al. 1988; Feldman et al. 1993). IL-6 concentrations in CSF and serum increased immediately following trauma whereas the acute-phase response appeared with a delay of 1 to 2 days. The acute-phase proteins CRP, α1-AT and fibrinogen increased rapidly following trauma, showing a peak within the first week. The maximal levels of these proteins correlated with the maximal values of IL-6 in serum, but not with IL-6 levels in CSF (Table 3). In contrast to other work (Young et al. 1988) albumin concentrations did not vary considerably in our patient group, possibly due to the parenteral substitution of albumin. With regard to the hematological pattern, leucocyte counts were always elevated throughout the study period with a peak during the first and second week. This feature may also be regulated by IL-6 since it has been shown to have a stimulatory effect on the bone marrow (van Snick 1990). The exact causes for the suppressed hemoglobin concentrations remain to be elucidated. While no concomitant injuries with severe blood loss occurred, occult bleeding into the gastrointestinal tract can not be excluded. Other factors may also influence hematopoiesis, or a dilution effect may occur due to the intensive volume therapy (Stocker et al. 1995). Variations of the thrombocyte counts appeared in all patients showing a dramatic decline in the early posttraumatic phase followed by a later increase. Such patterns have also been observed in burn patients (Nijsten et al. 1991). The initial decrease in thrombocytes may be due to sequestration, consumption, or to a dilution effect. In fact, the patients included in the study received massive volume substitution for circulatory support. Furthermore, it can be speculated that platelet activating factor plays a role, by inducing thrombocytopenia (Hosford and Braquet 1989). Although no statistical correlation was found between serum IL-6 concentrations and thrombocyte counts, IL-6 may be responsible for the later rise in total thrombocyte counts by inducing the maturation of megakaryocytes (Akira and Kishimoto 1992; Lotem et al. 1989). In addition, IL-6 was shown to be a potent thrombopoietic factor in mice (Ishibashi et al. 1989). The acute-phase reaction is characterized by increased body temperature and heart rate. These parameters were found elevated; however, in contrast to other findings (Young et al. 1988), they did not correlate with the IL-6 levels in either CSF or serum samples.

IL-1 is another cytokine found in ventricular CSF (McClain et al. 1987) which was assumed to be responsible for the acute-phase response (Young et al. 1988). In contrast to these results we could not detect any IL-1 in the CSF or serum in these individuals.

The role of the pleiotropic cytokine IL-6 in the events following traumatic brain injury may be of a multiple nature. IL-6 has a mitogenic effect on astrocytes (Selmaj et al. 1990), has a protective function on neurons (Hama et al. 1989) and can induce neuronal differentiation (Satoh et al. 1988). We could show an association between IL-6 and NGF. NGF was detected only in patients having high concentrations of IL-6 in CSF, and thus this factor may trigger NGF synthesis after brain injury. This hypothesis was supported by the in vitro results and suggests that cytokines act in synergism in vivo as already shown by others (Lindsay 1979; Awatsuji et al. 1993). The neuroprotective activity of IL-6 may also be exerted by its receptor which shares a common subunit, the protein gp 130, with the receptor of the ciliary neurotrophic factor (CNTF) (Kitamura et al. 1994).

In summary, the continuous presence of IL-6 was found in the CSF and serum following traumatic brain injury and since IL-6 in serum correlates with increased CRP, fibrinogen, and α1-AT in the systemic circulation, we suppose that IL-6 induces the acute-phase reaction. The higher IL-6 concentrations detected in CSF together with the initial BBB dysfunction, suggest that IL-6 may leak from the CNS into the systemic circulation inducing a general acute phase response. IL-6 may locally support neuroregenerative processes in the CNS either by its intrinsic activities or by the induction of neuroptrophic factors like NGF. IL-6 may also influence the general immunological status of the patients. IL-6 can display an additional protective effect since, as shown for monocytes, IL-6 inhibits the production of TNF-α (Aderka et al. 1989). This is of relevance for the nervous system, since this factor can have deleteri-

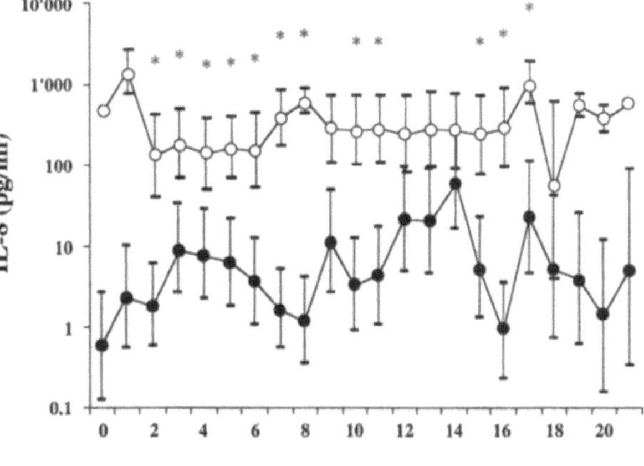

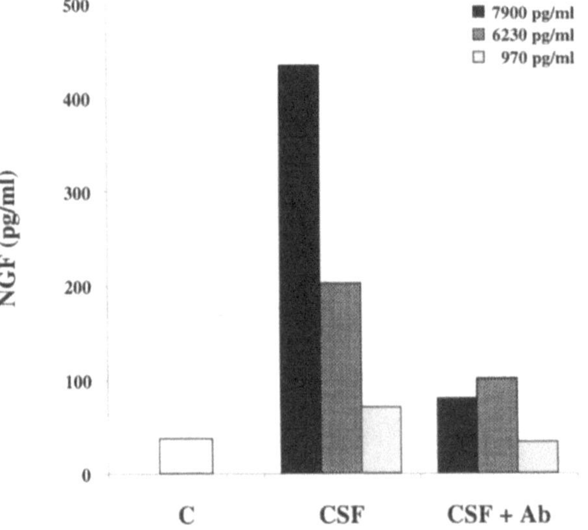

500
400
300
200
100
0
NGF (pg/ml)
7900 pg/ml
6230 pg/ml
970 pg/ml
C
CSF
CSF + Ab

Similarly to the IL-6 analysis, the higher IL-8 concentrations in the CSF suggest that this cytokine may be produced in the cerebral compartment following the traumatic impact. This is supported by the findings that astrocytes and microglia are capabable of producing IL-8 after challenge (Aloisi et al. 1992; Nitta et al. 1992; Mukaida and Matsushima 1992).

Discussion

Elevated levels of the pro-inflammatory cytokine IL-8 have been reported in numerous pathological conditions, including diseases of the CNS (Handa 1992; Nitta et al. 1992; van Meir et al. 1992; Halstensen et al. 1993; Seki et al. 1993; Tada et al. 1993; Mastroianni et al. 1994). IL-8 is produced by numerous cells including glial cells upon stimulation, and neutrophils (Bazzoni et al. 1991; Aloisi et al. 1992; Nitta et al. 1992). Cytokines such as TNF-α and IL-1 induce IL-8 in astrocytes, and the production of TNF-α, IL-1 and IL-6 has been demonstrated in experimental head injury models and in humans very early after the traumatic impact (Nieto-Sampedro and Berman 1987; Woodroofe et al. 1991; Taupin et al. 1993; McClain et al. 1987, 1991; Kossmann et al. 1995). In an animal model of shock induced by intravenous administration of endotoxin, the peak of IL-8 in serum was found succeeding the IL-1 and TNF-α peaks and occurring simultaneously with the IL-6 peak (Martich et al. 1991). Therefore, these cytokines, immediately released after head trauma, may promote the synthesis of later mediators such as IL-8 and IL-6.

IL-8 may display functions additional to its known regulation of the immune response such as the induction of neurotrophic factors. Up-regulation of NGF expression has been described following neurotrauma in animals as well as in humans (Nieto-Sampedro et al. 1982; Heumann et al. 1987; Patterson et al. 1993; Kossmann et al. 1996). NGF has the ability to favor the development and survival of cholinergic neurons (for review see Levi-Montalcini and Angeletti 1968). Much evidence supports a role for cytokines in the regulation of NGF synthesis (Lindholm et al. 1987, 1990; Gadient et al. 1990; Spranger et al. 1990; Carman-Krzan et al. 1991; Yoshida and Gage 1991; Kossmann et al. 1996). Enhanced NGF production has been shown following intrathecal injection of IL-1, TNF-α, and TGF-β (Spranger et al. 1990). This production is attributed predominantly to astrocytes and fibroblasts as a result of experiments performed in vitro (Furukawa et al. 1989; Gadient et al. 1990). However, we demonstrate for the first time that IL-8 also promotes the synthesis of NGF which may have beneficial consequences for the lesioned brain, since the administration of NGF was shown to result in increased neuronal survival (Kromer 1986; Apfel et al. 1991). This hypothesis is also supported by the findings that astrocytes and microglia express the IL-8 receptor, and therefore these cells are likely candidates for the production of NGF following challenge with IL-8 (Lacy et al. 1995). In addition, IL-8 itself has also been shown to promote the survival of hippocampal neurons (Araujo and Cotman 1993), possibly through the release of factors by astrocytes contaminating these cultures. The results together with the work of others indicate that IL-8 may act in synergy with other factors–cytokines as shown for IL-1 and TNF-α (Gadient et al. 1990). For this purpose, the CSF samples utilized for the culture experiments were tested for other cytokines (data not shown). IL-1 was not detected in any of the three samples, whereas IL-6 and TNF-α were found in small amounts. The IL-6 present in the CSF samples used for astrocyte stimulation may not be sufficient to promote NGF by itself, but contribute to a multifactorially regulated mechanism (Gadient et al. 1990; Kossmann et al. 1996). In addition, a greater cytokine concentration may be necessary in vitro to stimulate astrocytes since in vivo other cells such as fibroblasts may contribute to NGF production after brain injury (Furukawa et al. 1989). The functional significance of IL-8 production in the lesioned CNS remains to be elucidated. Although other studies found a correlation between IL-8 levels and clinical status in meningococcal infections of the CNS (Halstensen et al. 1993), IL-8 levels following head injury did not correlate with clinical status at admission nor with the outcome of the patients. This may depend on the pathophysiology of head trauma which considerably differs from the pathology of infectious diseases of the nervous system. However, IL-8 was found to be associated with a severe dysfunction of the BBB. Controversial opinions exist on the ability of cytokines to increase BBB permeability (Banks et al. 1991; Kim et al. 1992). The passage of cytokines across the BBB has been demonstrated in both directions, blood-to-brain and brain-to-blood, through a saturable active mechanism (Banks et al. 1995). In this analysis, patients with moderate to severe BBB damage had significantly higher CSF IL-8 concentrations than patients with only mild dysfunction or intact BBB. Although no data are available on the disruption of the BBB mediated by IL-8, the recruitment of neutrophils which may be promoted by IL-8, followed by the release of superoxyde radicals and other factors by these cells, may cause vascular damage and increase brain edema (Baggiolini et al. 1989; Chan et al. 1984; Shiga et al. 1991). This is supported by the fact that antibodies to the leucocyte intercellular adhesion molecule (ICAM)-1 reduce the neurological damage by inhibiting the adherence of neutrophils to the endothelium (Bowes et al. 1993).

In conclusion, IL-8 is found in the CSF and serum of brain-injured patients over several days after trauma and, apart from its pro-inflammatory properties, it may increase the permeability of the BBB. Furthermore, this cytokine may regulate regenerative processes through the induction of NGF synthesis by astrocytes.

TNF-α and IL-1

TNF-α was measured in CSF and serum in a group of 36 patients. The analysis for TNF-α showed elevated levels of this cytokine in serum and CSF, with concentration ranges from 0 to 757 pg/ml in CSF and from 0 to 157.5 pg/ml in serum (Fig. 9). In 27 patients the levels of TNF-α were found above 4.48 pg/ml, which is the mean concentration of TNF-α in CSF samples collected from 23 patients without brain injury. Differently from other cytokines which appeared very early after injury and remained elevated for some days, TNF-α patterns showed several peaks in both fluids with a different distribution for each patient. Serum TNF-α concentrations remained within the normal range (0–6.33 pg/ml) in 19 patients whereas in the other 17 they were elevated in 8%– 64% of all samples measured. In 29 patients CSF levels were higher than serum levels in 19%–100 % of all measurements of each patient. Of these, 11 had

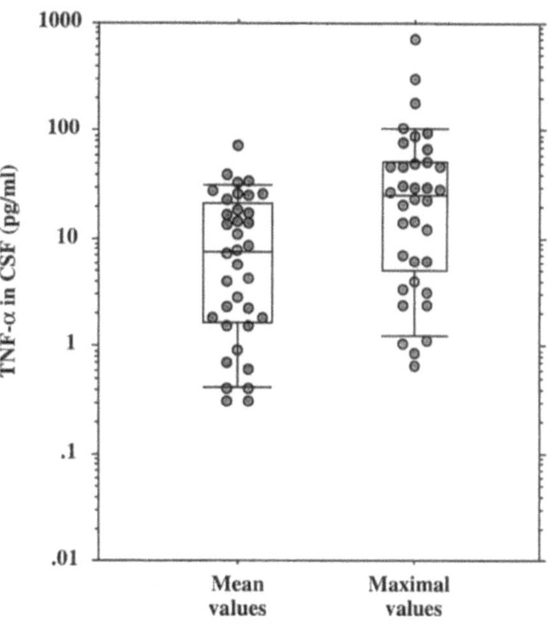

1000
100
10
1
.1
.01
TNF-α in CSF (pg/ml)
Mean values
Maximal values

Release of TGF-β in CSF and Serum of Brain Injured Patients

The presence of TGF-β was examined in the CSF and serum of 22 brain-injured patients (4 female, 18 male, 35.9 ± 3.4 years). Normal values for TGF-β were calculated as 95% reference interval from samples of 12 control subjects without any neuropatholgies: 6.6–69.1 ng/ml in serum and 11–112 pg/ml in CSF. TGF-β concentrations in CSF were increased in all patients except for one and in ten patients the values never dropped to the reference interval during the whole study period. Mean values of TGF-β in CSF were found increased during the whole study period showing a first peak at the day of trauma (498 pg/ml) and a second peak at day 8 (420 pg/ml), thereafter the levels of TGF-β decreased continuously. Seven patients showed increased concentrations in serum. Mean values in serum remained within the normal values (reference interval) during the whole study period, increasing steadily to a concentration of 58.5 ng/ml at day 21 (Fig. 10).

As the TGF-β concentrations in serum were 10 to 1000 times higher than in CSF the question arose as to whether this cytokine may cross the BBB due to leakage

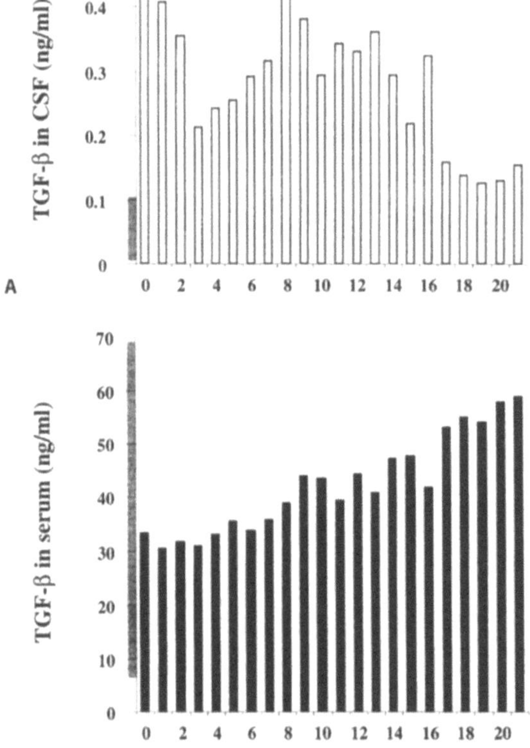

Fig. 10. Release of transforming growth factor-beta (*TGF*-β) into CSF and serum after brain injury. TGF-β concentrations (geometric mean) in the CSF (**A**) and serum (**B**) of 22 patients with severe traumatic brain injury over 21 days. In the CSF a first TGF-β peak appeared on the day of trauma and after a decrease a second peak followed at day 8. Concentrations of TGF-β in serum remained at levels between 30 and 40 ng/ml during the first week after trauma. Then a moderate increase was found until the end of the study period with a highest value at day 21. *Scattered bars* at the Y-axis indicate 95% confidence intervals

leading to an increase of intrathecal TGF-β. Therefore, the albumin ratio (Q_A) was used as a parameter for BBB function–dysfunction and was correlated with the corresponding TGF-β ratio (TGF-β_{CSF}/TGF-β_{serum} = Q_{TGF}-β). This revealed a significant correlation between maximal $Q_{TGF-\beta}$ and maximal Q_A with $r = 0.92$ and $p < 0.0001$ (Spearman Rank correlation). However, the maximal concentrations in CSF and serum did not show a significant correlation with each other ($r = 0.38$, $p = 0.08$; Spearman Rank correlation). This is also confirmed by the different TGF-β patterns in the two compartments which showed an opposite tendency, namely the increase in serum and a decrease in the CSF over time, the latter possibly caused by a restoration of the BBB to normal function.

Discussion

The analysis of the BBB function revealed that maximal albumin and TGF-β quotients correlate with each other, suggesting that an increased permeability of the BBB may allow the passage of this cytokine into the CSF. Locally, TGF-β may exert its multiple functions. Previously, it has been shown that astrocytes and microglia produce TGF-β and that this factor is up-regulated in CNS diseases (Wahl et al. 1991; Morganti-Kossmann et al. 1992b; Constam et al. 1992). The synthesis of TGF-β was demonstrated in infectious meningitis in mice and intraperitoneal injection of TGF-β2 resulted in the decrease of brain edema and the reduction of ICP (Frei et al. 1993). Previous studies have demonstrated the expression of TGF-β in experimental brain injury. The synthesis of TGF-β was found to be associated with macrophages and microglia following a stab wound as well as with astrocytes localized within the glial scar (Lindholm et al. 1992; Logan et al. 1992). TGF-β expression was also detected in a model of transient forebrain ischemia in regions of neuronal death rich in activated astrocytes and microglia (Wiessner et al. 1993). Reactive astrocytes and microglia are found at the lesioned site of the brain tissue and may perpetuate the cytokine cascade initiated by cells or factors which may have penetrated the nervous tissue. Cerebral overexpression of cytokines may cause neurological impairment therefore, downregulation of pro-inflammatory cytokine synthesis in the brain seems to be of fundamental importance (Morganti-Kossmann et al. 1992a). In experimental allergic encephalomyelitis TGF-β has shown the ability to suppress the activity of T-cells leading to an improvement of the outcome (Racke et al. 1991; Kuruvilla et al. 1991). The process of scarring may also be strongly modulated by TGF-β since its expression corresponded to the synthesis of fibronectin in GFAP-positive cells (Pasinetti et al. 1993). In addition to these properties, TGF-β may exert other protective activities due to its ability to prevent the neurotoxic effects of glutamate and to promote neuronal regeneration (Prehn et al. 1993; Lindholm et al. 1990; Spranger et al. 1990). The presence of TGF-β in the lesioned brain suggests that this cytokines may regulate the recruitment of blood cells during the inflammatory response induced by trauma as well as the healing process of the CNS.

In astrocytes TGF-β is regulated in both an autocrine and a paracrine fashion and has the ability to modulate cell growth and migration (Morganti-Kossmann et al.

1992b). It has been demonstrated that other cytokines like IL-1 trigger the synthesis of TGF-β in glial cells (da Cuhna et al. 1993). It remains to be elucidated whether or not resident cells of the CNS may contribute to TGF-β intrathecal production and whether cytokines, in particular IL-6, may trigger the synthesis of this mediator in glial cells as already suggested by others (Zhou et al. 1991). The impairment of the immune system described in patients with isolated head trauma may depend on the synthesis of TGF-β (Hoyt et al. 1990; Quattrocchi et al. 1991). Zhou et al. (1991) showed that the suppression of T-cell functions appeared to be mediated by TGF-β which is either promoted by IL-6 or activated by factors induced by IL-6 in macrophages. In our study, increasing levels of TGF-β were found in serum toward the end of the study period and may explain the immunosuppression observed often in these individuals.

Results and Discussion of the Experimental Study

A total number of 59 rats were used for the experimental model of diffuse brain injury. For each time point five rats were used with the exception of the group corresponding to the 4-h time point as shown in Table 2. For control, animals were sham operated and sacrificed at 2 and 24 h. Four animals died immediately or within 2 h after the traumatic impact to the head. Macroscopically, 24 animals showed skull fractures or instability of the sutures. Hemorrhages or small contusions were found in 18 animals.

Diffuse Axonal Injury Induces the Release of IL-6 into CSF and Serum

Significant release of IL-6 was detected in CSF and serum in these animals compared to sham operated animals (Fig. 11). IL-6 was found to be increased in the CSF already 1 h after injury and peaked at 4 h reaching a maximal concentration of 82 ng/ml. Thereafter, IL-6 levels returned to normal values between 16 to 24 h after trauma. The concentrations of IL-6 in CSF were significantly higher compared to the concentrations in serum after 2–8 h (paired t-test; $p < 0.0002$–$p < 0.05$). Differently from the CSF, IL-6 was detected in serum of all animals including the sham operated rats even though at low concentrations. A peak of IL-6 was also observed in serum after 4 h but at a much lower concentration (393 pg/ml) compared to IL-6 found in CSF.

Characterization and Distribution of Glial Cells After Brain Injury

Preliminary results on the immunohistochemistry performed on the brain tissue of the rats were obtained using the monoclonal antibodies OX-42 directed against the complement receptor type 3 which is expressed on activated macrophages and microglia, OX-6 directed against the MHC class II as a marker for cell activation, and GFAP, an antibody directed against the glial fibrillary acidic protein, a component of

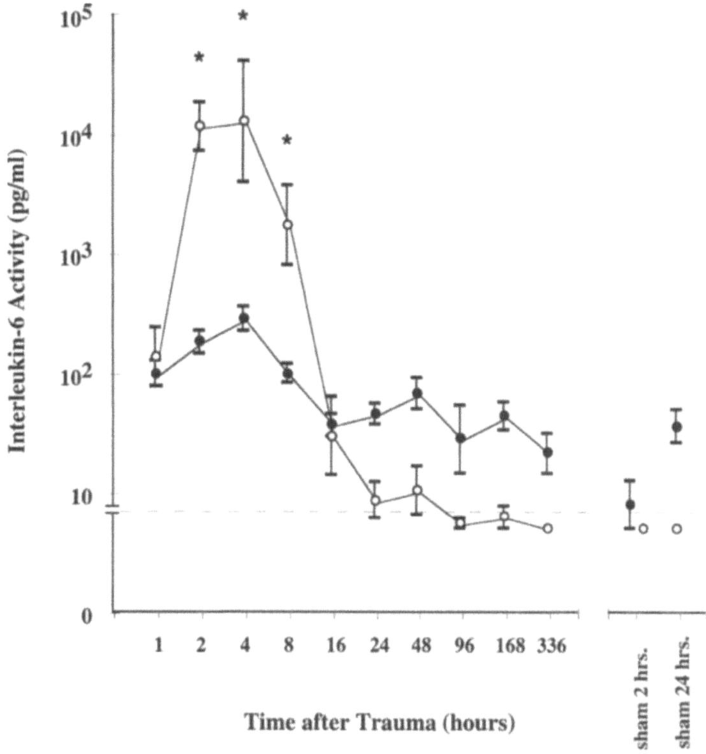

Fig. 11. Release of interleukin-6 (*IL-6*) in CSF and serum of animals after diffuse axonal injury. Concentrations (geometric means ± SEM) of IL-6 in CSF (*open circles*) and serum (*closed circles*) of rats following experimental brain injury. The number of animals for each time point are shown in Table 2. In CSF IL-6 concentrations were significantly higher (*) compared to serum during the first 8 h ($p < 0.05$; paired t-test)

the cytoskeleton, which was used as a marker for astrocytes. Brains were frozen immediately after removal and cryotom sections of 16 µm were cut. In this analysis the brains of three animals per time point were stained and a semiquantitative analysis was performed. The intensity of the staining of traumatized rat brains was always compared to the pattern seen in normal rat brain. The regions of the brain showing the major variations in the staining pattern are reported and summarized in Tables 5 and 6.

Discussion

The analysis of cytokine production in brain-injured patients revealed a profound inflammatory response in the peripheral as well as in the intrathecal compartments. The release of IL-6 in the CSF and serum of rats was analyzed in order to demonstrate the similarity of the clinical and the experimental settings. IL-6 levels in CSF showed similar kinetics compared to human CSF, however, this kinetic presented within a

Table 5. Semiquantitative evaluation of OX-42 and OX-6 immunoreactivity in various brain regions following a diffuse traumatic injury

Brain regions	OX-42	OX-6
Meninges	Decreased number of positive cells from 2h on (—) Mø-cells from 2h on (+), day 2 to 2 weeks (++) R-cells from day 2 up to 2 weeks (++)	Increase of positive cells from 2h, maximal from 48h–2 weeks (++)
Cortex: fronto-parietal	4h (+), 8–9 6h (++)	(+)
Cortex: basal	4h (+), from 8–96h (++)	Unchanged
Intraventricular	R-cells from 8–2h (++). No increase in cell number	Unchanged
Periventricular area	Mø-cell number up to 2 days (++) R-cells up to 1 week	(+/++)
Plexus choroideus	2h (+) Mø-like morphology, 8–96h (++)	24h–2 weeks (+++)
Hippocampus	Strong from 2h on (+++)	from 48h (+)
Hippocampal fimbriae	16h (+)	from 96h–2 weeks (++/+++)
Capsula interna	Unchanged	at 2h (+/++) and from 48h–2 weeks (+++)
Corpus callosum	16h–1 week (++)	48h–2 weeks (++)
Perivascular areas	2h (+), 8–16h (++)	96h–2 weeks (++)
Thalamus/ hypothalamus	2h–1 week in the hypothalamus (++)	from 48h–2 weeks (+)

Mø, cells with an activated macrophage-like type of morphology with a larger cell body; R, monocyte-like cells with a smaller round cell body.

shorter time period, between 8 and 24h, compared to several days as shown in humans (Fig. 1). This cytokine may be produced by resident cells of the CNS such as microglia, astrocytes and possibly by cells which migrate into the injured brain through a dysfunctional BBB.

Van den Brink et al. (1990), who established this rat model of diffuse axonal injury have observed that brain edema was already evident 6h after injury reaching a maximum after 24h. This study concluded that the brain edema was the consequence of either a very early patho-physiological dysfunction of the BBB or of cytotoxic edema. Pericapillary astrocytic swelling was also described in the cortex. The authors also described a similar degree of axonal injuries in the two groups of animals which were exposed to different impact forces (Foda and Marmarou 1994). The areas of injured neurons were rich in macrophages, possibly indicating phagocytosis of neuronal debris. In addition, a widespread activation of glial cells and and an infiltration of leukocytes may also be assumed (Giulian et al. 1989).

In order to investigate further the pathophysiological events following TBI at the cellular level, antibodies directed against macrophage–microglia, astrocytes and markers for cell activation (MHC class II antigens) were used. Diffuse brain injury caused an evident variation in the distribution of immunoreactivity of OX-42, OX-6 and GFAP compared to control brain tissue. The patterns of OX-42 and OX-6 did not always overlap, indicating that also other cells than microglia and macrophages such as astrocytes may be activated. Preliminary results indicate that monocytes which are positively stained with ED-1 (data not shown), a marker for monocytes–macrophages, may also be present in some regions. The most evident changes were noticed within the meninges, cortex, plexus, hippocampus, capsula interna and thalamus-hypothalamus.

The decrease of total cell number in the meninges and the relative increase of OX-42 positive cells in the cortex having a round amoeboid (R) as well as Mø-like morphology indicate that meningeal macrophages may migrate into the cortex and that microglia may become activated. The GFAP positivity below the meninges showed a decrease during the first 24 h which returned to a pattern comparable to normal brain later on. In the fronto-parietal sub-meningeal region astrocytes presented a more activated morphology, whereas in the basal sub-meningeal area a

Table 6. Semiquantitative evaluation of glial fibrillary acidic protein (GFAP)-positive cells in various brain regions following a diffuse traumatic injury

Brain Regions	GFAP
Meninges	Fronto-parietal area: decrease of GFAP intensity below the meninges within 24 h. Then light increase from 48 h to 1 week (+). The basal region showed swollen astrocytes from 48 h–1 week (+)
Cortex: frontoparietal	48 h–1 week (++)
Cortex: basal	2 h–2 weeks (+), stronger at 4 h and 96 h (++/+++)
Periventricular area	Decrease of stained cells within 16 h. At 24 h comparable to normal brain. Morphology: swollen from 24 h, maximum 48–96 h
Hippocampus: CA 1–3	4 days–1 week (+)
Hippocampus: gyrus dentatus	Loss of structural orientation from 8 h with maximum from 96 h–2 weeks
Hippocampal fimbriae	Light permanent decrease from 2 h up to 48 h (−). Similar to normal brain from 96 h–2 weeks
Corpus callosum	16 h–2 weeks (+/++)
Amygdala	Increased for 2 weeks, peaks at 4 h and 96 h (++)
Perivascular areas	2 h (++), 96 h–2 weeks (+++). Stronger staining in the basal cortex and amygdala
Thalamus	4 h (+), 8 h (++) 48 h–1 week (+++). Decrease at 2 weeks
Hypothalamus	8 h (+), 96 h–1 week (+++). Decrease at 2 weeks
Globus pallidus	48 h–2 weeks (+/++)
Putamen caudatum	24 h (+) 96 h–2 weeks (++)

rather swollen alteration was noticed. A traumatic impact usually causes a secondary injury to the opposite side of the brain (contrecoup injury) which may be revealed by degenerating astrocytes as observed in the basal cortex.

In the plexus and periventricular areas the patterns of OX-42 and OX-6 seem to be approximately similarly distributed. An intense OX-42 staining in the plexus already appeared after 2 h becoming stronger from 8 to 96 h. These cells also expressed MHC class II antigens from day 1 on. Interestingly, the increased OX-42 immunoreactivity found in the plexus and periventricular areas corresponded to the initial release of IL-6 in the CSF which occurred within the first 24 h after injury. This suggests that these cells may secrete cytokines into the ventricular fluid. The expression of MHC class II antigens appeared in most regions following a delay compared to the increased OX-42 positivity and lasted for the whole time period analyzed. The presence of OX-42 positive cells with R morphology was noticed in the ventricular spaces during the first 24 h. The periventricular area showed an initial loss of GFAP immunoreactivity which returned to normal after 1 day. In this area, swollen astrocytes were present from day 1 becoming enhanced between 2 and 4 days.

In the cortex, an increased number of OX-42 positive cells appeared during the first 96 h, whereas OX-6 positivity did not differ considerably from control brain. The accumulation of astrocytic clusters in the cortex suggests a possible proliferative activity from 4 days on up to 2 weeks. The intensity of GFAP immunoreactivity was more enhanced in the basal cortex compared to the fronto-parietal cortex.

A strong GFAP staining was also seen in the perivascular area of the basal cortex from 2 h to 2 weeks and was also accompanied by vasodilation. The number of microglia–macrophages in the perivascular area increased within the first 16 h, whereas OX-6 positivity was found to be more intense at later times from 4 to 14 days. It remains difficult to distinguish between blood derived cells which penetrated the brain tissue from the periphery and activated microglia located in the proximity of the vessels. Within the hippocampus the increase in microglia–macrophages remained constantly distributed from 2 h on within the CA-regions, whereas OX-6 positivity did not change considerably. A stronger OX-6 staining was evident in the hippocampal fimbriae from 4 days up to 2 weeks. The pattern of astrocytes in the hippocampus showed a variation in morphology and structural distribution rather than in cell number. In fact, the regular orientation of astrocytes in the gyrus dentatus was lost slightly after 8 h and more clearly from 4 to 14 days. Activation of microglia was noticed very early (2 h) in all the hippocampal areas, and the release of neurotoxic factors from these cells may lead to astrocytic alterations and neuronal loss.

A marked presence of reactive astrocytes was observed in the thalamic and hypothalamic regions and remained elevated from 2 h during the whole first week, whereas microglial cell activation only appeared in the hypothalamus lasting from 2 h through 7 days. In the capsula interna a marked increase of OX-6 positivity was noticed from 4 days and did not correlate with an increased OX-42 staining.

Overall, the increase of cellular activity found in the meninges, cortex and the perivascular areas was more enhanced in the basal regions compared to the frontal areas. This region may therefore represent the area where the impact produces its most severe effects.

The results presented above report an initial analysis of microglia and astrocyte activation following diffuse brain injury. Future experiments will examine the patterns of activated microglia and astrocytes and correlate these with the patterns of axonal injury, infiltration of T-cells, monocytes–macrophages and in situ cytokine expression.

Concluding Remarks

The inflammatory response initiated following a traumatic injury to the brain may have different consequences. Within the CNS the cooperation between recruited blood derived cells and activated glial cells may lead to a cytokine cascade and the release of other growth factors. In addition, our study supports the hypothesis that cytokines released intrathecally may also modulate systemic alterations as indicated by the acute phase reaction. The perpetuation of cytokine synthesis may be deleterious for the injured tissue by causing secondary damage as shown in chronic diseases of the CNS. Therefore, the release of anti-inflammatory cytokines down-regulating the inflammatory response may be beneficial and restore the homeostasis of the CNS and rather promote regeneration. The establishment of animal models will be used to elucidate and localize the complex immunological events which occur following the injury to the brain.

Acknowledgments. This study was supported by the Swiss National Fund No. 30-36375.92 and No. 31-42490.94.

References

Aarden LA, DeGroot EF, Schaap OL, Lansdorp PM (1987) Production of hybridoma growth factor by human monocytes. Eur J Immunol 17:1411–1416

Aderka D, Le J, Vilcek J (1989) IL-6 inhibits lipopolysaccharide-induced tumor necrosis factor production in cultured human monocytes, U937 cells and in mice. J Immunol 143:3517–3523

Akira S, Kishimoto T (1992) IL-6 and NF-IL6 in acute-phase response and viral infection. Immunol Rev 127:25–50

Alberico AM, Ward JD, Choi SC, Marmarou A, Young HF (1987) Outcome after severe head injury. Relationship to mass lesions, diffuse injury, and ICP course in pediatric and adult patients. J Neurosurg 67:648–656

Aloisi F, Care A, Borsellino G, Gallo P, Rosa S, Bassani A, Cabibbo A, Testa U, Levi G, Peschle C (1992) Production of hemolymphopoietic cytokines (IL-6, IL-8, colony stimulating factors) by normal human astrocytes in response to IL-1β and tumor necrosis factor-α. J Immunol 149:2358–2366

Apfel SC, Lipton RB, Arezzo JC, Kessler JA (1991) Nerve growth factor prevents toxic neuropathy in mice. Ann Neurol 29:87–90

Araujo DM, Cotman CW (1993) Trophic effects of interleukin-4, -7 and -8 on hippocampal neuronal cultures: potential involvement of glial derived factors. Brain Res 600:49–55

Awatsuji H, Furukawa Y, Hirota M, Murakami Y, Nii S, Furukawa S, Hayashi K (1993) Interleukin-4 and -5 as modulators of nerve growth factor synthesis/secretion in astrocytes. J Neurosci Res 34:539–545

Baggiolini M, Walz A, Kunkel SL (1989) Neutrophil-activating peptide-1/interleukin-8, a novel cytokine that activates neutrophils. J Clin Invest 84:1045–1049

Baggiolini M, Dewald B, Moser B (1992) Interleukin-8 and related chemotactic cytokines-CXC and CC chemokines. Adv Immunol 55:97–178

Banati RB, Gehrmann J, Schubert P, Kreutzberg GW (1993) Cytotoxicity of microglia. Glia 7:111–118

Banks WA, Ortiz L, Plotkin SR, Kastin AJ (1991) Human interleukin (IL) 1α, murine IL-1α and murine IL-1β are transported from blood to brain in the mouse by a shared saturable mechanism. J Pharmacol Exp Ther 259:988–996

Banks WA, Kastin AJ, Broadwell RD (1995) Passage of cytokines across the blood-brain barrier. Neuroimmunomodulation 2:241–248

Baumann H, Gauldie J (1994) The acute phase response. Immunol Today 15:74–80

Bazzoni F, Cassatella MA, Rossi F, Ceska M, Dewals B, Baggiolini M (1991) Phagocytosing neutrophils produce and release high amounts of neutrophil-activating peptide 1/interleukin-8. J Exp Med 173:771–774

Benveniste E (1995) The role of cytokines in multiple sclerosis/autoimmune encephalitis and other neurological disorders. In: Agarwal B, Puri R (eds) Human cytokines, their role in research and therapy. Blackwell, Boston/MA, pp 195–216

Bodmer S, Strommer K, Frei K, Siepl C, de Tribolet N, Heid I, Fontana A (1989) Immunosuppression and transforming growth factor-β in glioblastoma. J Immunol 143: 3222–3229

Bowes MP, Zivin JA, Rothlein R (1993) Monoclonal antibody to the ICAM-1 adhesion site reduces neurological damage in a rabbit cerebral embolism stroke model. Exp Neurol 119:215–219

Carman-Krzan M, Vige X, Wise BC (1991) Regulation by interleukin-1 of nerve growth factor mRNA expression in rat primary astroglial cultures. J Neurochem 56:636–643

Castell JV, Geiger T, Gross V, Andus T, Walter E, Hirano T, Kishimoto T, Heinrich PC (1988) Plasma clearance, organ distribution and target cells of interleukin-6/hepatocyte-stimulating factor in the rat. Eur J Biochem 177:357–361

Castell JV, Gómez-Lechón MJ, David M, Andus T, Geiger T, Trullenque R, Fabra R, Heinrich PC (1989) Interleukin-6 is the major regulator of acute phase protein synthesis in adult human hepatocytes. FEBS Lett 242:237–239

Chan PH, Schmidley JW, Fishman RA, Longar SM (1984) Brain injury, edema, and vascular permeability changes induced by oxygen derived free redicals. Neurology (NY) 34:315–320

Clark JM (1974) Distribution of microglial clusters in the brain after head injury. J Neurol Neurosurg Psychiatry 37:463–474

Constam DB, Philipp J, Malipiero UV, ten Dijke P, Schachner M, Fontana A (1992) Differential expression of transforming growth factor-β1, -β2 and -β3 by glioblastoma cells, astrocytes and microglia. J Immunol 148:1404–1410

Cortez SC, McIntosh TK, Noble LJ (1989) Experimental fluid percussion brain injury: vascular disruption and neuronal and glial alterations. Brain Res 482:271–282

Cross EM, Chaffin WW (1982) Use of the binomial theorem in interpreting results of multiple tests of significance. Educ Psychol Measurem 42:25–34

Da Cuhna A, Jefferson JA, Jackson RW, Vitovic L (1993) Glial specific mechanisms of TGF-β1 induction by IL-1 in cerebral cortex. J Neuroimmunol 42:71–86

Dinarello CA (1991) Interleukin-1 and interleukin-1 antagonism. Blood 77:1627–1652

Dixon CE, Lighthall JW, Anderson TE (1988) Physiologic, histopathologic, and cineradiographic characterization of a new fluid-percussion model of experimental brain injury in the rat. J Neurotrauma 5:91–104

Dubravec DB, Spriggs DR, Mannick JA, Rodrick ML (1990) Circulating human peripheral blood granulocytes synthesize and secrete tumor necrosis factor α. Proc Natl Acad Sci USA 87:6758–6761

Eddleston M, Mucke L (1992) Molecular profile of reactive astrocytes-implication for their role in neurologic disease. Neuroscience 54:15–36

Fabry Z, Raine CS, Hart MN (1994) Nervous tissue as an immune compartment: the dialect of the immune response in the CNS. Immunol Today 15:218–224

Feldman Z, Contant CF, Pahwa R, Goodman JC, Robertson CS, Narayan RK, Grossman RG (1993) The relationship between hormonal mediators and systemic hypermetabolism after severe head injury. J Trauma 34:806–816

Foda MA, Marmarou A (1994) A new model of diffuse brain injury in rats. II. Morphological characterization. J Neurosurg 80:301–313

Frankowski RF, Annegers JF, Whitman S (1985) The descriptive epidemiology of head trauma in US. In: Becker DP, Povlishock JT (eds) Central nervous system trauma. Status report. National Institutes of Health, Bethesda, pp 89–122

Frei K, Leist TP, Meager A, Gallo P, Leppert D, Zinkernagel RM, Fontana A (1988) Production of B cell stimulatory factor-2 and interferon-γ in the central nervous system during viral meningitis and encephalitis. J Exp Med 168:449–453

Frei K, Malipiero UV, Leist TP, Zinkernagel RM, Schwab ME, Fontana A (1989) On the cellular source and function of interleukin 6 produced in the central nervous system in viral diseases. Eur J Immunol 19:689–694

Frei K, Nadal D, Fontana A (1990) Intracerebral synthesis of tumor necrosis factor-α and interleukin-6 in infectious meningitis. Ann N Y Acad Sci 594:326–335

Frei K, Piani D, Pfister HW, Fontana A (1993) Immune-mediated injury in bacterial meningitis. Int Rev Exp Pathol 34:183–192

Frohman EM, Frohman TC, Dustin ML, Vayuvegula B, Choi B, Gupta A, van den Noort S, Gupta S (1989) The induction of intracellular adhesion molecule 1 (ICAM-1) expression on human fetal astrocytes by interferon-γ, tumor necrosis factor-α, lymphotoxin and interleukin-1: relevance to intracerebral antigen presentation. J Neuroimmunol 23:117–124

Furukawa Y, Tomioka N, Sato W, Satoyoshi E, Hayashi K, Furukawa S (1989) Catecholamines increase nerve growth factor mRNA content in both mouse astroglial cells and fibroblast cells. FEBS Lett 247:395–402

Gadient RA, Cron KC, Otten U (1990) Interleukin-1β and tumor necrosis factor-α synergistically stimulate nerve growth factor (NGF) release from cultured rat astrocytes. Neurosci Lett 117:335–340

Gallo P, Frei K, Rordorf C, Lazdins J, Tavolato B, Fontana A (1989) Human immunodeficiency virus type I (HIV-1) infection of the central nervous system: an evaluation of cytokines in cerebrospinal fluid. J Neuroimmunol 23:109–116

Gennarelli TA, Spielman GM, Langfitt TW, Gildenberg PL, Harrington T, Jane JA, Marshall LF, Miller JD, Pitts LH (1982) Influence of the type of intracranial lesion on outcome from severe head injury. J Neurosurg 56:26–32

Giulian D, Lachman LB (1985) Interleukin-1 stimulation of astroglial proliferation after brain injury. Science 228:4707–4717

Giulian D, Ingeman JE, George JK, Noponen M (1989) The role of mononuclear phagocytes in wound healing after traumatic brain injury to adult mammalian brain. J Neurosci 9:4416–1129

Halstensen A, Ceska M, Brandtzaeg P, Redl H, Naess A, Waage A (1993) Interleukin-8 in serum and cerebrospinal fluid from patients with meningococcal disease. J Infect Dis 167:471–475

Hama T, Miymoto M, Tsukui H, Nishio C, Hatanaka H (1989) Interleukin-6 as a neurotrophic factor for promoting the survival of cultured basal forebrain cholinergic neurons from postnatal rats. Neurosci Lett 104:340–344

Handa S (1992) Concentrations of interleukin-1β, interleukin-6, interleukin-8 and TNF-α in cerebrospinal fluid from children with septic or aseptic meningitis. Kurume Med J 39:257–265

Heumann R, Korshing S, Bandtlow C, Thoenen H (1987) Changes of nerve growth factor synthesis in non-neuronal cells in response to sciatic nerve transection. J Cell Biol 104:1623–1631

Hirano T, Taga T, Nakano N, Yasukawa K, Kashiwamura S, Shimizu K, Nakajima K, Pyun KH, Kishimoto T (1985) Purification to homogeneity and characterization of human B-cell differentiation factor (BCDF or BSFp-2). Proc Natl Acad Sci USA 84:5490–5494

Hosford D, Braquet P (1989) Potential role for platelet-activating factor and tumor necrosis factor in the immune impairments in shock and trauma. In: Faist E, Ninnemann J, Green D (eds) Immune consequences of trauma, shock and sepsis. Springer, Berlin, Heidelberg New York, pp 311–321

Hoyt DB, Ozkan N, Hansbrough JF, Marshall L, van Berkum-Clark M (1990) Head injury: an immunologic deficit in T-cell activation. J Trauma 30:759–767

Ishibashi T, Kimura H, Shikama Y, Uchida T, Kariyone S, Hirano T, Kishimoto T, Takatsuki F, Akiyama Y (1989) Interleukin-6 is a potent thrombopoietic factor in vivo in mice. Blood 74:1241–1244

Jennett B, Bond M (1975) Assessment of outcome after severe brain damage. Lancet 1:480–484

Kim KS, Wass CA, Cross AS, Opal SM (1992) Modulaton of blood-brain barrier permeability by tumor necrosis factor and antibody to tumor necrosis factor in the rat. Lymphokine Cytokine Res 11:293–298

Kitamura T, Ogorochi T, Miyajima A (1994) Multimeric cytokine receptors. Trends Endocrinol Metab 5:8–14

Kossmann T, Hans V, Imhof HG, Stocker R, Grob P, Trentz O, Morganti-Kossmann MC (1995) Intrathecal and serum interleukin-6 and the acute-phase response in patients with severe traumatic brain injuries. Shock 4:311–317

Kossmann T, Hans V, Imhof HG, Trentz O, Morganti-Kossmann MC (1996) Interleukin-6 released in human cerebrospinal fluid following traumatic brain injury may trigger nerve growth factor production in astrocytes. Brain Res 713:143–152

Kossmann T, Stahel PF, Lenzlinger PM, Redl H, Dubs RW, Trentz O, Schlag G, Morganti-Kossmann MC (1997) Interleukin-8 released into the cerebrospinal fluid after brain injury is associated with blood brain barrier dysfunction and nerve growth factor production. J Cereb Blood Flow Metab (in press)

Kromer LF (1986) Nerve growth factor treatment after brain injury prevents neuronal death. Science 235:214–216

Kuruvilla AP, Shah R, Hochwald GM, Liggitt HD, Palladino MA, Thorbecke GJ (1991) Protective effect of transforming growth factor $\beta1$ on experimental autoimmune diseases in mice. Proc Natl Acad Sci USA 88:2918–2921

Kushner I, Mackiewicz A (1987) Acute phase proteins as disease markers. Dis Markers 5:1–11

Lacy M, Jones J, Whittemore SR, Haviland DL, Wetsel RA, Barnum SR (1995) Expression of the receptors for the C5a anaphylatoxin, interleukin-8 and FMLP by human astrocytes and microglia. J Neuroimmunol 61:71–78

Leppert D, Frei K, Gallo P, Yasargil MG, Hess K, Baumgartner G, Fontana A (1989) Brain tumors: detection of B-cell stimulatory factor-2/interleukin-6 in the absence of oligoclonal bands of immunoglobulins. J Neuroimmunol 24:259–264

Levi-Montalcini R, Angeletti PU (1968) Nerve growth factor. Physiol Rev 48:534–569

Lindholm D, Heumann R, Meyer M, Thoenen H (1987) Interleukin-1 regulates synthesis of nerve growth factor in non neuronal cells of rat sciatic nerve. Nature 330:658–659

Lindholm D, Hengerer B, Zafra F, Thoenen H (1990) Transforming growth factor-$\beta1$ stimulates the expression of nerve growth factor in the rat CNS. Dev Neurosci 1:9–12

Lindholm D, Castren E, Kiefer R, Zafra F, Thoenen H (1992) Transforming growth factor-$\beta1$ in the rat brain: increase after injury and inhibition of astrocyte proliferation. J Cell Biol 117:395–400

Lindsay RM (1979) Adult rat brain astrocytes support survival of both NGF-dependent and NGF-insensitive neurons. Nature 282:80–82

Logan A, Frautschy SA, Gonzalez AM, Sporn MB, Baird A (1992) Enhanced expression of transforming growth factor-$\beta1$ in the rat brain after localized cerebral injury. Brain Res 587:216–225

Lotem J, Shabo Y, Sachs L (1989) Regulation of megakaryocyte development by interleukin-6. Blood 74:1545–1551

Maimone D, Gregory S, Arnason BGW, Reder AT (1991) Cytokine levels in the cerebrospinal fluid and serum of patients with multiple sclerosis. J Neuroimmunol 32:67–74

Marmarou A, Foda MA, van den Brink W, Campbell J, Kita H, Demetriadou K (1994) A new model of diffuse brain injury in rats. I. Pathophysiology and biomechanics. J Neurosurg 80:291–300

Marshall LF, Marshall SB, Klauber MR, Clarck MVB, Eisenberg HM, Jane JA, Luerssen TG, Marmarou A, Foulkes M (1991) A new classification of head injury based on computerized tomography. J Neurosurg 75:S14–S20

Martich GD, Danner RL, Ceska M, Suffredini AF (1991) Detection of interleukin-8 and tumor necrosis factor in normal humans after intravenous endotoxin: the effect of antiinflammatory agents. J Exp Med 173:1021–1024

Marucha PT, Zeff RA, Kreutzer DL (1990) Cytokine regulation of IL-1β gene expression in the human polymorphonuclear leukocyte. J Immunol 145:2932–2937

Mastroianni CM, Paoletti F, Rivosecchi RM, Lancella L, Ticca F, Vullo V, Delia S (1994) Cerebrospinal fluid interleukin-8 in children with purulent bacterial and tuberculous meningitis. Pediatr Infect Dis J 13:1008–1010

Mathiesen T, Andersson B, Loftenius A, von Holst H (1993) Increased interleukin-6 levels in cerebrospinal fluid following subarachnoid hemorrhage. J Neurosurg 78:562–567

McClain CJ, Cohen D, Ott L, Dinarello C, Young B (1987) Ventricular fluid interleukin-1 activity in patients with head injury. J Lab Clin Med 110:48–54

McClain C, Cohen D, Phillips R, Ott L, Young AB (1991) Increased plasma and ventricular fluid interleukin-6 levels in patients with head injury. J Lab Clin Med 118:226–231

Morganti MC, Taylor J, Pesheva P, Schachner M (1990) Oligodendrocyte-derived J1–160/180 extracellular matrix glycoproteins are adhesive or repulsive depending on the partner cell type and time of interaction. Exp Neurol 109:98–110

Morganti-Kossmann MC, Kossmann T (1995) The immunology of brain injury. In: Rothwell NJ (ed) Immune responses in the nervous system. Bios Scientific, Oxford, pp 159–187

Morganti-Kossmann MC, Kossmann T, Wahl SM (1992a) Cytokines and neuropathology. Trends Pharmacol Sci 13:286–291

Morganti-Kossmann MC, Kossmann T, Brandes ME, Mergenhagen SE, Wahl SM (1992b) Autocrine and paracrine regulation of astrocyte function by transforming growth factor-β. J Neuroimmunol 39:163–174

Morita M, Kasahara T, Mukaida N, Matsushima K, Nagashima T, Nishizawa M, Yoshida M (1993) Induction and regulation of interleukin-8 and MCAF production in human brain tumor cell lines and brain tumor tissues. Eur Cytokine Netw 4:351–358

Mosmann T (1983) Rapid cholorimetric assay for cellular growth and survival: application to proliferation and cytotoxicity assay. J Immunol Methods 65:55–63

Mukaida N, Matsushima K (1992) Regulation of interleukin-8 production and the characteristics of the receptors for interleukin-8. Cytokines 4:41–53

Nieto-Sampedro M, Berman MA (1987) Interleukin-1 like activity in rat brain: sources, targets and effects of injury. J Neurosci Res 17:214–219

Nieto-Sampedro M, Lewis ER, Cotman CW, Manthorpe M, Skaper SD, Barbin G, Longo FM, Varon S (1982) Brain injury causes a time-dependent increase in neuronotrophic activity at the lesion site. Science 217:860–861

Nijsten MWN, Hack CE, Helle M, ten Duis HJ, Klasen HJ, Aarden LA (1991) Interleukin-6 and its relation to the humoral immune response and clinical parameters in burned patients. Surgery 109:761–767

Nitta T, Allegretta M, Okumura K, Sato K, Steinman L (1992) Neoplastic and reactive human astrocytes express interleukin-8 gene. Neurosurg Rev 15:203–207

Okada M, Sakaguchi N, Yoshimura N, Hara H, Shimizu K, Yoshida N, Yoshizaki K, Kishimoto S, Yamamura Y, Kishimoto T (1983) B cell growth factors and B cell differentiation factor from human T hybridomas: two distinct kinds of B cell growth factors and their synergism in B cell proliferation. J Exp Med 157:583–590

Pasinetti GM, Nichols NR, Tocco G, Morgan T, Laping N, Finch CE (1993) Transforming growth factor β1 and fibronectin messenger RNA in rat brain: responses to injury and cell type localization. Neuroscience 54:893–907

Patterson SL, Grady MS, Bothwell M (1993) Nerve growth factor and fibroblast growth factor-like neurotrophic activity in cerebrospinal fluid of brain injured human patients. Brain Res 605:43–49

Prehn JHM, Peruche B, Unsicker K, Krieglstein J (1993) Isoform specific effects of transforming growth factor-β on degeneration of primary neuronal cultures induced by cytotoxic hypoxia or glutamate. J Neurochem 60:1665–1672

Quattrocchi KB, Frank EH, Miller CH, Amin A, Issel BW, Wagner FC Jr (1991) Impairment of helper T-cell function and lymphokine-activated killer cytotoxicity following severe head injury. J Neurosurg 75:766–773

Racke MK, Jalbut SD, Cannella B, Albert PS, Raine CS, McFarlin DE (1991) Prevention and treatment of chronic relapsing experimental allergic encephalomyelitis by transforming growth factor-β1. J Immunol 146:3012–3017

Reiber H, Felgenhauer K (1987) Protein transfer at the blood cerebrospinal fluid barrier and the quantitation of the humoral immune response within the central nervous system. Clin Chim Acta 163:319–328

Satoh T, Nakamura S, Taga T, Matsuda T, Hirano, Kishimoto T, Kairo Y (1988) Induction of neuronal differentiation in PC 12 cells by B cell stimulatory factor-2/interleukin-6. Mol Cell Biol 8:3546–3549

Seki T, Joh K, Oh-ishi T (1993) Augmented production of interleukin-8 in cerebrospinal fluid in bacterial meningitis. Immunology 80:333–335

Selmaj KW, Farooq M, Norton WT, Raine CS, Brosnan CF (1990) Proliferation of astrocytes in vitro in response to cytokines. A primary role for tumor necrosis factor. J Immunol 144:129–135

Selmaj KW, Raine CS, Farooq M, Norton WT, Brosnan CF (1991) Cytokine cytotoxicity against oligodendrocytes apoptosis induced by lymphotoxin. J Immunol 147: 1522–1529

Shackford SR, Mackersie RC, Davis JW, Wolf PL, Hoyt DB (1989) Epidemiology and pathology of traumatic deaths occurring at a level I trauma center in a regionalized system: the importance of secondary brain injury. J Trauma 29:1392–1397

Shiga Y, Onodera H, Kogure K, Yamasaki Y, Yashima Y, Syozuhara H, Sendo F (1991) Neutrophil as a mediator of ischemic edema formation in the brain. Neurosci Lett 125:110–112

Spranger M, Lindholm D, Bandtlow C, Heumann R, Gnahn H, Naeher-Noe M, Thoenen H (1990) Regulation of nerve growth factor (NGF) synthesis in the rat central nervous system: comparison between the effects of interleukin-1 and various growth factors in astrocyte cultures and in vivo. Eur J Neurosci 2:69–76

Stocker R, Bernays R, Kossmann T, Imhof H-G (1995) Monitoring and treatment of acute head injury. In: Goris RJA, Trentz O (eds) The integrated approach to trauma care. Springer, Berlin Heidelberg New York, pp 197–210

Tada M, Suzuki K, Yamakawa Y, Sawamura Y, Sakuma S, Abe H, van Meir E, de Tribolet N (1993) Human glioblastoma cells produce 77 amino acid interleukin-8. J Neuro Oncol 16:25–34

Taupin V, Toulmond S, Serrano A, Benavides J, Zavala F (1993) Increase in IL-6, IL-1 and TNF levels in rat brain following traumatic lesion. J Neuroimmunol 42:177–186

Teasdale G, Jennett B (1974) Assessment of coma and impaired consciousness. A practical scale. Lancet 2:81–84

Terebuh PD, Otterness IG, Strieter RM, Lincoln PM, Danforth JM, Kunkel SL, Chensue SW (1992) Biologic and immunhistochemical analysis of interleukin-6 expression in vivo. Am J Pathol 140:649–657

Van Damme J, De Ley M, van Snick J, Dinarello C, Billiau A (1987) The role of interferon-β1 and the 26 kDa protein (interferon-β2) as mediators of the antiviral effect of interleukin-1 and tumor necrosis factor. J Immunol 139:1867–1872

Van den Brink WA, Marmarou A, Avezaat CJ (1990) Brain oedema in experimental closed head in jury in the rat. Acta Neurochir Suppl (Wien) 51:261–262

Van Meir E, Ceska M, Effenberger F, Walz A, Grouzmann E, Desbaillets I, Frei K, Fontana A, de Tribolet N (1992) Interleukin-8 is produced in neoplastic and infectious diseases of the human central nervous system. Cancer Res 52:4297–4305

Van Snick J (1990) Interleukin-6: an overview. Annu Rev Immunol 8:253–278

Wahl SM (1994) Transforming growth factor beta (TGF-β) in inflammation: a cause and a cure. J Clin Immunol 12:61–74

Wahl SM, Allen JB, McCartney-Francis N, Morganti-Kossmann MC, Kossmann T, Ellingsworth L, Mai UEH, Mergenhagen SE, Orenstein JM (1991) Macrophage- and astrocyte-derived transforming growth factor-β as a mediator of central nervous system dysfunction in acquired immunodeficiency syndrome. J Exp Med 173:981–991

Wiessner C, Gehrmann J, Lindholm D, Toepper R, Kreutzberg GW, Hossmann KA (1993) Expression of transforming growth factor-β1 and interleukin-1β mRNA in rat brain following transient forebrain ischemia. Acta Neuropathol (Berl) 86:439–446

Woodroofe MN, Sarna GS, Wadhwa M, Hayes GM, Loughlin AJ, Tinker A, Cuzner ML (1991) Detection of interleukin-1 and interleukin-6 in adult rat brain, following mechanical injury by in vivo microdialysis: evidence of a role for microglia in cytokine production. J Neuroimmunol 33:227–236

Yoshida K, Gage FH (1991) Fibroblast growth factors stimulate nerve growth factor synthesis and secretion by astrocytes. Brain Res 538:118–126

Young AB, Ott LG, Beard D, Dempsey RJ, Tibbs PA, McClain CJ (1988) The acute-phase response of the brain-injured patient. J Neurosurg 69:375–380

Zhou D, Munster A, Winchurch RA (1991) Pathologic concentrations of interleukin-6 inhibit T
cell responses via induction or activation of TGF-β. FASEB J 5:2582–2585

Discussion 1

Traber:
In your presentation you mention the fact that IL-8 was producing changes in permeability of the blood–brain barrier. What indices did you use to determine that the blood–brain barrier function had changed?

Kossmann:
We were looking at the albumin quotient in these patients, so we assume – we have still to prove it by an experimental protocol – we could find a correlation between the levels of IL-8, and the dysfunction of the blood–brain barrier. This is at the moment the only parameter to judge the blood–brain barrier function, by measuring the albumin levels in CSF and serum.

Traber:
Do you control for bleeding, or do you control your albumin level with, for instance, hemoglobin level to ensure that your albumin was not there as a result of hemorrhage?

Kossmann:
It is frequent to have patients with bleeding in the CSF. But what we do is to analyze the CSF thoroughly to exclude that we have any blood.

Morganti-Kossmann:
I would also like to add that sometimes at the beginning the CSF looks hemolytic, but in many cases the CSF does not. This shows that there is not a severe bleeding, therefore we would exclude that in many cases a bleeding into the CSF occurred.

Traber:
Another question is: Do you have any normal data, and samples from normals as to what the cytokines are in normal individuals to control for this?

Morganti-Kossmann:
Yes, this is published. In fact, the albumin quotient in normals is between 0.005 and 0.007 and above this range is pathological.

Traber:
I was referring to cytokine levels: How do your cytokine levels that you are getting at day 0 compare with normals?

Kossmann:
This issue we actually discussed yesterday, when I asked where you get your normal controls from. This is still a problem, because it is very difficult to get intraventricular CSF from a normal patient. So we have CSF from lumbar puncture or CSF from shunt patients. And there we do not find detectable cytokine levels.

Prough:
One of the things that is hard for me to figure out from looking at your data is the extent to which the systemic inflammatory response syndrome might constitute a confounding variable. Most head-injured patients, particularly head-injured patients that have other injuries, who stay in the ICU for 2, 3 or 4 days, become colonized with bacteria, begin to at least act infected, may or may not become frankly septic, may develop pneumonia. I wonder to what extent these variables might confound your observations?

Kossmann:
I know what you are referring to. It is known from experimental data that injection of IL-6 into the brain is sufficient to induce an acute-phase reaction. That is why we suppose that the IL-6 which is very high in the beginning, triggers the acute phase reaction. And what you are referring to comes later on, according to my experience. In fact, infections may appear at later days. But when we are looking at the acute-phase reaction the onset is much earlier. The raise of acute phase proteins occurs after 1 or 2 days already, so we believe that there might be an interrelationship between intrathecal IL-6 and the acute-phase response, and that the trigger might come from the brain.

Kochanek:
You might just consider separating out your multiple trauma patients from your pure head injury patients. I expect you may have already done that.

Kossmann:
These patients had only isolated head injuries and we are currently looking into the multiple or polytraumatized patients with and including those without severe head injury.

Kochanek:
Maybe Don and I were a little confused by that, because your initial presentation was with a large number of polytraumatized patients.

Kossmann:
Yes, however we only concentrated on isolated head injury.

Kochanek:
Obviously this is a beautiful presentation, I was wondering, what are you using to measure human NGF?

Morganti-Kossmann:
It is an ELISA from Boehringer-Mannheim. The protocol is given by the manufacturer and was changed a little. We concentrate the CSF in order to detect NGF.

Kochanek:
And it is an anti-human NGF?

Morganti:
No, it actually is anti-mouse, but it cross reacts with human NGF as well. The homology between human, rat and mouse NGF is very high.

Shackford:

I congratulate you on a nice presentation. It appears that you worked very hard to get these data. My question deals with, first, your high craniotomy rate: You had 99 craniotomies in 300 patients – that is almost a 30% craniotomy rate. In the US, in most trauma centers it is around 10%. Do you have a referral center? Are these patients first seen in other hospitals and then referred to you?

Kossmann:

Since we are a trauma I center and also a neurotrauma center in the region, most of the head traumas come directly to us.

Shackford:

And what is the time from injury to the time you get the catheter in?

Kossmann:

This depends on the transport. Since Switzerland is a small country, we get them very quickly, between the accident and the admission. This means about 1–2 h coming to our center, another 1.5 h for diagnostics, so we are ranging somewhere between 4 and 6 h until we have the catheter. When we looked in our treatment protocols from a N-methyl-D-aspartate (NMDA) receptor antagonist phase II study in which we are involved, we were one of the quickest centers for the therapeutic window and we are ranging somewhere from 8–8.5 h, but this means the patient was already on the ICU at this time. These were severely head-injured patients, and all of them had an ICP monitoring device.

Shackford:

So you think it is about 8 h from the time of injury to the time you have your catheter in and you are getting your first sample?

Kossman:

Yes, 8–12 h.

Shackford:

And it looked to me (I may have misread that on some of your data slides) that the first measurement was not the highest measurement? It appeared that maybe it was the second or third, which would mean that perhaps in some cases it was 24–48 h before you saw the peaks?

Kossmann:

Right.

Shackford:

Which might mean that this was a secondary, rather than the primary trauma.

Kossmann:

We cannot exclude this at the end. This is a very heterogeneous patient group and to have exact data now, whether this is a diffuse axonal injury or a focal injury, we need many more patients to figure out the type of injury. We can only do the zero measurements by taking what we have. This is not controlled like in an experimental standardized model.

Shackford:
Just one more question, just to follow up, and it relates to the stratification that we are talking about, as you gather more patients, because this is very interesting. The work that Dr. Zornow showed us yesterday about looking at MRIs and edema formation would be a nice correlation between your albumin flux data and the generation of edema. Then going back and looking at the images, compared to what your cytokines are showing you, would give you some continuity. I think it is fascinating work and encourage you to continue.

Morganti-Kossmann:
Thanks, I would also like to add that the cytokines like IL-6 and IL-8 belong to the secondary cytokine cascade and this might also explain why we do not measure any IL-1 due to the delay in collection of CSF samples. In animal models such as percussion injury it has been shown that IL-1 is detected within a few hours.

Bolton:
I think the investigations are very important and tell us a lot about the mechanism of secondary effects from brain injury. This might ultimately lead to some form of treatment. One key to what is happening is in the blood–brain barrier. Further investigations of this and correlation with your results will be very important. Investigators at the University of Missouri, the department of neurosurgery, are doing interesting experiments on severe burns in rats. Blood vessels on the surface of the brain are looked at under high magnification. There is an immediate increase in the permeability of blood vessels with exudation into the tissue. I suspect that trauma itself is having an immediate and severe effect on the blood–brain barrier.

Kossmann:
Yes, I agree with this, and actually now, you will see that we did not only focus on the patients, and we have to wait for the next contribution. Since it is very difficult sometimes to interpret the data we get, we try now to clarify the relationship of these different mediators by establishing experiments in cell cultures and also an experimental head trauma model, where we have controlled circumstances. So we started actually from the bed, going to the bench, in the in vitro experimental system.

Kochanek:
One other point: Head injury has somewhat led the way in this; I think these cytokines and any of these inflammatory mediators are undoubtedly produced in stroke, cardiac arrest, asphyxia and all of the other important CNS diseases. I think we have only been able to examine head injury because of the CSF analysis available in traumatic brain injury.

Kossmann:
As I mentioned in my talk, when we first began our project a lot of our colleagues thought we were wasting time doing something very elaborate, but it seems that the analysis of the CSF is becoming more and more important. I have talked to several of the people in the audience, asking them what is actually in the CSF? This is because we have absolutely no idea of all the therapeutical protocols we are applying which may affect the brain and, if it is affecting, how it is affecting. To elucidate the penetration

of drugs into the brain we are measuring different kinds of drugs in the CSF since there is no data on this issue.

Young:
Did your patients receive corticosteroids?

Kossmann:
No.

Young:
I also want to ask about your thoughts on brain injury and the blood–brain barrier breakdown playing a role in the systemic serum concentrations of these various cytokines. Because of the blood–brain barrier breakdown, there may be a back diffusion from brain into blood. Do you relate the blood–brain barrier breakdown to the serum concentrations of cytokines in pure head injury (as opposed to multi-system trauma)?

Kossmann:
That is a difficult issue. What is known by publications from Banks, he had shown that there are transport mechanisms for TNF-α, IL-1 and IL-6 through the blood–brain barrier. The blood–brain barrier is not easily judged only by the albumin levels. This is somehow a very rough measurement you can do, and we are focussing on the blood–brain barrier function by describing more of what is happening with the different cytokines. What we actually emphasize is that there may be an exchange, so when there is high concentration inside the CSF, we think there is a leakage out and vice-versa. But to judge this we have to use many more experimental head trauma models to get the right answer before we really can judge it.

Kochanek:
I have one more question: I think another potential avenue related to your findings and our findings would be the use of the ventricular space as a port for drug delivery. I think it has only been utilized so far for the administration of antibiotics. This is another potentially important site for delivering agents, whether it is to manipulate inflammation or to manipulate other aspects of head injury.

Kossmann:
I absolutely agree with that. You see, as a trauma surgeon it is very difficult. We, for example, regard the head as a closed box which we are not allowed to open. So when we have, for example, a bleeding in another cavity, like in the thorax or the abdomen, what do we do as surgeons? We go in, we take out the clot, we wash it and so on. We do a lot of things in the other compartments, but we are somehow very anxious about doing anything inside the brain, beside evacuating major mass lesions. But there is, I think, big potential in what we can do by either injecting drugs directly inside the CNS or other things.

Discussion 2

Prough:
You are finding these changes in animals that are behaviorally normal?

Morganti:
Yes, they go back to their cage, they eat and drink and they walk, sometimes they show a little bit of disorientation at the beginning, after trauma, but after some time they recover almost completely.

Kossmann:
Just in addition to this: We were only allowed to do a non-lethal trauma model, and not a more severe head trauma. Of course, if you apply more force to these animals, there would be much more damage to the brain, but also higher lethality.

Morganti:
Marmarou, who established this model, has also varied the weight, obtaining up to a 50% death rate. But we did not want to do that. We wanted to have a standardized model which we can study, since we want to analyze changes in terms of cytokines, cell activation, and in situ cytokine production at different intervals after trauma.

Kochanek:
I would like to thank you for a very comprehensive presentation. I think you would be somewhat incorrect in saying that these animals are normal. They look normal in their cage; however, the functional outcome studies that have been done by other investigators basically show that they have very marked motor deficits (if you do balance beam testing, beam walking testing). It is not visually apparent to an animal walking around in its cage, however, you are right, Don, that these animals do not have a cognitive impairment. If you test them in the Morris water maze they do not have a defect. I do not know that the time course of cytokine production is contracted in the rat. And it may not be that, it may be that if you had a more severe head injury model you would see a more protracted time course, more analogous to the human.

Morganti:
It has been shown that there are differences in the immune response, comparing different animal strains.

Kochanek:
I recognize that, I just think it would be interesting to know, if you had a rat injury model which produced sustained coma, where it would be necessary to keep the animals mechanically ventilated like you would with humans, what would the CSF cytokine pattern look like?

Shackford:
I congratulate you on some very nice work. Just a methodologic question: How did you know that those were astrocytes in your cell culture work? How did you know that that was a pure culture of astrocytes? Did you exclude the possibility of endothelial cells?

Morganti:

We stained them for GFAP. The purity is about 95%. There are always contaminating microglial cells. There is a method to remove microglia since they adhere to the top of astrocytes. By shaking the flask, they come off and it is possible to remove most of the microglial cells by changing the medium.

Shackford:

Just one more question: Something that we have done with cerebral microvascular endothelial cells is to build a percussion device, and actually percuss them and see what happens in the supernatant. There is some fascinating information. For example, endothelial cells express a procoagulant when they are percussed. So you might want to try that. Also, another suggestion: Since you do have such a high craniotomy rate, it would be nice to get human astrocytes, perhaps from the specimens, if they are removing any brain.

Morganti:

Yes, very interesting. There are some human glioma cell lines which have been used a lot in in vitro experiments. Of course they are transformed cells, and therefore they are not really the same.

Young:

I also want to congratulate the doctors Kossmann for their very nice work. I think it is very interesting. The regional distribution of the astrocytosis, especially in the hippocampus, seems especially relevant because we so commonly see posttraumatic memory impairment as a consequence of even moderate head injury. I wondered also if you had used a more stressful type of learning task, like the radial arm maze, for testing the rats, if you could find some cognitive problems. I wanted to ask you, if you concluded that the astrocytosis is due to the cytokine phenomenon and not due to the excitatory amino acid toxicity with astrocytosis secondary to neuronal death. Do you think that this is purely a cytokine-mediated phenomenon or do you think there is still a role for excitatory aminoacids in the pathology that you found?

Morganti:

Yes, absolutely. I think that excitatory aminoacids can play an important role. It is difficult to say. First of all, astrocytosis has been shown to be induced by, for example, IL-1 and other cytokines injected in the brain, obtaining increased astrocyte growth. The increase in GFAP staining was thought to be due to the fact that astrocytes change their morphology, but now the message for GFAP is found increased after trauma. Glutamate and other toxic factors are metabolized by astrocytes, and maybe, if they are released in an abundant concentration, can lead to damage of the astrocytes. I do not know if this has been shown already, because most of the work has concentrated on neurons, but it would be very interesting to do. With regard to the regions showing damage, one hypothesis is the contre-coup effect on the basal cortex. This may be an explanation for that. Probably there are some regions which are more sensitive to trauma. On the other hand there are changes in the sub-meningeal parietal cortex, which may be explained by the fact that the impact is deliverd on these regions.

Kochanek:

One other question: Have you looked at the brain stem or spinal cord in this model? Several investigators suggest that the damage in the white matter tracts that may account for the motor deficit produced by this model, may occur (at least in part) in the brain stem or spinal cord.

Morganti:

Actually, no. But it is an interesting thing to do.

Enhanced Osteogenesis: Systemic Consequence of Traumatic Brain Injury

R. Wildburger, N. Zarkovic, S. Borovic, K. Zarkovic, and Z. Kejla

Background

Already in 1918, Dejerine and Ceillier [9] described for the first time the appearance of abundant osseous neoformations near joints and bones in patients with injuries of the spinal cord. Calandriello in 1964 [7] and Roberts in 1968 [28] were the first authors to describe the phenomenon in patients with traumatic brain injury (TBI). The advantage of this phenomenon is early consolidation of the fractures, while an extreme disadvantage is extensive periarticular calcification that could, in spite of the spontaneous ending of the process, lead to complete ankylosis of the affected joint (Figs. 1, 2).

However, in spite of a relatively long history of studies on the phenomenon, the mechanism of enhanced osteogenesis in patients with traumatic injury of the central nervous system (CNS) is not understood [27,35,40]. Probably, the main reason for that is the lack of knowledge on very challenging topics: (1) regulative mechanisms of the tissue regeneration or wound healing, and (2) mechanisms of systemic reaction to trauma.

The lack of general knowledge on these topics, particularly on the role of CNS in growth control and wound healing, as well as possible practical usefulness of the study of the phenomenon, were the reasons for the joint research study of the University Clinic of Traumatology in Graz and Ruđer Bošković Institute in Zagreb supported by the AO/ASIF Foundation. In this joint research study the sera of three groups of patients have been examined and compared with the sera of healthy subjects.

Group I comprised the patients with fractures of long bones and/or large joints only, group II included patients with TBI only and, group III those with combined injury, i.e., fractures of long bones or large joints together with TBI. All the patients with TBI, alone or combined with bone fractures, were in coma for 9–14 days but recovered completely without neurological deficits. Only two of them required neurosurgical treatment during the initial post-traumatic period. The groups comprised 9–11 patients, with equal incidence of male and female subjects, who were on average 20 years old.

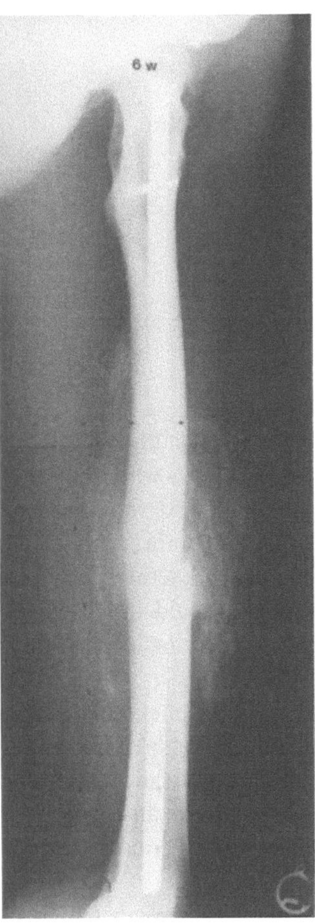

Fig. 1. X-ray image of the hypertrophic callus formed at the site of a femur fracture in a patient with traumatic brain injury after a traffic accident (photograph taken 6 weeks after the accident). Patient: male, aged 18; diagnosis: moderate subdural and intracerebral hemorrhages, unconscious for 11 days, fracture of the nose, femur fracture; treatment: conservative treatment, intubation for 6 days, intramedullary nailing of the femur; outcome: full neurological recovery, hypertrophic callus already formed after 4 weeks

Defined Parameters of Enhanced Osteogenesis in Patients with TBI

The results obtained during the last few years, combined with the results of the other authors, are summarized in Table 1.

Evaluation of post-traumatic dynamic change of various serum components revealed that the reliable predictive parameters of the enhanced osteogenesis could be: (1) alkaline phosphatase (ALP) and its bone isoenzyme, whose activity correlates with the intensity of bone mineralization [10], and (2) carboxyterminal propeptide of type I procollagen (PICP), whose serum level reflects synthesis of type I collagen [19] which accounts for more than 90% of the organic matrix of bone [6]. ALP, its bone isoenzyme, and PICP were slightly increased in the sera of patients with isolated fractures as well as in patients with TBI alone, but in patients with combined TBI and fractures of long bones associated by the hypertrophic callus formation, these parameters were already dramatically increased during the first 2 weeks after injury and were significantly different from the values observed for the patients with isolated trauma [41].

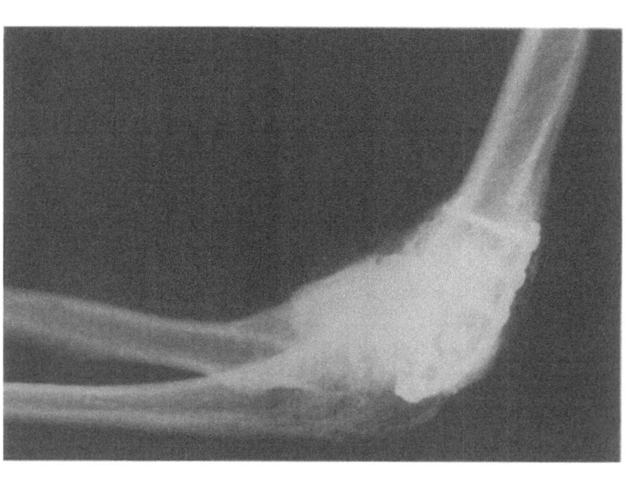

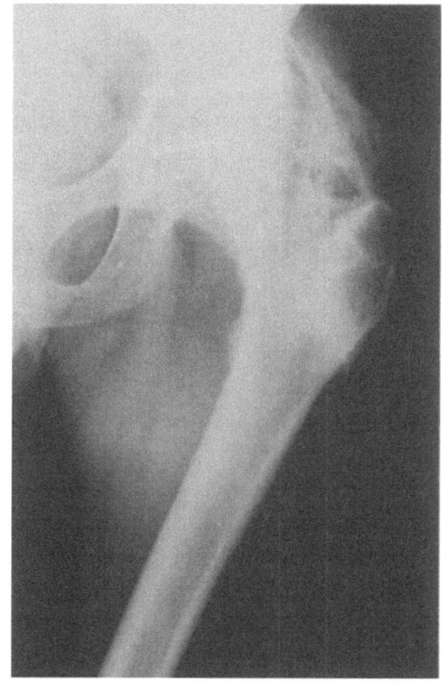

Table 1. Parameters of the phenomenon of enhanced osteogenesis in patients with traumatic brain injury (TBI)

Parameter	Description	Specificity	Relevance
Traumatic event	Traumatic brain injury combined with fractures of the long bones or big joints	Heterotopic ossifications develop in patients with spinal cord injury too, even if there is no bone fracture, but hypertrophic callus does not	Full neurological recovery and faster healing of the fractures leading to invalidity due to ankylosis of the affected joints
Serum alkaline phosphatase – bone isoenzyme	Remarkable increase of the key enzyme of bone remodeling and mineralization, particularly between the second and the third week after injury	Significantly above normal values or values obtained for patients with TBI alone or bone fractures alone	Early prediction of the phenomenon of enhanced osteogenesis and prediction of the callus volume
Serum alkaline phosphatase – liver isoenzyme	Transient and moderate increase	Unspecific, similar to the patients with TBI alone or bone fractures alone	Uncertain
C-terminal propeptide of type I procollagen (PICP)	Remarkable increase of the marker of bone matrix synthesis, particularly during the 1st and second week after injury	Significantly above normal values or values obtained for patients with TBI alone or bone fractures alone	Early prediction of the phenomenon of enhanced osteogenesis, but not so much for prediction of callus volume
Hormone levels – cortisol, ACTH, GH, PTH	Transient and moderate increase	Unspecific similar to patients with TBI alone or bone fractures alone	Uncertain
Hormone levels – prolactin	Initial decrease followed by gradual and transient increase peaking at the end of the first month after injury	Specific for patients with combined TBI and bone fractures. In other patients transient increase not different from the other hormones	Uncertain

Basic fibroblast growth factor (bFGF)	Remarkable increase during the first-second, fourth, and seventh eighth week after injury interrupted by decrease to normal values	Specific for patients with combined TBI and bone fractures. In other patients transient increase during the first 2 weeks only	Uncertain, but probably related to the systemic reaction to polytrauma or to phenomenon
Titer or antibodies against oxidized low density lipoproteins (oLDL)	Initial decrease followed by the gradual increase at the end of the 1st month	Unspecific – similar to the patients with TBI alone or bone fractures alone	Suggests involvement of the oxidative stress in the post-traumatic recovery
Effects of the serum on the growth of the cultured cells – DNA synthesis in L929 fibroblasts	Stimulative effects during the first week, afterwards inhibition	Unspecific, similar to the patients with TBI alone or bone fractures alone	Uncertain, indicates that there is no causative relationship between bFGF values and the development of enhanced osteogenesis
Effects of the serum on the growth of the cultured cells – reactivity of the human peripheral mononuclear cells to the PHA mitogen in vitro	Immunosuppressive effects of serum – decrease of reactivity to PHA	Unspecific, similar to the patients with TBI alone or bone fractures alone	Uncertain – indices for the engagement of the immune system in post-traumatic recovery
Effects of the serum on the growth of the cultured cells – effects on the growth of the bone cells in vitro	Initial bone resorption followed by intensive bone remodeling and new bone production in vitro	Initial bone resorption, unspecific. New bone synthesis, specific for patients with TBI	Possible causative relationship with the enhanced osteogenesis in patients with TBI indicating humoral nature of the phenomenon

ACTH, adrenocorticotropic hormone; GH, growth hormone; PTH, parathyroid hormone; PHA, phytohemagglutinin.

"Unspecific" Parameters of the Phenomenon

Enhanced osteogenesis could be a very particular example of unspecific systemic consequences of (multiple) trauma affecting CNS. In favor of this possibility are findings of unspecific hormonal changes of standard "stress hormones", adrenocorticotropic hormone (ACTH) and cortisol, after injury equal in patients with TBI alone, bone fractures alone or combined injury [44].

The exceptions were values of prolactin which decreased below the normal values during the first week after injury only in the sera of patients with TBI and bone fractures. Afterwards prolactin concentrations gradually increased, peaking at the end of the first month, i.e., at the time of hypertrophic callus formation. Since an increase of serum prolactin values was also described as "non-specific" post-traumatic change during the first few hours after fracture of the long bone or large joints [32], it can be assumed that this particular hormone is somehow related to the systemic reaction to trauma, but also to the phenomenon of impaired bone fracture healing.

Similarly, it seems that "non-specific" oxidative stress could be of importance in the development of enhanced osteogenesis in patients with TBI. Due to the post-traumatic subarachnoidal bleeding in patients with TBI [as verified by computed tomography (CT) scanning], oxidative stress of the brain should develop and have prominent biological, mainly harmful, consequences [1,5,17,26,29,39]. Moreover, abundant bleeding in patients with multiple trauma (acute loss of up to 2 l of blood), particularly at the site of bone fracture, could cause transient hemorrhagic shock which will induce general oxidative stress affecting the brain as well [17,39]. Hence, possible relevance of the post-traumatic oxidative secondary brain injury for the phenomenon of enhanced osteogenesis should be studied further.

Further study on the pathophysiology of oxidative stress at the site of bone fracture, caused by the resorption of hematoma, also seems necessary. Namely, beside the physical compression of hematoma on the healing tissue and the release of the growth factors due to the resorption of hematoma, a certain role in impaired fracture healing might be played by "second toxic messengers of the oxygen free radicals" such as 4-hydroxynonenal (HNE) [50], which is not only a cytotoxic product of lipid peroxidation but also shows cell growth modifying activity dependent on the un-known serum factors [53,54]. Such a study should be of particular interest also for the practical surgical management of the fracture since the mediators of the oxidative stress are involved in the control of bone growth and remodeling [14,15].

Irrespective of the pathophysiological bases of the oxidative stress in traumatized patients, an important consequence of it could be the generation of oxidatively modi-fied lipids. Of particular interest can be effects of oxidative stress on low density and high density lipoproteins (LDL and HDL, respectively), since LDL is a source of free fatty acids and cholesterol necessary for cell growth and proliferation [16,36], and is intensively metabolized by proliferating cells, thus probably, together with HDL, even influencing the control of their growth [36,49,51,52]. Oxidatively modified LDL (oLDL) can induce the generation of auto-antibodies against "novel" epitopes on oLDL [2,12,24,30]. Hence, intensive oxidative stress could influence both the lipopro-tein metabolism and the immune system function, particularly production of the anti-oLDL autoantibodies as was shown for the diseases associated with ischemia-reperfusion type of injuries [11,33,38] and recently also for patients with bone fractures and/or TBI [4]. Due to the effects of oLDL on the functional activity of monocytes and T-lymphocytes [13,18,21,37] its possible involvement in the function of the immune system and in the systemic reaction to trauma should be analysed.

Another reason for such an analysis is the fact that the role of the immune system (both cellular and humoral components) in the control of the healing process and systemic reaction to injury is not understood, although it seems to be of great importance [8,23,34]. Of particular interest could be the possible role of interleukins and prostaglandins which affect the function of the immune competent cells as well as the metabolism of the bone cells [22,25,31,48].

On the other hand, in septic baboons the dynamic change of serum cytokines during the onset of sepsis could be abolished by the use of the proper anti-cytokine antibodies [20]. That could not, however, abolish the early immunosuppressive effects of the sera of septic baboons as defined by their inhibiting effects on the reactivity of the normal human peripheral blood mononuclear cells to phytohemagglutinin (PHA) in vitro [20]. Similarly, the preliminary findings indicate that the sera of patients with bone fractures and/or TBI could have very similar and long lasting immunosuppressive effects (even more than 1 month after injury) [46]. That could indicate a similar "unspecific" cascade of events affecting immune-competent cells in sepsis and in TBI which should be further evaluated.

Thus, humoral mechanisms either specific (depending on the type of trauma or the affected organs) or unspecific (as a general systemic reaction to trauma) could play a role in the phenomenon of enhanced osteogenesis in patients with TBI.

The Humoral Nature of Enhanced Osteogenesis in Patients with TBI

It seems that among the humoral growth factors related to the phenomenon, basic fibroblast growth factor (bFGF) could be of particular importance. In the sera of patients exerting enhanced osteogenesis periods of high bFGF concentration (up to 20 times higher than the normal values) observed during weeks 2, 4, and 7–8 after injury were interrupted by sudden decreases even to the normal values (during weeks 3 and 5–6 after injury) [42]. However, it is uncertain if such a pattern of dynamic change of the serum bFGF is causatively related to the phenomenon of enhanced osteogenesis in patients with TBI. The results of our study did not indicate a relationship between the phenomenon of enhanced osteogenesis in patients with TBI and the serum levels of bFGF [45,47]. Namely, irrespective of the type of trauma and the content of bFGF, the sera of injured subjects stimulated in vitro growth of L929 fibroblasts only if taken during the first week after injury [45]. If the serum was prepared from the blood taken afterwards (weekly during the following 2 months) addition of the serum inhibited the growth of fibroblasts [45].

Hence, the change of serum bFGF and the phenomenon of enhanced osteogenesis could both be consequences of some systemic reaction to the intensive injury, probably also manifested by the increased toxicity of the serum from the second week after injury. Evaluation of this hypothesis should not only aid the understanding of the phenomenon of enhanced osteogenesis in patients with TBI, but also the understanding of the systemic reaction to injury and regulation of the tissue regeneration.

Thus, although enhanced osteogenesis in patients with TBI is without doubt a consequence of the impaired systemic reaction to trauma and local regulation of the bone fracture healing, even the humoral nature of the phenomenon is uncertain. Bidner [3] described in 1990 that in the sera of patients with severe head injury and bone fractures who develop hypertrophic callus formation, growth stimulating activity, which probably enhances osteogenesis, is increased. In contrast, in 1994, Renfree et al. [27] described a transient, unspecific, growth-inhibiting effect of the injured patients' sera during the initial post-traumatic week followed afterwards by unspecific growth-promoting activity.

Hence, to obtain further data on the humoral nature of the phenomenon, we started pilot experiments using cultures of human bone cells isolated from the head

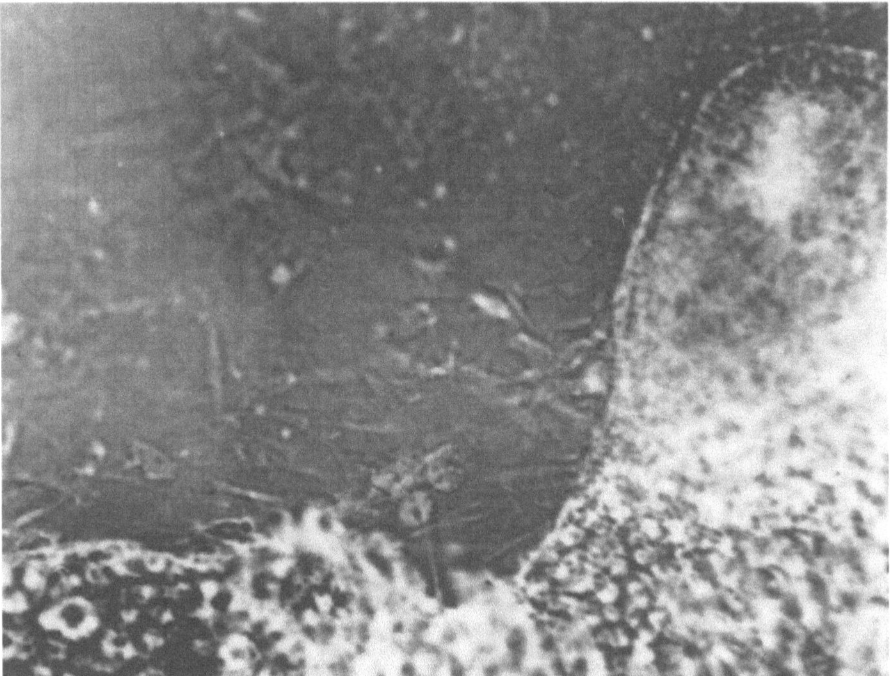

Fig. 3. Primary culture of human bone cells. Mechanical destruction of the head of the femur of a middle-aged male patient obtained after surgical removal of the bone (for the implantation of hip protesis) was combined with partial digestion of the tissue by collagenase and pronase solutions. Thus obtained particles were incubated for 10 days at 37°C in a humidified air atmosphere with 5% CO_2 in dMEM-F12 Ham's solution supplemented with 10% fetal calf serum. Migration of the bone cells from the bone particle into the culture medium and development of a gentle monolayer cell culture at the bottom of the flask can be seen. The same cells were afterwards used for the "bone-tissue" cultures, by implanting the cells into the bovine bone matrix (see Figs. 4–7)

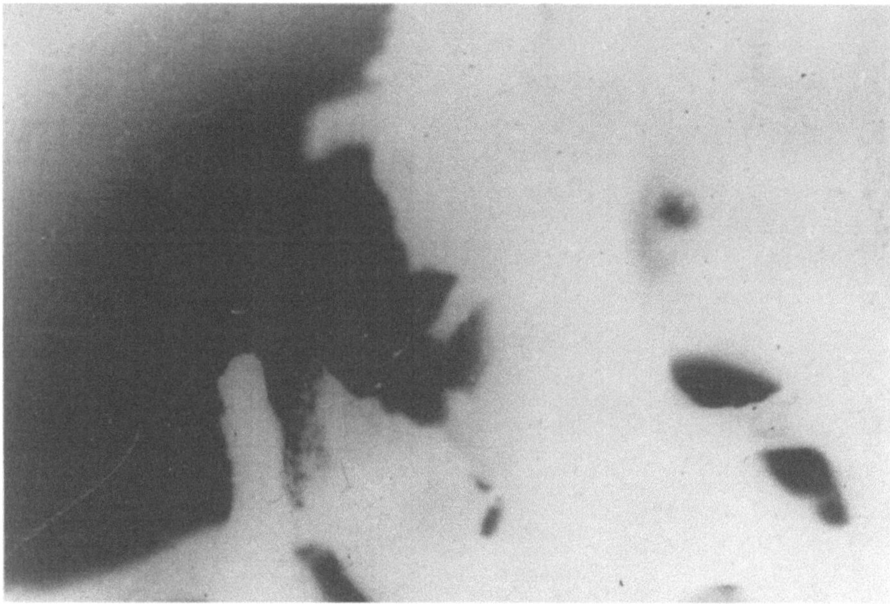

Fig. 4. Culture of human bone cells incubated for 1 week in bovine bone tissue matrix in the presence of 1% serum obtained during the first week after injury from the blood of patients with traumatic brain injury (TBI) and bone fractures (pool prepared from the blood of ten donors). Marginal parts of the bone matrix were resorbed by the bone cells resulting in the tissue "defects" (*left* and *central part* of the photograph). The same phenomenon was also observed for cells cultured in the presence of normal human serum or sera of patients with bone fractures only or TBI only

of the femur. The cells are not only incubated as monolayer cultures (Fig. 3) for the analysis of the cellular DNA synthesis or proliferation rate, but also as "tissue cultures". For that purpose, the cells are cultured in vitro in the bovine bone matrix which is used for bone plastic surgery as a replacement for destroyed tissue. The cells are cultured either in normal human serum (obtained from the pool of ten donors) or in pooled sera of the injured patients suffering from TBI alone, bone fractures alone or polytrauma, respectively. The samples of sera are replaced weekly following the time schedule of blood withdrawal from injured patients for the sera preparation. Hence, bone tissue cultures of injured patients are exposed in vitro to the sera of injured patients in consecutive weekly intervals according to the post-traumatic recovery of the patients.

The use of normal human serum, as well as the sera of injured patients obtained during the first week after injury, did not differ much from each other regarding their influence on cell growth behavior. For all the cultures obvious resorption of the bone matrix could be seen (Figs. 4, 5). However, replacing the "first week" serum with those obtained during consecutive weeks resulted in intensive synthesis of new bone material which even resulted in reintegration of the previously resorbed bone particles (Figs. 6, 7). This phenomenon of bone remodeling resembled phenomenon of enhanced osteogenesis in patients with TBI since it could be observed only if

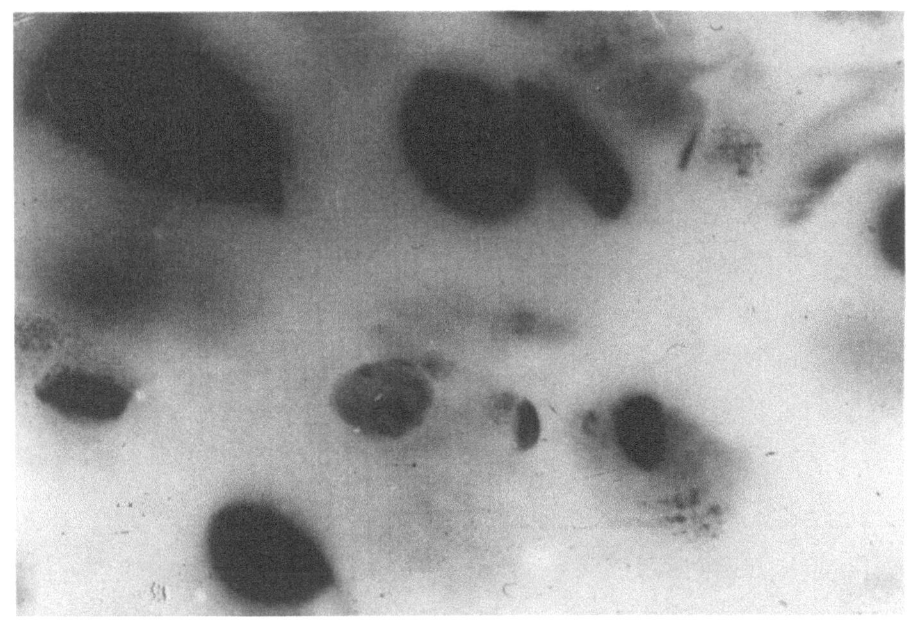

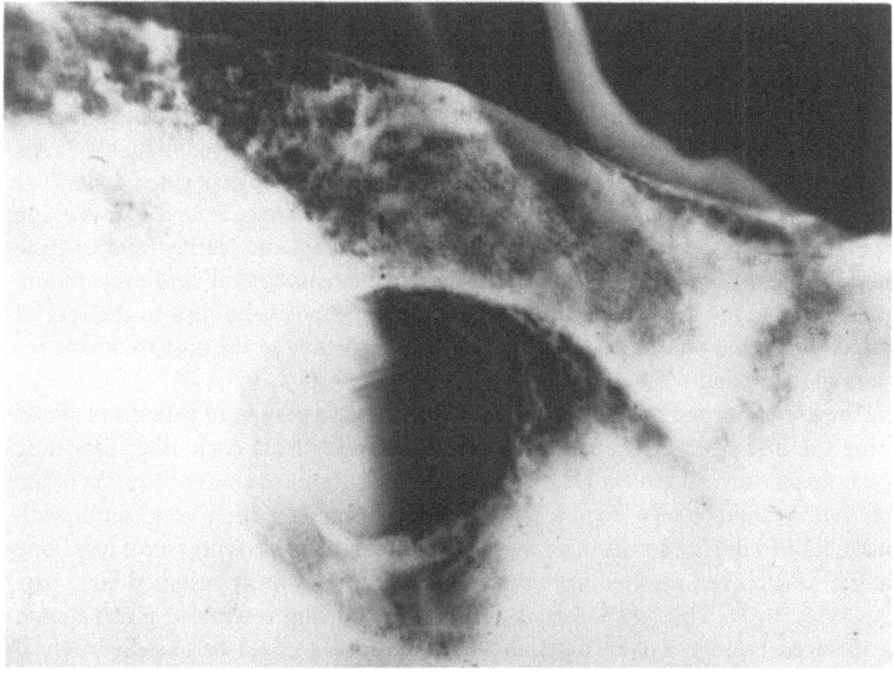

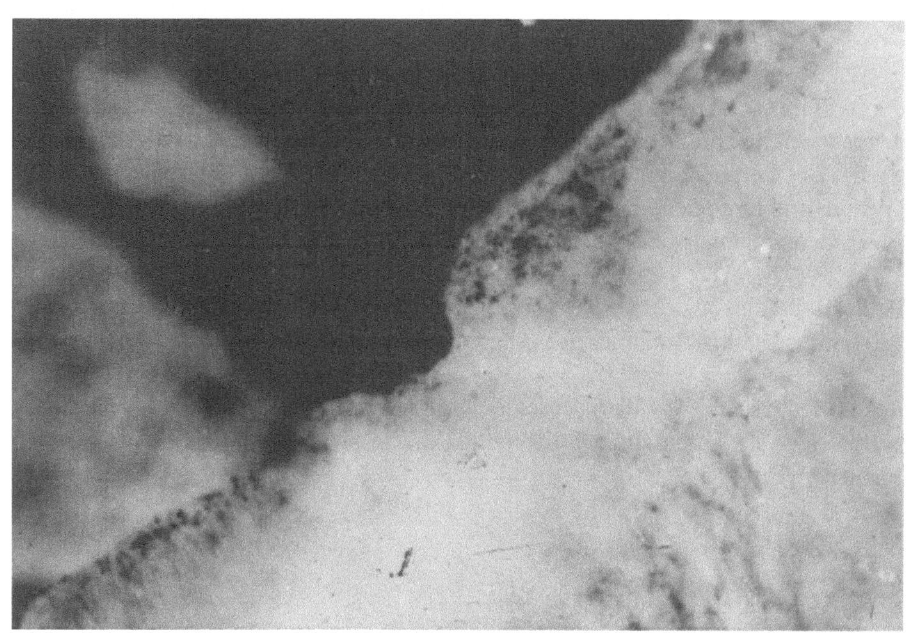

the sera of patients with TBI alone or TBI combined with bone fractures were used in vitro.

Thus, we assume that the brain plays an important, but not understood, role in the central control of growth and wound healing which should be further studied to define the nature of the humoral factors involved in growth control. For that purpose studies on the phenomenon of enhanced osteogenesis after TBI analyzing such a precious and rare phenomenon could be very useful and should be intensified by the experimental models both in vivo and in vitro.

Dedication. This article is dedicated to the memory on the late Professor Walter Petek whose enthusiasm and ideas encouraged us to do the study described.

Acknowledgments. The data presented are results of the research study supported by the AO/ASIF Foundation, Switzerland, and in part by the Croatian Ministry of Science.

References

1. Anderson DK, Means ED (1983) Lipid peroxidation in spinal cord: FeCl2 induction and protection with antioxidants. Neurochem Pathol 1:249–264
2. Bellomo G, Maggi E, Poli M, Agosta FG, Bollati P, Finardi G (1995) Autoantibodies against oxidatively modified low-density lipoproteins in NIDDM. Diabetes 44:60–66
3. Bidner SM (1990) Evidence for a humoral mechanism for enhanced osteogenesis after head injury. J Bone Joint Surg [Am] 72:1144–1149
4. Borović S, Žarković N, Wildburger R, Tatzber F, Jurin M (1995) Post-traumatic differences in titer of autoantibodies against oxidised low density lipoproteins (oLDL) in the sera of patients with traumatic bone fractures and brain injury. Period Biol 97:289–293
5. Braughler JM, Hall ED (1989) Central nervous system trauma and stroke. I. Biochemical considerations of oxygen radical formation and lipid peroxidation. Free Radic Biol Med 6:289–301
6. Burgeson RE (1988) New collagens, new concepts (Review). Annu Rev Cell Biol 4:551–557
7. Calandriello B (1964) Callus formation in severe brain injuries. Bull Hosp Jt Dis Orthop Inst 25:170–175
8. Chaudry IH, Ayala A, Meldrum A, Ertel W (1993) Hemorrhage-induced alterations in cell mediated immune function. In: Faist E, Meakins J, Schildberg FW (eds) Host defense dysfunction in trauma, shock and sepsis. Springer, Berlin Heildelberg New York, pp 149–160
9. Dejerine ME, Ceillier MA (1918) Para-ostéo-arthropathies des paraplégiques par lésion médullaire. Ann Med 5:497
10. Diduch DR, Coe MR, Joyner C, Owen ME, Balian G (1993) Two cell lines from bone marrow that differ in terms of collagen synthesis, osteogenic characteristics and matrix mineralization. J Bone Joint Surg [Am] 75:92–105
11. Eber B, Schumacher M, Tatzber F, Kaufmann P, Lupha O, Esterbauer H, Klein W (1994) Autoantibodies to oxidized low density lipoproteins in restonosis following coronary angioplasty. Cardiology 84:310–315
12. Esterbauer H, Waeg G, Puhl H (1993) Lipid peroxidation and its role in atherosclerosis. Br Med Bull 49:566–576
13. Frostegard J, Wu R, Giscombe R, Holm G, Lefvert AK, Nilsson J (1992) Induction of T-cell activation by oxidized low density lipoprotein. Arterioscler Thromb 12:461–467
14. Garret LR, Boyce BF, Oreffo ROC, Bonewski L, Poser J, Mundy GR (1990) Oxygen-derived free radicals stimulate osteoclastic bone resorption in rodent bone in vitro and in vivo. J Clin Invest 85:632–639

15. Göktürk E, Turgut A, Baycu C, Günal I, Seber, S, Gülbas Z (1995) Oxygen-free radicals impair fracture healing in rats. Acta Orthop Scand 66:473–475
16. Gotto AM Jr (ed) (1987) Plasma lipoproteins. Elsevier, Amsterdam
17. Hall ED, Braughler JM (1989) Central nervous system trauma and stroke. II. Physiological and pharmacological evidence for involvement of oxygen radicals and lipid peroxidation. Free Radic Biol Med 6:289–301
18. Huber LA, Böck G, Jürgens G, Trail KN, Schönitzer D, Wick G (1990) Increased expression of high affinity LDL receptors on human T-blasts. Int Arch Allergy Appl Immunol 93:205–211
19. Joerring S, Jensen LT, Andersen GR, Johansen JS (1992) Types I and III procollagen extension peptides in serum respond to fracture in humans. Arch Orthop Trauma Surg 111:265–267
20. Junger WG, Hoyt DB, Redl H, Liu FC, Loomis WH, Davies J, Schlag G (1995) Tumor necrosis factor antibody treatment of septic baboons reduces the production of sustained T-cell suppressive factors. Shock 3:173–178
21. Jürgens G, Xu Q, Huber LA, Böck G, Howanietz H, Wick G, Trail KN (1989) Promotion of lymphocyte growth by high density lipoproteins (HDL). J Biol Chem 264:8549–8556
22. Kawaguchi H, Pilbeam CC, Harrison JR, Raisz LG (1995) The role of prostaglandins in the regulation of bone metabolism. Clin Orthop 313:36–46
23. Miller-Graziano CL, Szabo G, Koyds K, Metha B (1993) Interactions of immunopathological mediators (tumor necrosis factor α, -β, prostaglandin E_2) in traumatized individuals. In: Faist E, Meakins J, Schildberg FW (eds) Host defense dysfunction in trauma, shock and sepsis. Springer, Berlin Heidelberg New York, pp 637–650
24. Parums DV, Brown DL, Mitchinson MJ (1990) Serum antibodies to oxidised LDL and ceroid in chronic periaartitis. Arch Pathol Lab Med 114:383–387
25. Raisz LG (1988) Bone metabolism and its hormonal regulation: an update. Triangle 27:5–10
26. Redl H, Gasser H, Hallstrom S, Schlag G (1993) Radical related cell injury. In: Schlag G, Redl H (eds) Pathophysiology of shock, sepsis, and organ failure. Springer, Berlin Heildelberg New York, pp 92–110
27. Renfree KJ, Banovac K, Hornicek FJ, Lebwhol NH (1994) Evaluation of serum osteoblast mitogenic activity in spinal cord and head injury in patients with acute heterotopic ossification. Spine 19:740–746
28. Roberts PH (1968) Heterotopic ossification complicating paralysis of intracranial origin. J Bone Joint Surg [Br] 50:70–77
29. Sadrzadeh SMH, Eaton JW (1992) Hemoglobin-induced oxidant damage to the central nervous system. In: Moslaen MT, Smith CV (eds) Free radical mechanisms of tissue injury. CRC, Boca Raton, pp 24–34
30. Salonen JT, Ylä-Hertuala S, Yamamoto R, Butler S, Korpela H, Salonen R, Nyssönnen K, Palinski W, Witzum JL (1992) Autoantibody against oxidised LDL and progression of carotid atherosclerosis. Lancet 339:883–887
31. Schlag G, Redl H, Baharami S, Davies J, Smuts P , Marzi I (1993) Trauma and cytokines. In: Schlag G, Redl H, Traber DL (eds) Shock, sepsis, and organ failure. Springer, Berlin Heidelberg New York, pp 128–156 (Third Wiggers Bernard Conference-Cytokine Network)
32. Schnai E, Lamprey JM, Viljoen MJ, Joffe BI, Seftel HC (1987) The early biochemical and hormonal profile in patients with long bone fractures at risk of fat embolism syndrome. J Trauma 27:309–311
33. Schumacher M, Eber B, Tatzber F, Kaufmann P, Halwachs G, Fruhwald FM, Zweiker R, Esterbauer H, Klein W (1995) Transient reduction of autoantibodies against oxidized LDL in patients with acute myocardial infarction. Free Radic Biol Med 18:1087–1091
34. Schutze S (1993) Humoral and neural mediators of systemic response to surgery. Dan Med Bull 40:365–377
35. Sobus KML, Alexander MA, Harcke HT (1993) Undetected musculosceletal trauma in children with traumatic brain injury or spinal cord injury. Arch Phys Med Rehabil 74:902–904
36. Spiegel RJ, Schaefer EJN, Magrath IT, Edwards BK (1982) Plasma lipid alteration in leukemia and lymphoma. Am J Med 72:775–782

37. Trail KN, Huber LA, Wick G, Jürgens G (1990) Lipoprotein interactions with T cells: an update. Immunol Today 11:411–417
38. Virella G, Virella I, Leman RB, Pryor MB, Lopes-Virella MV (1993) Anti-oxidised low-density lipoprotein antibodies in patients with coronary heart disease and normal healthy volunteers. Int J Clin Lab Res 23:95–101
39. Waterfall AH, Singh G, Fry JR, Marsden CA (1995) Detection of the lipid peroxidation product malondyaldehide in the rat brain in vivo. Neurosci Lett 200:69–72
40. Wildburger R, Žarković N (1995) Enhanced osteogenesis in patients with traumatic brain injury (Editorial). Period Biol 97:281–288
41. Wildburger R, Žarković N, Dobnig H, Petek W, Hofer HP (1994) Post-traumatic dynamic change of carboxyterminal propeptide of type I procollagen, alkaline phosphatase and its isoenzymes as predictors for enhanced osteogenesis in patients with severe head injury. Res Exp Med 194:247–259
42. Wildburger R, Žarković N, Egger G, Petek W, Žarković K, Hofer HP (1994) Basic fibroblast growth factor (bFGF) immunoreactivity as a possible link between head injury and impaired bone fracture healing. Bone Miner 27:183–192
43. Wildburger R, Žarković N, Petek W, Dobnig H, Leopold-Wildburger U, Schweighofer F, Hofer HP (1995) A possible early quantitative prediction of bone fracture callus volume according to the post-traumatic increase in the serum alkaline phosphatase and procollagen I. Med Sci Res 23:219–223
44. Wildburger R, Tonković G, Žarković N (1995) Posttraumatske promjene vrijednosti hormona u serumu: Prolaktin kao veza izmedu kraniocerebralne ozljede i fenomena pojacane osteogeneze. Lijec Vjesn 117 [Suppl 1]: 13
45. Wildburger R, Žarković N, Egger G, Petek W, Mainitzer A, Borović S, Žarković K, Li L, Stipančić I, Trbojević-Čepe M, Čvoriščec D, Doko M (1995) Comparison of the values of basic fibroblast growth factor determined by an immunoassay in the sera of patients with traumatic brain injury and enhanced osteogenesis and the effects of the same sera on the fibroblast growth in vitro. Eur J Clin Chem Clin Biochem 33:693–698
46. Wildburger R, Žarković N, Borović S, Žarković K, Stipančić I, Kejla Z, Golubić J, Li L, Tonković G, Škorić T, Jurin M (1995) The effects of sera of injured patients on the growth of human peripheral blood mononuclear cells: possible involvement of the immune system in the phenomenon of enhanced osteogenesis in patients with traumatic brain injury (TBI). Period Biol 97 [Suppl 1]:58
47. Wildburger R, Žarković N, Petek W, Egger G, Leopold U, Schweighofer F (1996) Hypertrophe Kallusformation und Schädel-Hirn-Trauma: Frühdiagnostik und das Verhalten des basischen Fibroblastenwachstumsfaktors. Unfallchirurg 99:17–23
48. Williams TJ, Peck MJ (1977) Role of prostaglandin-mediated vasodilatation in inflammation. Nature 270:530–531
49. Xu Q, Jürgens G, Huber LA, Böck G, Wolf H, Wick G (1992) Lipid utilization by human peripheral blood lymphocytes correlates to their high density lipoprotein binding site activity. Biochem J 285:105–112
50. Zollner H, Schaur RJ, Esterbauer H (1991) Biological activities of 4-hydroxyalkenals. In: Sies H (ed) Oxidative stress. Academic, London, pp 337–369
51. Žarković N, Salzer B, Hrženjak M, Ilić Z, Pifat G, Stipančić I, Vučković I, Jurin M (1991) The effects of gallium arsenide laser irradiation and partial hepatectomy on murine skin wound healing and lipoprotein composition. Period Biol 93:359–361
52. Žarković N, Pifat G, Salzer B (1992) The influence of liver regeneration and tumor growth on serum lipoprotein composition in mice. Period Biol 94:53–58
53. Žarković N, Ilić Z, Jurin M, Schaur RJ, Puhl H, Esterbauer H (1993) Stimulation of HeLa cell growth by physiological concentrations of 4-hydroxynonenal. Cell Biochem Funct 11:279–286
54. Žarković N, Schaur RJ, Puhl H, Jurin M, Esterbauer H (1994) Mutual dependence of growth modifying effects of 4-hydroxynonenal and fetal calf serum in vitro. Free Radic Biol Med 16:877–884

Springer
and the
environment

At Springer we firmly believe that an international science publisher has a special obligation to the environment, and our corporate policies consistently reflect this conviction.

We also expect our business partners – paper mills, printers, packaging manufacturers, etc. – to commit themselves to using materials and production processes that do not harm the environment. The paper in this book is made from low- or no-chlorine pulp and is acid free, in conformance with international standards for paper permanency.

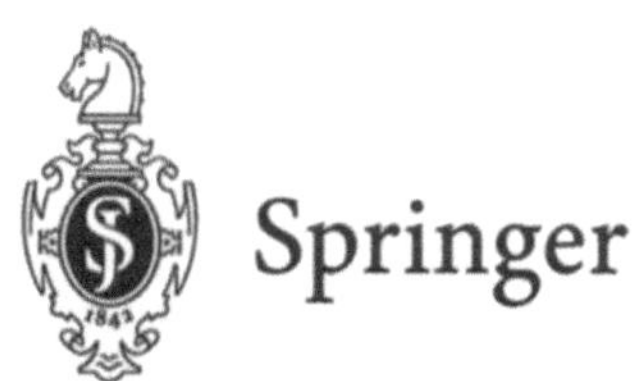

Springer

MIX
Papier aus verantwortungsvollen Quellen
Paper from responsible sources
FSC® C105338

If you have any concerns about our products,
you can contact us on
ProductSafety@springernature.com

In case Publisher is established outside the EU,
the EU authorized representative is:
**Springer Nature Customer Service Center GmbH
Europaplatz 3, 69115 Heidelberg, Germany**

Printed by Libri Plureos GmbH
in Hamburg, Germany